# Electrical Neuroimaging

# Electrical Neuroimaging

Edited by

Christoph M. Michel

Thomas Koenig

Daniel Brandeis

Lorena R.R. Gianotti

Jiří Wackermann

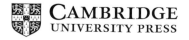

CAMBRIDGE UNIVERSITY PRESS
Cambridge, New York, Melbourne, Madrid, Cape Town,
Singapore, São Paulo, Delhi

Cambridge University Press
The Edinburgh Building, Cambridge CB2 8RU, UK

Published in the United States of America
by Cambridge University Press, New York

www.cambridge.org
Information on this title: www.cambridge.org/9780521879798

© Cambridge University Press 2009

First published 2009

Printed in the United Kingdom
at the University Press, Cambridge

*A catalogue record for this publication is available from the British
Library*

*Library of Congress Cataloguing in Publication data*
Electrical neuroimaging / edited by Christoph M. Michel ...
[et al.].
    p. ; cm.
Includes bibliographical references and index.
ISBN 978-0-521-87979-8 (hardback)
1. Brain – Imaging.    2. Electroencephalography.
3. Evoked potentials (Electrophysiology)    I. Michel, Christoph
M., 1959–    II. Title.
[DNLM: 1. Brain – physiology.    2. Brain Mapping – methods.
3. Electroencephalography – methods.
4. Evoked Potentials. WL 335 E38 2009]
QP376.6.E44    2009
616.8′047547 – dc22        2009009343

ISBN 978-0-521-87979-8 hardback

Dedicated to
Dietrich Lehmann, our teacher, mentor
and friend

# Contents

*List of contributors*   viii
*Preface*   ix

1  **From neuronal activity to scalp potential fields**   1
Daniel Brandeis, Christoph M. Michel and Florin Amzica

2  **Scalp field maps and their characterization**   25
Thomas Koenig and Lorena R.R. Gianotti

3  **Imaging the electric neuronal generators of EEG/MEG**   49
Roberto D. Pascual-Marqui, Kensuke Sekihara, Daniel Brandeis and Christoph M. Michel

4  **Data acquisition and pre-processing standards for electrical neuroimaging**   79
Christoph M. Michel and Daniel Brandeis

5  **Overview of analytical approaches**   93
Thomas Koenig and Jiří Wackermann

6  **Electrical neuroimaging in the time domain**   111
Christoph M. Michel, Thomas Koenig and Daniel Brandeis

7  **Multichannel frequency and time-frequency analysis**   145
Thomas Koenig and Roberto D. Pascual-Marqui

8  **Statistical analysis of multichannel scalp field data**   169
Thomas Koenig and Lester Melie-García

9  **State space representation and global descriptors of brain electrical activity**   191
Jiří Wackermann and Carsten Allefeld

10  **Integration of electrical neuroimaging with other functional imaging methods**   215
Daniel Brandeis, Christoph M. Michel, Thomas Koenig and Lorena R.R. Gianotti

*Index*   233

# Contributors

**Carsten Allefeld**
Institute for Frontier Areas of Psychology
and Mental Health
Freiburg im Breisgau, Germany

**Florin Amzica**
Department of Stomatology
Université de Montreal
Montreal, Canada

**Daniel Brandeis**
Department of Child and Adolescent
Psychiatry
University of Zürich
Switzerland
and Central Institute of Mental Health
Mannheim, Germany

**Lorena R.R. Gianotti**
The KEY Institute for Brain-Mind Research
University Hospital of Psychiatry
University of Zürich
Zürich, Switzerland

**Thomas Koenig**
Department of Psychiatric
Neurophysiology
University Hospital of Psychiatry
University of Bern
Bern, Switzerland

**Lester Melie-García**
Neuroinformatics Department
Cuban Neuroscience Center
Havana, Cuba

**Christoph M. Michel**
Functional Brain Mapping Laboratory
Neurology Clinic, University Hospital
and Fundamental Neuroscience
Department
University Medical School
University of Geneva
Geneva, Switzerland

**Roberto D. Pascual-Marqui**
The KEY Institute for Brain-Mind Research
University Hospital of Psychiatry
University of Zürich
Zürich, Switzerland

**Kensuke Sekihara**
Department of Systems Design and
Engineering
Tokyo Metropolitan University
Tokyo, Japan

**Jiří Wackermann**
Institute for Frontier Areas of Psychology
and Mental Health
Freiburg im Breisgau, Germany

# Preface

In 1929, Hans Berger, the founding father of electroencephalography (EEG), described EEG as a "window into the brain," because EEG appeared to be a sensitive indicator of mental states. Eighty years later, recording and analysis methods exist that have made EEG a widespread and validated tool to observe the spatial and temporal dynamics of brain network activity during a large variety of mental states and processes in a completely noninvasive fashion. This has been made possible by significant technological advances that now allow the simultaneous recording of an EEG from a large number of electrodes at a high sampling rate, and the application of space-domain oriented approaches to the analysis of these recordings. This book gives an overview of these methods. Illustrated by various examples from experimental and clinical studies, the book is a tutorial on how to use EEG as a modern functional imaging method with the advantage of directly recording neuronal activity with millisecond temporal resolution, an approach called electrical neuroimaging.

Electrical neuroimaging has enormous potential if properly applied, but it can also easily lead to erroneous conclusions if its basic principles are not properly understood. This book intends to give a comprehensive introduction to the basics of multichannel recording of EEG and event-related potential (ERP) data, and to spatio-temporal analysis of the potential fields. All chapters include practical examples from clinical and experimental research. The book enables a researcher to measure valid data, select and apply appropriate analysis strategies and draw the correct conclusions when analyzing and interpreting multichannel EEG/ERP data. It informs the research community about the possibilities opened by these space-domain oriented strategies to the analysis of brain electrical activity, and of their potential for multimodal integration with other (structural, metabolic, etc.) data.

Electrical neuroimaging is decisively different from the traditional analysis of EEG and ERP data, which is based upon waveform morphology and/or frequency characteristics of recordings at certain electrode positions. Electrical neuroimaging exclusively considers the spatial properties of electric fields and the temporal dynamics of these fields. It uses these to conclude on putative generators in the brain that gave rise to these recorded fields on the scalp. The approach therefore fills an important gap that has not been covered by other comprehensive textbooks on the analysis of EEG and ERP.

The book begins with an introduction of what the EEG on the scalp surface actually records. It comprises the basics of what we know about the generation of electric fields in the brain, which can be measured noninvasively at the scalp, and about the generation of oscillatory activity at different frequency ranges. This basic knowledge is needed for understanding the following chapter on how electric potential fields on the scalp are generated and how they are characterized. Knowing the generators in the brain and the expression of these activities on the scalp surface allows the key issue of estimating putative generators in the brain to be addressed. The book therefore contains a thorough discussion of the methods available to solve the electromagnetic inverse problem, focusing mainly on distributed inverse solutions that impose minimal a priori constraints. It is followed by a rather practical chapter on the basic requirements for recording high-density EEG and preparing these data for electrical neuroimaging. The subsequent chapters show with many practical examples how to assess the many different facets of time- and frequency-domain EEG. The knowledge and methods presented here are strictly based on well-established facts about the relation between generators in the brain and scalp-surface recordings. The results obtained by these methods thus have simple and unique interpretations in terms of intracerebral brain electric activity. Finally, the emerging field of multimodal integration is discussed, with special emphasis on the combination of EEG-based neuroimaging and functional MRI.

The book will be of great utility to cognitive neuroscientists, but also clinical neurophysiologists, neurologists and psychiatrists, as we emphasize with many practical examples the usefulness of these methods for developmental and clinical applications. The first attempts in the early 1990s to introduce quantitative EEG mapping into clinical applications were hampered by severe technical difficulties. This is not the case any more. High resolution EEG with up to 256 channels is very easy and fast to apply in clinical routine in adults as well as in children, allowing the application of the analysis methods described in this book to pathological alterations of brain function that continue to intrigue clinical neurophysiologists. It should provide them with a new tool to critically increase the sensitivity, specificity and interpretability of the measure they have used for over half of a century, which is the electroencephalogram.

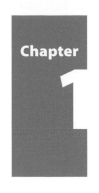

Chapter

1

# From neuronal activity to scalp potential fields

Daniel Brandeis, Christoph M. Michel and Florin Amzica

## Introduction

The EEG, along with its event-related aspects, reflects the immediate mass action of neural networks from a wide range of brain systems, and thus provides a particularly direct and integrative noninvasive window onto human brain function. During the 80 years since the discovery of the human scalp EEG[1], our neurophysiological understanding of electrical brain activity has advanced at the microscopic and macroscopic level and has been linked to physical principles, as summarized in standard textbooks[2-5]. The present introduction builds upon these texts but focuses on spatial aspects of EEG generators, many of which are applicable to both spontaneous and event-related activity[6-8]. In particular, it is critical for the purpose of electrical neuroimaging to know which neural events are detectable at which spatial scales. As we will show, the spatial characterization of the neural EEG generators, and the advances in spatial signal processing and modeling converge in important aspects and provide a sufficiently sound basis for electrical neuroimaging. Because of the unique high temporal resolution of the EEG, electrical neuroimaging not only concerns the possible neuronal generator of the scalp potential at one given moment in time, but also the possible generators of rhythmic oscillations in different frequency ranges. In fact, understanding the intrinsic rhythmic properties of cortical or subcortical–cortical networks can help to constrain electrical neuroimaging to certain frequency ranges of interest and to perform spatial analysis in the frequency domain[9-10]. This is why this chapter not only discusses the general aspects of the generators of the potential fields on the scalp, but it also discusses the mechanisms underlying the genesis of the oscillatory behavior of the EEG.

## Spikes and local field potentials

Invasive neurophysiological studies, mainly in animals, have proven crucial in clarifying the principles of neural activation and transmission at different spatial scales. Since the physics of currents and potential fields ensures their linear superposition, some understanding at both the microscopic and the macroscopic levels is essential for understanding spatio-temporal properties and constraints of the EEG generators. *Intracellular recordings* from individual neurons in animals demonstrate that the dominant electrical events at the microscopic level are focal, large and fast action potentials depolarizing the cell's resting potential by more than 80 mV (from −70 mV to positive values and back in less than 2 ms) when measured across the few nanometers of the cell membranes. These action potentials frequently originate at the soma (axon hillock) and propagate within < 1 ms to the axonal terminals. Nearby

*Electrical Neuroimaging*, ed. Christoph M. Michel, Thomas Koenig, Daniel Brandeis, Lorena R.R. Gianotti and Jiří Wackermann. Published by Cambridge University Press. © Cambridge University Press 2009.

*extracellular recordings* reveal corresponding spikes, which resemble the first temporal derivative of their intracellular counterparts and can reach at least 600 µV. The *multi-unit activity* filtered to include only frequencies above 300 Hz is dominated by these spikes which mainly reflect neuronal output, while the slower local field potentials ($< 300\,\text{Hz}$) reflect mainly postsynaptic potentials and thus neuronal input. However, in general both signals strongly correlate with local intracellular spiking as well as with metabolic demand[11]. Spatial aspects of such activity are revealed by multichannel intracranial recordings with regularly spaced electrodes. These recordings confirm that spike amplitudes fall off rapidly to a tenth ($< 60\,\mu\text{V}$) outside a 50 µm radius[12], which limits their spatial spread to the sub-millimeter scale. This property thus prevents the fields due to individual spikes becoming potentially measurable as "far fields" in the EEG, i.e. at the scalp, which is at least 2 cm away from brain tissue. Also, the short spike duration makes summation in time less likely. As a consequence, individual spikes or action potentials propagating along the axons, and more generally electric events in white matter structures such as large fiber bundles, can be neglected as direct EEG generators. A possible exception are very small ($< 0.5\,\mu\text{V}$), fast (latency under 20 ms), high frequency oscillations (above 100 Hz) which may contribute to the heavily averaged evoked patterns measured at the scalp such as the early auditory brain-stem potentials[13] or early somatosensory oscillations[14].

Spiking correlates with the less focal, and typically slower and weaker extracellular field potentials[15]. These reflect neural mass activity due to linear superposition of those fields which do not form closed field current loops. In brain regions such as the neocortex, this extracellular activity is synchronized well beyond the sub-millimeter scale and reflects summation of excitatory or inhibitory postsynaptic potentials in space and time. Such neural mass action occurs if neurons are both arranged in parallel over some distance, and receive synchronized synaptic input in a certain layer as typical for the neocortex with its aligned pyramidal cells. Although the EEG of patients with focal epilepsy is dominated by slow frequencies, very strong high-frequency oscillations (fast ripples, 100–500 Hz) can be recorded intracranially from the seizure onset zone. These oscillations typically extend over a few millimeters[16,17], which suggests that they reflect synchronized field potentials rather than spikes. Their focality, and the fact that they are typically accompanied by more widespread and even stronger lower-frequency oscillations limit their detectability in scalp recordings.

## Sinks and sources

The major generators of the scalp EEG are extended patches of gray matter, polarized through synchronous synaptic input either in an oscillatory fashion or as transient evoked activity, which reflects additional generators rather than just phase reorganization of ongoing oscillations[18]. In the cortex, such patches contain thousands of cortical columns, where large pyramidal cells are aligned perpendicularly to the cortical surface, and where the different layers are characterized by synaptic connections from different structures. The extracellular currents which flow between the layers of different polarity are matched by reverse intracellular currents. Models which consider the realistic cell geometries suggest that not only apical but also basal dendrites may contribute to EEG[19]. Such variable generator regions are consistent with the variety of laminar potential and current density distributions. While evoked activity often starts with prominent current sinks in cortical layer IV[20,21], more variable laminar distributions are found for later components of the evoked potentials as well as for epileptic activity[22]. Unfortunately, there are only rough indirect estimates regarding the degree (defined by the local dipole strength and the percentage of neuronal elements contributing) and the spatial extent (area) of polarization due to neural synchronization, particularly for the healthy human brain.

The relation of intracortical activity to surface-recorded EEG is far from simple. The surface EEG does not allow distinguishing between the various possible arrangements of sinks and sources in the different cortical layers[20]. This is due to the fact that the scalp potentials represent only the open field dipolar component of the complex multipolar current generators within the different cortical layers[23]. It has already been mentioned above that the scalp EEG reflects not only the activity of the uppermost parts of the apical dendrites, but also activities in deeper layers or structures. In addition, there have been studies showing that early surface evoked potential components can be related to presynaptic activation of the thalamocortical afferents and excitatory postsynaptic potentials on the stellate cells in area 4C[23,24]. This questions the generally held notion that only cortical pyramidal cells are generating open fields that can be detected by the EEG. Additional concerns are raised by the possibility that glial cells, if organized along an axis parallel to the apical dendrites, could constitute a powerful dipole which could constitute a source of EEG activities. This aspect is discussed in detail below with respect to the generators of delta rhythms. The difficulty of relating the scalp potential to a specific distribution of sources and sinks in the different layers of the cortex is illustrated in Figure 1.1. It shows the scalp evoked potentials recorded from 32 epicranial electrodes in anesthetized mice during whisker stimulation as well as the intracranial evoked potentials and the current source density profile from a multi-electrode probe inserted in the S1 barrel cortex[25]. A complex distribution of sinks and sources in the different layers can be seen in the intracranial recording that drastically changes across time. The initial activation at around 10 ms is dominated by sinks in layers II–III and layer V and sources in layers I, IV and VI. A nearly reverse distribution is seen at around 40 ms. Despite this very different source/sink distribution at the two time points, the same positive potential is measured on the epicranial electrode and nearly similar configurations of the potential maps are seen. Thus, the scalp potential represents a weighted sum of all active currents within the brain that generate open fields (for a detailed discussion and comparison with human evoked potentials see Megevand et al., 2008)[25]. The sum of all these open field generators forms what is often called an equivalent dipole generator[26]. The current dipoles are thus used as simple, idealized models describing strength, orientation and localization of the sum of the volume-conducted open field activity of all layers of the cortex (see also Chapter 3).

## Equivalent current dipoles

Current dipoles of 10 nA are considered typical when modeling evoked activity at the scalp in normal physiological conditions; this holds for the EEG as well as for the MEG (magnetoencephalogram) which reflects the magnetic field generated by the same current dipoles[19,27]. This estimate is also consistent with laminar recording of current source density. However, estimates regarding degree and spatial extent of postsynaptic neural synchronization represented by such a dipole vary considerably. They range from just 50 000 pyramidal neurons[19] to 1 million synapses in a cortical area of 40–200 mm²[27], which would mean that less than 1% of the synapses contribute to the EEG at any given moment. Stronger activity is observed during spontaneous oscillations, and the largest activities exceeding 500 µV are observed during epileptic seizures and during slow-wave sleep, particularly in children; whether this

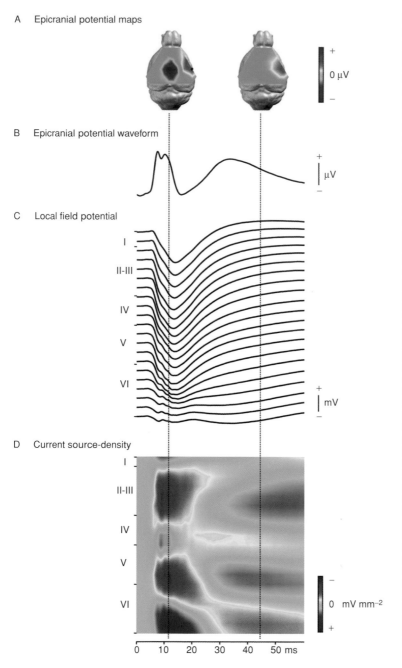

A  Epicranial potential maps

B  Epicranial potential waveform

C  Local field potential

D  Current source-density

**Figure 1.1** Time course of epicranial and intracranial potentials evoked by left whisker stimulation in anesthetized mice. A. Epicranial potential maps recorded from 32 electrodes placed in equidistance over the whole cortex. Maps are selected at two time points (12 and 45 ms). Note the positive potential on the electrode over the S1 barrel cortex for both time points. B. Evoked potential waveform for the electrode over S1 (marked in the map in A), showing two positive components at around 8–14 ms and 30–50 ms. C. Intracranial local field potential recorded from a multi-electrode probe in the cortex underlying the S1 electrode, spanning all cortical layers. Note the negative potential over all electrodes during the first component, and the positive potential during the second component. D. Current source density (CSD) profile calculated from the intracranial local field potentials (red = sink, blue = source). Note the nearly inverted source/sink distribution between the first and second component. (Modified from Megevand et al.[25] with permission from Elsevier. Copyright © 2008 Elsevier Inc.)

is due to a larger extent or a larger degree of synchronization is essentially open. Simplifying assumptions, such as that the EEG generators reflect mainly surface negativity of cortical patches due to excitatory postsynaptic input at the apical dendrites, are thus not supported.

To qualify as major EEG generators, patches of consistently polarized brain tissue also need an approximately planar geometry to ensure that linear summation produces a net

**Figure 1.2**
Electroencephalography
and MEG sources.
Volume currents due to
mass activity of
synchronized, aligned
pyramidal neurons can
be modeled as
point-like polarization
dipoles and
corresponding EEG and
MEG maps. Maps with
0.2 µV (EEG) and 50 fT
(MEG) contour spacing.
Red for positive, blue
for negative electric
potential and magnetic
field. Dipole model
with 20 nA peak
strength.

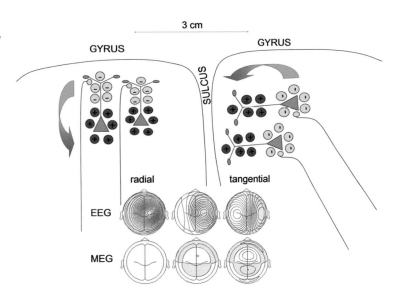

polarization or "far field" along the dominant or mean orientation. This typically holds for activity on the cortical gyri (parallel to the skull, with radial polarization), but also on the walls of cortical sulci (with tangential polarization) or in deeper structures like the cingulate gyrus. Both radial and tangential polarizations give rise to characteristic but distinct scalp EEG maps, while radial polarization generates no MEG maps, as illustrated in Figure 1.2. Closely folded brain structures only generate "closed fields" which cancel within a few millimeters due to nearby sources with random or opposite orientations. Although some structures like the cerebellum were historically considered to generate only closed fields and no EEG, recent MEG findings of consistent cerebellar activation[28-30] strongly suggest that the cerebellum can also generate scalp EEG. The same is true for mesial temporal structures such as the hippocampus and the amygdala as demonstrated in EEG and MEG studies with simulations[31] as well as with recordings in patients with mesial temporal lobe epilepsy[32,33].

Forward solutions of the electric scalp field can be computed in an accurate and unambiguous fashion from the intracranial electrical distribution, provided the geometric and electric properties of the head (i.e. the shape and conductivity of all compartments) are known (see Figure 1.2 and Chapter 3). However, a full description of the electrical distribution at all spatial scales, starting at the microscopic level with its large intracellular voltages, is obviously beyond reach. Spatial considerations which constrain this description to potential EEG generators are thus critical.

Electroencephalography sources generate field potentials which still fall off steeply within the brain, but far less so if measured through the scalp. This is because the lower conductivity of the skull compared with the brain causes spatial blurring at the scalp. Superficial sources are thus attenuated more strongly than deep ones, as confirmed by recordings of the intracranial and scalp distribution induced by intracranial stimulation in patients[34] which closely matched predictions from dipole models. Accordingly, scalp voltages generated by the deepest sources in the center of the head still reach 20–52% of the voltages generated by the most superficial sources of the same source strength; this percentage would be considerably reduced (to only 4–15%) with equal skull and brain conductivities.

The important consequence for electrical neuroimaging is that the EEG displays a considerable sensitivity to deep sources which is more pronounced than for the MEG (Figure 1.2) and is often underestimated. Neglecting the contribution of deep sources to the EEG is thus generally not justified. Another consequence is that the relative sensitivity to superficial versus deep sources depends critically upon the conductivity of the skull. The systematic developmental changes in relative conductivity thus need to be considered in electrical neuroimaging[35]. Higher conductivity of infant skulls leads to less spatial blurring which emphasizes superficial sources and lowers spatial correlations[36]. The issue of conductivity and spatial blurring is discussed in detail in Chapter 4.

## Spatial smoothness

The spatial extent and the spatial smoothness of the synchronized polarization in EEG generators is another crucial but only partly resolved issue for electrical neuroimaging. The most direct knowledge about the spatial extent of human EEG generators comes from the few studies where intracranial and scalp recordings in epilepsy patients were combined for diagnostic purposes. Despite the caveat that the coverage with intracranial electrodes is typically very limited, and that the epileptic EEG is not typical of normal oscillatory or event-related activity but characterized by particularly strong and synchronized EEG events, these findings provide crucial constraints for source models, and illustrate the different scales of spatial smoothness and resolution which govern intracranial and scalp EEG. Intracranial recordings find that interictal spike activity reaches 50–500 $\mu$V and is often limited to 2–3 cm (i.e. to 2–3 contacts of multicontact electrodes with typical spacing), with sharp fall-offs beyond the active region (to under 10% at the next contact)[37], or to less than 6 cm$^2$ on an electrode grid. These focal spikes are usually hard to detect in the scalp EEG, even despite considerable intracranial amplitude and averaging based on an intracranial channel[37–40]. Similarly, strong synchronization (using coherence estimates, see Chapter 7) between neighboring electrodes of intracortical grids is typically limited to well-demarcated regions of 2–5 cm diameter[41]. This corresponds well to historical estimates based on a cadaver model, where at least 6 cm$^2$ of a model generator is needed to contribute for scalp amplitudes of 25 $\mu$V[42], and to models suggesting that at least 4–6 cm$^2$ need to be activated synchronously[19,27,43]. More recent work with epilepsy patients even suggests that for such epileptiform activity, synchronization of at least 10 cm$^2$ is required, and that synchronization of under 6 cm$^2$ does not generate visually detectable scalp amplitudes[39], but such estimates may be somewhat inflated due to the use of isolating grids[44]. Intracranial recordings of spontaneous rhythmic activity are particularly rare. They provide evidence for a similar spatial extent over a few centimeters, with some polarity reversals between adjacent occipital electrodes spaced about 1 cm apart[45].

What amplitude is detectable in the scalp EEG clearly depends on both the detection method and the signal-to-noise ratio. Typically, epilepsy potentials above 10–20 $\mu$V at the scalp exceed the level of spontaneous activity and noise in some EEG channels and become reliably visible. Averaging can also retrieve much smaller activities at the scalp ($< 0.5$ $\mu$V as for the brain-stem potentials) provided they are systematically time locked to external (or larger intracranial) events.

Taken together, evidence from basic neurophysiology and from intracranial recordings suggests that the main source of the EEG is the dynamic, synchronous polarization of spatially aligned neurons in extended gray matter networks, due to postsynaptic rather than action potentials. Important constraints regarding the spatial extent and the maximal physiological polarization of effective EEG generators can be derived from this evidence. However, further constraints regarding orientation and depth of EEG generators are rarely justified. Recent evidence rather suggests that a wider range of active brain structures than previously thought may contribute to the EEG. This point is particularly relevant with respect to some of the potential generators of EEG oscillatory rhythms that are discussed in the following section.

## Oscillations in brain networks

An important question for electrical neuroimaging is whether spatial aspects of the activated networks can be derived from frequency characteristics of the scalp-recorded oscillations. The characteristic rhythms in cortical structures have long been thought to be mainly under thalamic control, and thus to involve an entire thalamocortical network in both normal[46,47] and pathological conditions[48,49]. However, recent research emphasizes, on the one hand, the intrinsic rhythmic properties of cortical networks[50] (for review, see Amzica & Steriade, 1999[51]); on the other hand, it is known that some of the rhythms recorded at the EEG level are exclusively generated within specific structures: either the cortex alone, or the thalamus alone, or outside the thalamocortical system, in the hippocampus.

An EEG analysis is often made according to the spectral content of the recording signals (see Chapter 7). Although this might confer certain advantages, it also contains numerous pitfalls that prevent correct conclusions. This is mainly due to the fact that a given frequency band may ambiguously reflect various conditions, or phenomena originating at different locations. We will organize this section according to the frequency bands traditionally encountered in the EEG praxis, however, emphasizing the possible sources of haziness related to the interpretation of EEG signals. The reader should keep in mind, when extrapolating from cellular data to EEG, that:

(1) Cellular recordings are almost exclusively performed in animals, whose phylogenetic development, behavioral and structural peculiarities are often neglected.

(2) The study of the intrinsic properties of cells is mostly carried out in vitro or in cultures, preparations that are as far as one can imagine from the complex reality of the whole brain, both in terms of network linkages and physiological state. At best, these preparations would correspond to a deeply comatose brain.

(3) The study of the network interactions, however multisite they might be, are still based on recordings from spatially discrete and limited locations rather than continuous.

(4) Anesthesia is often unavoidable in animal studies and the elimination of the pharmacological effect is more complicated than a mere subtraction.

## Slow, delta rhythms

Grey Walter[52] was the first to assign the term "delta waves" to particular types of slow waves recorded in the EEG of humans. Although Walter introduced the term delta waves in correspondence to pathological potentials due to cerebral tumors, with time delta activities became more related to sleep and anesthesia. The IFSECN[53] defines delta waves as waves with a duration of more than 1/4 s (which implies a frequency band between 0 and 4 Hz). There have been various studies aiming at disclosing the relationship between cellular activities and EEG and the sources of delta activities[54,55]. In the following it will be emphasized that the 0–4 Hz frequency range reflects more than one phenomenon and that definitions based exclusively on frequency bands may conceal the underlying mechanism. Studies have unveiled the electrophysiological substrates of several distinct activities in the frequency range below 4 Hz during sleep and anesthesia. Their interaction within corticothalamic networks yields to a complex pattern whose reflection at the EEG level takes the shape of polymorphic waves.

It should also be stressed from the beginning that delta activities cover two EEG phenomena: waves and oscillations with some regularity of the variation, with no clear separations between the two, as far as spectral analysis is concerned.

As for now, there are at least two sources of delta activities: one originating in the thalamus and the other one in the cortex.

*Thalamic delta* oscillations have been found in a series of in vitro studies. They revealed that a clock-like oscillation within the delta frequency range (1–2 Hz) is generated by the interplay of two intrinsic currents of thalamocortical cells. Whereas most brain oscillations are generated by interactions within networks of neurons, but also glial cells, the thalamic delta oscillation is an intrinsic oscillation between two inward currents of thalamocortical cells: the transient calcium current ($I_t$) underlying the low-threshold spike (LTS) and a hyperpolarization-activated cation current ($I_h$)[56,57].

This oscillation was also found in vivo, in the thalamocortical neurons of the cat, after decortications[58]. Thalamocortical neurons from a variety of sensory, motor, associational and intralaminar thalamic nuclei were able to display a clock-like delta rhythm either induced by imposed hyperpolarizing current pulses or spontaneously. However, in intact preparations, with functional cortico-thalamic loops, the regular thalamic delta oscillation was absent or largely prevented by the ongoing cortical activity[59]. This raises concerns as to the emergence of this intrinsically generated thalamic rhythm at the level of the EEG.

The existence of *cortical delta* was suggested on the basis that delta waves, mainly at 1–2 Hz, survive in the EEG of athalamic cats[60]. Whether such procedures generate a physiological or a pathological pattern remains an open question; nonetheless, they create a deafferentation of the cortex. Extracellular recordings of cortical activity during pathological delta waves (as obtained by lesions of the sub-cortical white matter, the thalamus or the mesencephalic reticular formation) have shown a relationship between the firing probability and the surface-positive (depth-negative) delta waves, whereas the depth-positive waves were associated with a diminution in discharge rates[61]. These field-unit relationships led to the assumption that the depth-positive component of delta waves reflects maximal firing of inhibitory interneurons. However, this has not been found. It was suggested that EEG delta waves are rather generated by summation of long-lasting after-hyperpolarizations produced by a variety of potassium currents in deep-lying pyramidal neurons[62].

A third type of delta patterns appeared with the discovery of a novel oscillation dominating sleep EEG activities (around, but generally below 1 Hz)[63-68]. Its thorough investigation at the cellular level (see below) set the basis for revisiting the cellular basis of delta rhythms. The frequency of this slow oscillation depends on the anesthetic used and the behavioral state: it is slower under anesthesia than during natural sleep. It is found in both animals[63,68] and humans[64-68]. The slow oscillation is generated within the cortex because it survives after thalamectomy[69], is absent from the thalamus of decorticated animals[70] and is present in cortical slices[71]. At the intracellular level, the slow oscillation showed that cortical neurons throughout layers II to VI displayed a spontaneous oscillation recurring with periods of 1–5 seconds, depending on the anesthetic/sleep stage, and consisting of prolonged depolarizing and hyperpolarizing components (Figure 1.3A). The long-lasting depolarizations of the

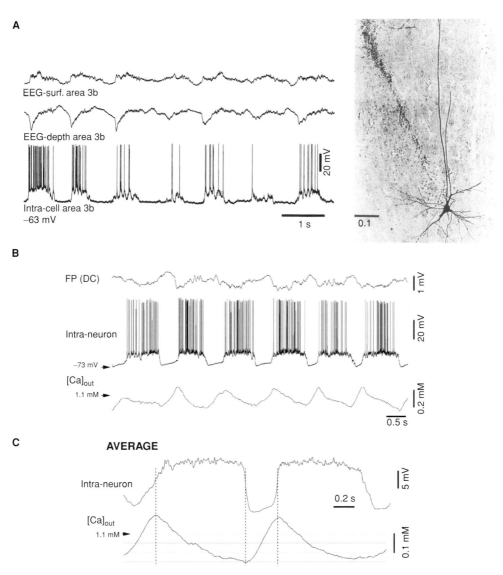

**Figure 1.3** A. Pyramidal cell from the somatosensory cortex (area 3b) during the slow (< 1 Hz) oscillation. The left panel shows intracellular recordings and simultaneously recorded EEG in the vicinity (~1 mm) of the cell. The EEG was recorded by means of coaxial electrodes located on the surface and at a depth of ~0.6 mm. The cell oscillated at 0.9 Hz with depolarizing phases corresponding to depth-EEG negative (surface-positive) potentials. The right panel shows the corresponding cell stained with Neurobiotin (calibration bar in mm). (Modified from[41].)
B. Fluctuations during the slow oscillation. Relationships between intracellular membrane potential, extracellular calcium ([Ca]$_{out}$) and field potential. Periodic neuronal depolarizations triggering action potentials were interrupted by periods (300–500 ms) of hyperpolarization and silenced synaptic activity. [Ca]$_{out}$ dropped by about 0.25 mM during the depolarizing phase reaching a minimum just before the onset of the hyperpolarization. Then, [Ca]$_{out}$ rose back until the beginning of the next cycle. C. Thirty cycles were averaged (spikes from the neuronal signal were clipped) after being extracted around the onset of the neuronal depolarization. The vertical dotted lines tentatively indicate the boundaries of the two phases of the slow oscillation. (Modified from Massimini & Amzica[74] with permission from the American Physiological Society. Copyright © 2001.)

slow oscillation consisted of EPSPs, fast prepotentials and fast IPSPs reflecting the action of synaptically coupled GABAergic local-circuit cortical cells[72]. The long-lasting hyperpolarization, interrupting the depolarizing events, is associated with network disfacilitation in the cortex[73] achieved by a progressive depletion of the extracellular calcium ions during the depolarizing phase of the slow oscillation[74] (Figure 1.3B–C).

All major cellular classes in the cerebral cortex display the slow oscillation[72,75]. During the depth-positive EEG wave they are hyperpolarized, whereas during the sharp depth-negative EEG deflection cortical neurons are depolarized (Figure 1.3). The spectacular coherence between all types of cortical neurons and EEG waveforms mainly relies on the integrity of intracortical synaptic linkages, but other projections, possibly cortico-thalamo-cortical, as well as networks of gap junctions (see below) might contribute to the synchronizing of the slow oscillation.

The better comprehension of the mechanisms determining the pacing of the slow oscillations came from experiments considering the possible dialogue between neurons and glial cells. Dual simultaneous intracellular recordings from neurons and adjacent glial cells explored the possibility that glia may not only passively reflect, but also influence, the state of neuronal networks[76]. The behavior of simultaneously recorded neurons and glia is illustrated in Figure 1.4. During spontaneously occurring slow oscillations, the onset of the glial depolarization did, in the vast majority of the cases, follow the onset of the neuronal depolarization with an average time lag around 90 ms (Figure 1.4). This time lag is, however, longer than the one obtained from pairs of neurons (around 10 ms in Amzica & Steriade[77]). The glial depolarization reflects with virtually no delay the potassium uptake[78]. Toward the end of the depolarizing phase, the glial membrane begins to repolarize before the neurons (Figure 1.4)[79]. Glial cells might thus control the pace of the oscillation through changes in the concentration of extracellular potassium[78].

The overall synchronization of the slow oscillation in the cortex is also assisted by glial cells, which are embedded in a gap junction-based network, through the phenomenon of spatial buffering[80,81]. Spatial buffering evens local increases of extracellular potassium by transferring it from the extracellular milieu to the neighboring glial cells, then through gap junctions and along the potassium concentration gradient, at more distant sites with lower concentrations of potassium, where it is again expelled into the extracellular space. The local spatial buffering during slow oscillations might play two roles: (i) it contributes to the steady depolarization of neurons during the depolarizing phase of the slow oscillation, and (ii) it modulates the neuronal excitability. The latter mechanism could favor the synaptic interaction within cortical networks at the onset of the depolarizing phase of the slow oscillation, but it could equally induce a gradual disfacilitation.

The same cortical glial cells, if organized along an axis parallel to the apical dendrites, could constitute a powerful dipole, which, together with the already existing dipole of arterioles plunging into the cortex from the pial surface, could constitute a source of EEG activities. This aspect of utmost importance still remains to be investigated.

The complex electrographic pattern of slow-wave sleep results from the coalescence of the slow oscillation with spindle (see below) and delta oscillations[82]. The weight of each of these major components is dynamically modulated during sleep by synaptic coupling, local circuit configurations and the general behavioral state of the network. Through its rhythmic occurrence at a frequency that is lower than that of other sleep rhythms (spindles and delta), and due to its wide synchronization at the cortical level, the cortical slow oscillation

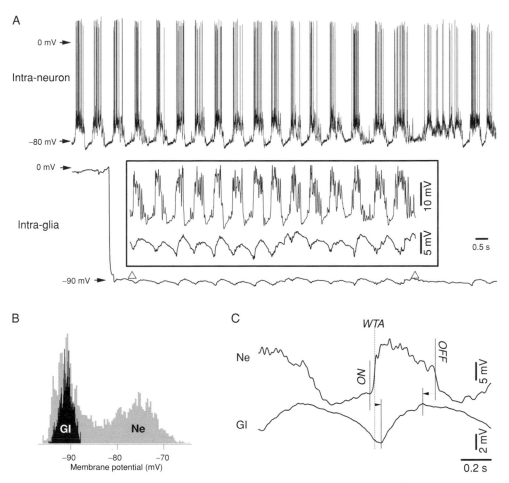

**Figure 1.4** Simultaneous recording of a neuron–glia pair in the cortex of the cat during slow oscillatory patterns. A. Relationship between neuronal and glial depolarizations on the one hand, and between neuronal hyperpolarization and glial repolarizations, on the other hand (note enlargement within the box). The glial impalement occurred during this period of the recording and is depicted as a brisk drop of the potential from the extracellular (0 mV) to the intracellular (−90 mV) level. B. Histogram of membrane potential variations in the neuron (in gray) and glial cell (in black). C. Typical time relationship between the onset and offset moments of the two phases of a slow oscillatory cycle. Note that the onset of the depolarizing phase starts in the neuron, but that the end of this period is anticipated in the glia. (Modified from Amzica & Massimini[79] by permission of Oxford University Press.)

provides a synchronous input to thalamic neurons, thus triggering and/or grouping sequences of spindles or delta oscillations.

## Theta rhythms

Theta waves are usually in the 4–7 Hz frequency range. The normal theta activity should not be confused with pathological theta waves[83], described as a slowing down of alpha activity, expressed during cerebral blood flow reduction[84], or metabolic encephalopathies[85].

In humans and monkeys[86], locally generated intracranial theta activity is prominent in anterior midline and cingulate regions during working memory tasks[87,88]. It is often phase locked to high frequency gamma activity[89] (see below), giving rise to an "oscillatory hierarchy."

Theta activity appears conspicuously in rodents such as rabbits (first description of the rhythm by Green & Arduini, 1954[90]) and rats (see below) in relation with sensory processing and the control of different types of movements[91]. In cats, theta oscillations occur almost exclusively during REM sleep[92].

These theta waves have been described in the cortical limbic system (hippocampus, entorhinal cortex and cingular areas) where they display, according to species and conditions, rhythmic activities extending from 3–4 Hz to 10 Hz, which is somehow larger than the conventional range of the theta rhythm (4–7 Hz). The search for a theta pacemaker has led to controversial results: on the one hand, it was claimed that the septo-hippocampal cholinergic system, driven by the brain-stem reticular core, is the pacemaker of the theta[93,94]. On the other hand, a dipole of theta activity was found in the entorhinal cortex, with two amplitude maxima, one superficial in layers I–II and the other in layer III[95-97]. Another theta dipole is set up by inhibitory currents on the soma of pyramidal cells[98,99] generated by hippocampal local circuit inhibitory cells. Different dipoles have been found in restrained and freely moving animals[100-102]. The presence of such well-organized dipoles in the hippocampus, together with the very dorsal location of the hippocampus in the brain of rodents is one of the reasons for the overt expression of theta activity in the EEG of these animals.

The theta oscillation is considered to be the result of an interaction within neuronal networks. The first intracellular recordings reported that 85% of the pyramidal cells of the hippocampus CA1 and CA2 areas were synchronous with the field potentials and that this was due to rhythmic excitatory synaptic potentials (EPSPs)[103]. The latter observation received formal confirmation from Nuñez and colleagues[104], who also mentioned the contribution of calcium-mediated slow spikes to the depolarizing events.

## Alpha rhythms

This section summarizes the few elements presently known about the mechanism(s) and origin(s) of alpha rhythm occurring in the frequency range of 8–13 Hz, mainly around 10 Hz. Its initial description also marked the beginning of EEG. A more recent and exhaustive review of different EEG patterns of alpha rhythms in the waking adult can be found in Niedermeyer[105]. However, with few exceptions, the study of the cellular behavior was prevented mainly by the fact that alpha oscillations appear only during wakefulness and no valid anesthesia model was established. The fact that the alpha band overlaps with another EEG phenomenon, the sleep spindles (or sigma rhythms, see below) led to a legitimate, although failed attempt to study it under barbiturate anesthesia[106]. Thus, most of our present knowledge is based on scalp recordings in humans and laminar profiles of cortical field potentials in animals.

Occipital alpha waves usually occur during reduced visual attention. However, there are reports of their enhancement by attention tasks[107,108]. In a series of prolific and elegant experimental studies performed on dogs, Lopes da Silva and colleagues established that alpha rhythms originate in the cerebral cortex, mostly in the visual areas, although they can also be recorded in the visual thalamus (lateral geniculate and pulvinar nuclei)[109]. In the visual cortex, alpha waves are generated by an equivalent dipole layer centered at the level of the somata and basal dendrites of pyramidal neurons in layers IV and V[110]. Furthermore, the coherence of alpha waves within the visual cortex was not dependent on the thalamic coherence measured in the same animal[110,111] leading to the conclusion that horizontal intracortical linkages are essential to the spread of alpha activities, with only moderate implication of the thalamus.

## Spindle (sigma) rhythms

Classically, spindles have been regarded as one of the first signs of EEG synchronization during the early stage of quiescent sleep. This type of oscillation is defined by the presence of two distinct rhythms: waxing and waning spindle waves at 7–14 Hz within sequences lasting for 1–2 seconds, and the periodic recurrence of spindle sequences with a slow rhythm, generally 0.2–0.5 Hz. Spindles are generated within the thalamus because they survive in the thalamus after decortications and high brainstem transsection[112]. Sleep spindles have been mostly studied in cats (in vivo) and ferrets (in vitro). Humans and cats have similar sleep cycles, EEG patterns and ultrastructural organization of their thalamus. Both intrinsic properties of various thalamic neurons[113] and network linkages (for review, see Steriade[114]) contribute to the patterning of spindles.

The thalamic circuits comprise two main structures: (a) the dorsal thalamus, made of several nuclei, each of them containing both relay (thalamo-cortical) and local circuit (inter-) neurons, and (b) the nucleus reticularis thalami (RE). The latter is a thin sheet of GABA-ergic neurons that covers the rostral, lateral and ventral surfaces of the thalamus[115]. It mainly receives inputs from the cerebral cortex and dorsal thalamus, but also from the rostral sector of the brainstem and basal forebrain. The RE-thalamic-cortical-RE loop constitutes a resonating circuit that reinforces the spindle oscillation. Moreover, spindles generated within the RE nucleus travel along the dorsal thalamic relay pathway en route to the cortex, which probably is responsible for the genesis of the dipole that allows them to surface in the EEG. Interestingly, no spindles are recorded in the EEG of kittens during the first 6–7 days of life, although they are already present in thalamic recordings 3–4 hours after birth[116], suggesting that no viable dipole is generated in the thalamus. The brainstem and basal forebrain projections exert activating effects on the above-mentioned circuit with the result of inhibiting spindles.

The RE nucleus has been pointed out as the pacemaker for spindle oscillations because spindles were abolished in the dorsal thalamus after disconnection from the RE[117]. Similarly, spindles are absent in the cingular cortex[118] and habenular nuclei, other structures that are devoid of RE inputs.

A fundamental question concerns the triggering factor of a spindle. Steriade and colleagues[119] have assumed that any excitatory drive stimulating RE cells would start the process. In an intact sleeping brain, the reticulo-thalamic network undergoes periodic, synchronized excitatory inputs from the cortex such as K-complexes (see above), which then shape and modulate the duration of spindles[120]. Moreover, the synchronization of spindles in the thalamus was widespread, with virtual zero time-lag, in intact preparations, but dropped drastically after decortications[121,122].

A final observation concerns the overlapping frequency range of spindles and alpha waves. It should be emphasized that topography[123] as well as behavioral context and mechanisms are dissimilar. Alpha waves generally occur during relaxed wakefulness and, in some studies they are considered to regulate afferent and efferent signals[124]. Spindle oscillations, however, occur during unconsciousness, thus making the idea of an alpha-to-spindle continuum obsolete.

# Faster (beta, gamma) rhythms

At the opposite side of the EEG spectrum of slow sleep rhythms are fast ($> 15\,Hz$) oscillations associated with wakefulness and paradoxical (REM) sleep. The brain substrate of EEG activation upon arousal has been increasingly understood since the pioneering work of Moruzzi and Magoun[125]. They reported an "activation" response to the stimulation of brainstem structures consisting of the suppression of spindles and slower EEG rhythms. The cellular mechanisms of this suppressing mechanism have recently been analyzed: the blockage of spindles occurs at the very site of their genesis (the RE nucleus) through the action of acetylcholine, serotonin and norepinephrine. Acetylcholine hyperpolarizes RE[126,127], the last two depolarize it[128], but the combined action of these neurotransmitters is far from being understood. The intrinsically generated thalamic delta oscillation is blocked through the depolarizing action of both acetylcholine[58] and monoamines ([118,129]). Finally, slow cortical delta activities are prevented by cholinergic actions of the nucleus basalis neurons[130,131].

The disappearance of slow-sleep waveforms during the activating response is also accompanied by the appearance of peculiar fast rhythms characterizing wakefulness[132]. This study reported, in addition to the ocular syndrome of arousal, a clear-cut enhancement in amplitude of the spontaneous EEG rhythms and their regular acceleration to 40–45 Hz instead of the until-then observed flattening of the cortical EEG. Since then, several papers have mentioned the presence of 20–40 Hz waves in various cortical areas, during different conditions of increased alertness. For instance, fast rhythms were observed in a canine subject in the occipital cortex while the dog paid intense attention to a visual stimulus[133]; during accurate performance of a conditioned response to a visual stimulus in a monkey[134]; during tasks requiring fine finger movements and focused attention in monkey motor cortical cells[135]; and during behavioral immobility associated with an enhanced level of vigilance while a cat was watching a visible but unseizable mouse[136]. Other studies have described stimulus-dependent oscillations at 25–45 Hz of the focal EEG and/or neuronal firing in the olfactory system[137] and visual cortex[138–142].

The main functional implication of these rhythms in the cortex was proposed to rely on the degree of spatial and temporal synchronization, thus allowing, at a given moment, the aggregation of various cortical areas with the purpose of creating global and coherent properties of patterns, a prerequisite for scene segmentation and figure-ground distinction[143]. The issue of this "feature binding" is controversial, especially in view of the fact that such fast rhythms are coherent within thalamocortical and cortical networks during states such as sleep and deep anesthesia reputed for the absence of any conscious behavior[144]. The latter studies were performed in myorelaxed animals therefore precluding any contamination from muscle or movement-related activities, as such interferences were described[145].

The genesis of fast (beta-gamma) activities lies at the crossroads of intrinsic and network properties. Cortical neurons generate upon depolarization intrinsic oscillations in the range around 40 Hz[146,147]. This is equally valid for a subclass of rostral intralaminar thalamic neurons[148], a property that is in line with their implication in fast oscillations during activated states associated with neuronal depolarizations, waking and REM sleep. Intralaminar nuclei are particularly fit for wide-range synchronization due to their widespread projections to the cerebral cortex[115] including the visual areas[149].

In spite of these intrinsic properties that make neurons prone to generate fast oscillations, their embedding in complex, especially cortical, circuits, is required for the short- and long-range synchronization, in order to make the rhythm emerge at the EEG level. Freeman[137] postulated that the generation of 40–80 Hz activity in the olfactory bulb depends on feedback inhibitory circuits involving local-circuit GABAergic neurons acting on output elements, the mitral cells. Rat somatosensory slices with slightly reduced inhibition, however, displayed activities around 37 Hz generated by networks of intrinsically pyramid-shaped (excitatory) cells[150].

With particular consequences for the presence of fast (beta-gamma) activities in the EEG is the fact that, under anesthesia, they do not show field reversal at any depth of the cortex[63]. Volume conduction was precluded because the negative field potentials of the fast oscillations were systematically associated, at all depths, with neuronal firing and were not observable in the underlying white matter. The absence of potential reversal was explained by the fact that local currents mainly result from transmembrane components, while vertically distributed currents are weaker because current-source-density analyses show alternatively distributed microsinks and microsources[151].

The thalamus also participates in the genesis of fast oscillations. It was proposed that corticothalamic axons drive RE neurons, which further lead to the production of IPSP-rebound sequences at 40 Hz in thalamocortical relay cells thus reinforcing cortical activity[152]. If so (data still lacking), during the waking state when fast rhythms are supposed to occur preferentially, the inhibitory input from RE thalamic neurons would sculpt the tonic firing of thalamocortical cells, and rhythmic spike trains would be transmitted back to the cortex. It is nevertheless established that thalamocortical cells do oscillate within the beta-gamma frequency range and this occurs coherently with field potentials recorded from the related cortical areas (Figure 1.5).

Despite their presence during sleep and under anesthesia, fast (beta-gamma) oscillations are mainly associated with increased levels of alertness, thus closely following the onset of activity in cholinergic aggregates of the brainstem and basal forebrain. The cholinergic activation induces a twofold increase of cortical EEG waves around 40 Hz. Beyond the depolarizing effect exerted by acetylcholine on thalamocortical and cortical neurons, this neurotransmitter when tested in vivo hyperpolarized most of the glial cells, in parallel with an overall decrease in the extracellular potassium concentration[153]. This effect was also accompanied by an increase of cerebral blood flow, leading to the interpretation that the glial hyperpolarization is due to a boosted transport of potassium across capillary membranes. This is further supported by the fact that EEG activation, when recorded with DC amplifiers, generally displays a persistent positive DC shift[152]. In addition, brain activation was accompanied in glial cells by a reduced membrane capacitance suggesting that the interglial syncytium shuts down during wakefulness, preventing nonspecific synchronization through spatial buffering mechanisms (as described in the section on slow waves). This feature may thus leave the synchronization of beta-gamma activities strictly to synaptic networks, achieving a more specific aggregation of the neuronal populations involved.

## Conclusions

The scalp EEG can reflect mass activity from a much wider range of brain structures and cellular types than previously thought. Selected preparations (anesthesia in animals) and certain states (slow-wave sleep) or activation patterns (e.g. early cortical responses) are rather well understood with regard to their laminar and cellular correlates. These models can bridge the gap between cellular and macroscopic scalp events and have proven essential to validate electrical neuroimaging assumptions and source models as discussed in Chapter 4. However, for most human scalp EEG patterns of interest, solid evidence regarding their cellular,

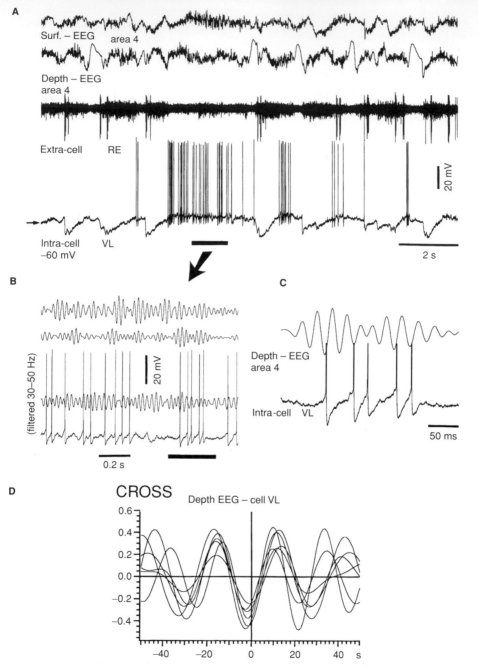

**Figure 1.5** Episodes of tonic activation are associated with coherent fast rhythms (40 Hz) in cortical EEG and intracellularly recorded thalamocortical neuron. Cat under ketamine-xylazine anesthesia. A. Four traces represent simultaneous recordings of surface and depth EEG from motor cortical area 4, extracellular discharges of neuron from the rostrolateral part of the thalamic reticular (RE) nucleus, and intracellular activity of thalamocortical neuron from ventrolateral (VL) nucleus. Electroencephalogram, RE and VL cells displayed a slow oscillation (0.7–0.8 Hz) during which the sharp depth-negative (excitatory) EEG waves led to IPSPs in VL cell, presumably generated by spike bursts in a cortically driven GABAergic RE neuron. Part marked by horizontal bar, taken from a short-lasting period of spontaneous EEG activation, is expanded in B (arrow), with EEG waves and field potentials from the RE nucleus filtered between 30 and 50 Hz; part marked by horizontal bar in this panel is further expanded in C to illustrate relations between action potentials of VL cell and depth-negative waves in cortical EEG at a frequency of 40 Hz. D. Cross-correlation (CROSS) between action potentials and depth-EEG shows clear-cut relation, with opposition of phase, between intracellularly recorded VL neuron and EEG waves. (Modified from Seignew *et al.*[153] with permission.)

laminar and regional correlates is still mostly lacking. Given the multiple generator mechanisms for several EEG frequencies, the uncertain spatial extent of synchronization, and the lack of simple one-to-one correspondence between surface and laminar activity, inferring specific circuits, cell types and laminar activities from EEG frequencies and surface polarities is certainly not warranted.

# References

1. Berger H. Über das Elektroenkephalogramm des Menschen. *Archiv für Psychiatrie und Nervenkrankheiten* 1929;**87**:527–570.

2. Niedermeyer E, Lopes da Silva F. *Electroencephalography*. Philadelphia: Lippincott Williams & Wilkins; 2005.

3. Kandel ER. *Principles of Neural Science*. 4th edn. New York: McGraw-Hill; 2000.

4. Zschocke S. *Klinische Elektroenzephalographie*. Berlin: Springer; 1995.

5. Nunez PL, Srinivasan R. *Electric Fields of the Brain*. 2nd edn. New York: Oxford University Press; 2006.

6. Lehmann D. Principles of spatial analysis. In Remond A, Gevins A (eds.), *Handbook of Electroencephalography and Clinical Neurophysiology. Vol. 1: Methods of Analysis of Brain Electrical and Magnetic Signals*. Amsterdam: Elsevier, 1987, pp. 309–354.

7. Brandeis D, Lehmann D. Event-related potentials of the brain and cognitive processes: approaches and applications. *Neuropsychologia* 1986;**24**:151–168.

8. Lehmann D, Skrandies W. Reference-free identification of components of checkerboard-evoked multichannel potential fields. *Electroencephalography and Clinical Neurophysiology* 1980;**48**:609–621.

9. Lehmann D, Ozaki H, Pal I. Averaging of spectral power and phase via vector diagram best fits without reference electrode or reference channel. *Electroencephalography and Clinical Neurophysiology* 1986;**64**:350–363.

10. Lehmann D, Michel CM. Intracerebral dipole source localization for FFT power maps. *Electroencephalography and Clinical Neurophysiology* 1990;**76**:271–276.

11. Logothetis NK, Pauls J, Augath M, Trinath T, Oeltermann A. Neurophysiological investigation of the basis of the fMRI signal. *Nature* 2001;**412**:150–157.

12. Henze DA, Borhegyi Z, Csicsvari J et al. Intracellular features predicted by extracellular recordings in the hippocampus in vivo. *Journal of Neurophysiology* 2000;**84**:390–400.

13. Scherg M, Von Cramon D. A new interpretation of the generators of BAEP waves I–V: Results of a spatio-temporal dipole model. *Electroencephalography and Clinical Neurophysiology* 1985;**62**: 290–299.

14. Gobbele R, Buchner H, Scherg M, Curio G. Stability of high-frequency (600 Hz) components in human somatosensory evoked potentials under variation of stimulus rate – evidence for a thalamic origin. *Clinical Neurophysiology* 1999; **110**:1659–1663.

15. Steriade M, McCormick DA, Sejnowski TJ. Thalamocortical oscillations in the sleeping and aroused brain. *Science* 1993; **262**:679–685.

16. Bragin A, Wilson CL, Staba RJ et al. Interictal high-frequency oscillations (80–500 Hz) in the human epileptic brain: entorhinal cortex. *Annals of Neurology* 2002;**52**:407–415.

17. Jirsch JD, Urrestarazu E, LeVan P et al. High-frequency oscillations during human focal seizures. *Brain* 2006;**129**:1593–1608.

18. Shah AS, Bressler SL, Knuth KH et al. Neural dynamics and the fundamental mechanisms of event-related brain potentials. *Cerebral Cortex* 2004;**14**:476–483.

19. Murakami S, Okada Y. Contributions of principal neocortical neurons to magnetoencephalography and electroencephalography signals. *Journal of Physiology* 2006;**575**:925–936.

20. Mitzdorf U. Current source-density method and application in cat cerebral cortex: investigation of evoked potentials

and EEG phenomena. *Physiological Reviews* 1985;**65**:37–100.

21. Schroeder C, Mehta A, Givre S. A spatiotemporal profile of visual system activation revealed by current source density analysis in the awake macaque. *Cerebral Cortex* 1998;**8**:575–592.

22. Ulbert I, Heit G, Madsen J, Karmos G, Halgren E. Laminar analysis of human neocortical interictal spike generation and propagation: current source density and multiunit analysis in vivo. *Epilepsia* 2004; **45 Suppl.** 4:48–56.

23. Tenke CE, Schroeder CE, Arezzo JC, Vaughan HG, Jr. Interpretation of high-resolution current source density profiles: a simulation of sublaminar contributions to the visual evoked potential. *Experimental Brain Research* 1993;**94**:183–192.

24. Steinschneider M, Tenke CE, Schroeder CE *et al.* Cellular generators of the cortical auditory evoked potential initial component. *Electroencephalography and Clinical Neurophysiology* 1992;**84**: 196–200.

25. Megevand P, Quairiaux C, Lascano AM, Kiss JZ, Michel CM. A mouse model for studying large-scale neuronal networks using EEG mapping techniques. *Neuroimage* 2008;**42**:591–602.

26. Scherg M, Vajsar J, Picton TW. A source analysis of the late human auditory evoked potential. *J Cogn Neurosci* 1989;**1**:336–355.

27. Hämäläinen MS, Hari R, Ilmoniemi RJ, Knuutila JE, Lounasmaa OV. Magnetoencephalography – theory, instrumentation, and applications to noninvasive studies of the working human brain. *Review of Modern Physics* 1993;**65**: 413–497.

28. Ioannides AA, Fenwick PBC. Imaging cerebellum activity in real time with magnetoencephalographic data. *Progress in Brain Research* 2004;**148**:139–150.

29. Martin T, Houck JM, Pearson Bish J *et al.* MEG reveals different contributions of somatomotor cortex and cerebellum to simple reaction time after temporally structured cues. *Human Brain Mapping* 2006;**27**:552–561.

30. Timmermann L, Gross J, Dirks M *et al.* The cerebral oscillatory network of parkinsonian resting tremor. *Brain* 2002; **126**:199–212.

31. Attal Y, Bhattacharjee M, Yelnik J *et al.* Modeling and detecting deep brain activity with MEG & EEG. *Conference Proceedings of the IEEE Engineering in Medicine and Biology Society* 2007;**2007**:4937–4940.

32. Lantz G, Grave de Peralta R, Gonzalez S, Michel CM. Noninvasive localization of electromagnetic epileptic activity. II. Demonstration of sublobar accuracy in patients with simultaneous surface and depth recordings. *Brain Topography* 2001;**14**:139–147.

33. Michel CM, Lantz G, Spinelli L *et al.* 128-channel EEG source imaging in epilepsy: clinical yield and localization precision. *Journal of Clinical Neurophysiology* 2004;**21**:71–83.

34. Smith DB, Sidman RD, Henke JS *et al.* Scalp and depth recordings of induced deep cerebral potentials. *Electroencephalography and Clinical Neurophysiology* 1983;**55**:145–150.

35. Lai Y, van Drongelen W, Ding L *et al.* Estimation of in vivo human brain-to-skull conductivity ratio from simultaneous extra- and intra-cranial electrical potential recordings. *Clinical Neurophysiology* 2005; **116**:456–465.

36. Grieve PG, Emerson RG, Fifer WP, Isler JR, Stark RI. Spatial correlation of the infant and adult electroencephalogram. *Clinical Neurophysiology* 2003;**114**:1594–1608.

37. Lantz G, Holub M, Ryding E, Rosen I. Simultaneous intracranial and extracranial recording of interictal epileptiform activity in patients with drug resistant partial epilepsy: patterns of conduction and results from dipole reconstructions. *Electroencephalography and Clinical Neurophysiology* 1996;**99**:69–78.

38. Nayak D, Valentin A, Alarcon G *et al.* Characteristics of scalp electrical fields associated with deep medial temporal epileptiform discharges. *Clinical Neurophysiology* 2004;**115**:1423–1435.

39. Tao JX, Ray A, Hawes-Ebersole S, Ebersole JS. Intracranial EEG substrates of scalp EEG interictal spikes. *Epilepsia* 2005;**46**: 669–676.

40. Zumsteg D, Friedman A, Wennberg RA, Wieser HG. Source localization of mesial temporal interictal epileptiform discharges: Correlation with intracranial foramen ovale electrode recordings. *Clinical Neurophysiology* 2006;**117**:562–571.

41. Schevon CA, Cappell J, Emerson R *et al.* Cortical abnormalities in epilepsy revealed by local EEG synchrony. *NeuroImage* 2007; **35**:140–148.

42. Cooper R, Winter AL, Crow HJ, Walter WG. Comparison of subcortical, cortical and scalp activity using chronically indwelling electrodes in man. *Electroencephalography and Clinical Neurophysiology* 1965;**18**:217–228.

43. Kobayashi K, Yoshinaga H, Ohtsuka Y, Gotman J. Dipole modeling of epileptic spikes can be accurate or misleading. *Epilepsia* 2005;**46**:397–408.

44. Zhang Y, Ding L, van Drongelen W *et al.* A cortical potential imaging study from simultaneous extra- and intracranial electrical recordings by means of the finite element method. *Neuroimage* 2006; **31**:1513–1524.

45. Perez-Borja C, Chatrian GE, Tyce FA, Rivers MH. Electrographic patterns of the occipital lobe in man: a topographic study based on use of implanted electrodes. *Electroencephalography and Clinical Neurophysiology* 1962;**14**:171–182.

46. Amzica F, Steriade M. Integration of low-frequency sleep oscillations in corticothalamic networks. *Acta Neurobiologiae Experimentalis (Warszawa)* 2000;**60**:229–245.

47. Steriade M, Contreras D. Relations between cortical and thalamic cellular events during transition from sleep patterns to paroxysmal activity. *Journal of Neuroscience* 1995;**15**:623–642.

48. Sarnthein J, Morel A, von Stein A, Jeanmonod D. Thalamocortical theta coherence in neurological patients at rest and during a working memory task.

49. Steriade M, Contreras D, Amzica F. Synchronized sleep oscillations and their paroxysmal developments. *Trends in Neuroscience* 1994;**17**:199–208.

50. McCormick DA, Contreras D. On the cellular and network bases of epileptic seizures. *Annual Review of Physiology* 2001;**63**:815–846.

51. Amzica F, Steriade M. Spontaneous and artificial activation of neocortical seizures. *Journal of Neurophysiology* 1999;**82**:3123–3138.

52. Walter G. The location of cerebral tumors by electro-encephalography. *Lancet* 1936; **8**:305–308.

53. IFSECN. A glossary of terms most commonly used by clinical electroencephalographers. *Electroencephalography and Clinical Neurophysiology* 1974;**37**:538–548.

54. Kellaway P, Gol A, Proler M. Electrical activity of the isolated cerebral hemisphere and isolated thalamus. *Experimental Neurology* 1966;**14**:281–304.

55. Rappelsberger P, Pockberger H, Petsche H. The contribution of the cortical layers to the generation of the EEG: field potential and current source density analyses in the rabbit's visual cortex. *Electroencephalography and Clinical Neurophysiology* 1982;**53**:254–269.

56. McCormick DA, Pape HC. Properties of a hyperpolarization-activated cation current and its role in rhythmic oscillation in thalamic relay neurones. *Journal of Physiology* 1990;**431**:291–318.

57. Leresche N, Jassik-Gerschenfeld D, Haby M, Soltesz I, Crunelli V. Pacemaker-like and other types of spontaneous membrane potential oscillations of thalamocortical cells. *Neuroscience Letters* 1990;**113**:72–77.

58. Steriade M, Dossi RC, Nunez A. Network modulation of a slow intrinsic oscillation of cat thalamocortical neurons implicated in sleep delta waves: cortically induced synchronization and brainstem cholinergic suppression. *Journal of Neuroscience* 1991;**11**:3200–3217.

59. Nita DA, Steriade M, Amzica F. Hyperpolarisation rectification in cat

48. ... *International Journal of Psychophysiology* 2005;**57**:87–96.

lateral geniculate neurons modulated by intact corticothalamic projections. *Journal of Physiology* 2003;**552**:325–332.

60. Villablanca J. Role of the thalamus in sleep control: sleep-wakefulness studies in chronic diencephalic and athalamic cats. In Petre-Quadens O, Schlag J, eds. *Basic Sleep Mechanisms.* New York: Academic Press; 1974, pp. 51–81.

61. Ball GJ, Gloor P, Schaul N. The cortical electromicrophysiology of pathological delta waves in the electroencephalogram of cats. *Electroencephalography and Clinical Neurophysiology* 1977;**43**:346–361.

62. Steriade M, Gloor P, Llinas RR, Lopes de Silva FH, Mesulam MM. Report of IFCN Committee on Basic Mechanisms. Basic mechanisms of cerebral rhythmic activities. *Electroencephalography and Clinical Neurophysiology* 1990;**76**:481–508.

63. Steriade M, Amzica F, Contreras D. Synchronization of fast (30–40 Hz) spontaneous cortical rhythms during brain activation. *Journal of Neuroscience* 1996;**16**:392–417.

64. Amzica F, Steriade M. The K-complex: its slow (< 1-Hz) rhythmicity and relation to delta waves. *Neurology* 1997;**49**:952–959.

65. Achermann P, Borbely AA. Low-frequency (< 1 Hz) oscillations in the human sleep electroencephalogram. *Neuroscience* 1997;**81**:213–222.

66. Molle M, Marshall L, Gais S, Born J. Grouping of spindle activity during slow oscillations in human non-rapid eye movement sleep. *Journal of Neuroscience* 2002;**22**:10941–10947.

67. Simon NR, Manshanden I, Lopes da Silva FH. A MEG study of sleep. *Brain Research* 2000;**860**:64–76.

68. Massimini M, Rosanova M, Mariotti M. EEG slow (approximately 1 Hz) waves are associated with nonstationarity of thalamo-cortical sensory processing in the sleeping human. *Journal of Neurophysiology* 2003;**89**:1205–1213.

69. Steriade M, Nunez A, Amzica F. Intracellular analysis of relations between the slow (< 1 Hz) neocortical oscillation and other sleep rhythms of the electroencephalogram. *Journal of Neuroscience* 1993;**13**:3266–3283.

70. Timofeev I, Contreras D, Steriade M. Synaptic responsiveness of cortical and thalamic neurones during various phases of slow sleep oscillation in cat. *Journal of Physiology* 1996;**494 (Pt 1)**:265–278.

71. Sanchez-Vives MV, McCormick DA. Cellular and network mechanisms of rhythmic recurrent activity in neocortex. *Nature Neuroscience* 2000;**3**:1027–1034.

72. Steriade M, Nunez A, Amzica F. A novel slow (< 1 Hz) oscillation of neocortical neurons in vivo: depolarizing and hyperpolarizing components. *Journal of Neuroscience* 1993;**13**:3252–3265.

73. Contreras D, Timofeev I, Steriade M. Mechanisms of long-lasting hyperpolarizations underlying slow sleep oscillations in cat corticothalamic networks. *Journal of Physiology* 1996;**494 (Pt 1)**:251–264.

74. Massimini M, Amzica F. Extracellular calcium fluctuations and intracellular potentials in the cortex during the slow sleep oscillation. *Journal of Neurophysiology* 2001;**85**:1346–1350.

75. Contreras D, Steriade M. Cellular basis of EEG slow rhythms: a study of dynamic corticothalamic relationships. *Journal of Neuroscience* 1995;**15**:604–622.

76. Amzica F, Neckelmann D. Membrane capacitance of cortical neurons and glia during sleep oscillations and spike-wave seizures. *Journal of Neurophysiology* 1999;**82**:2731–2746.

77. Amzica F, Steriade M. Short- and long-range neuronal synchronization of the slow (< 1 Hz) cortical oscillation. *Journal of Neurophysiology* 1995;**73**:20–38.

78. Amzica F, Massimini M, Manfridi A. Spatial buffering during slow and paroxysmal sleep oscillations in cortical networks of glial cells in vivo. *Journal of Neuroscience* 2002;**22**:1042–1053.

79. Amzica F, Massimini M. Glial and neuronal interactions during slow wave and paroxysmal activities in the neocortex. *Cerebral Cortex* 2002;**12**:1101–1113.

80. Orkand RK, Nicholls JG, Kuffler SW. Effect of nerve impulses on the membrane potential of glial cells in the central

nervous system of amphibia. *Journal of Neurophysiology* 1966;**29**:788–806.

81. Kettenmann H, Ransom BR. Electrical coupling between astrocytes and between oligodendrocytes studied in mammalian cell cultures. *Glia* 1988;**1**:64–73.

82. Steriade M, Amzica F. Coalescence of sleep rhythms and their chronology in corticothalamic networks. *Sleep Research Online* 1998;**1**:1–10.

83. Sarnthein J, Morel A, von Stein A, Jeanmonod D. Thalamocortical theta coherence in neurological patients at rest and during a working memory task. *International Journal of Psychophysiology* 2005;**57**:87–96.

84. Ingvar DH, Sjolund B, Ardo A. Correlation between dominant EEG frequency, cerebral oxygen uptake and blood flow. *Electroencephalography and Clinical Neurophysiology* 1976;**41**: 268–276.

85. Saunders MG, Westmoreland BF. The EEG in evaluation of disorders affecting the brain diffusely. In Klass DW, Daly DD, eds. *Current Practice of Clinical Electroencephalography*. New York: Raven Press; 1979; pp. 343–379.

86. Tsujimoto T, Shimazu H, Isomura Y. Direct recording of theta oscillations in primate prefrontal and anterior cingulate cortices. *Journal of Neurophysiology* 2006;**95**:2987–3000.

87. Raghavachari S, Lisman JE, Tully M *et al.* Theta oscillations in human cortex during a working-memory task: evidence for local generators. *Journal of Neurophysiology* 2006;**95**:1630–1638.

88. Meltzer JA, Zaveri HP, Goncharova, II *et al.* Effects of working memory load on oscillatory power in human intracranial EEG. *Cerebral Cortex* 2008;**18**:1843–1855.

89. Lakatos P, Shah AS, Knuth KH *et al.* An oscillatory hierarchy controlling neuronal excitability and stimulus processing in the auditory cortex. *Journal of Neurophysiology* 2005;**94**:1904–1911.

90. Green JD, Arduini AA. Hippocampal electrical activity in arousal. *Journal of Neurophysiology* 1954;**17**:533–557.

91. Buzsaki G. The hippocampo-neocortical dialogue. *Cerebral Cortex* 1996;**6**:81–92.

92. Jouvet M. Paradoxical sleep – a study of its nature and mechanisms. In Akert K, Bally C, Schadé JP, eds. *Progress in Brain Research, Vol. 18, Sleep Mechanisms.* Amsterdam: Elsevier; 1965, pp. 20–57.

93. Petsche H, Gogolak G, Vanzwieten PA. Rhythmicity of septal cell discharges at various levels of reticular excitation. *Electroencephalography and Clinical Neurophysiology* 1965;**19**:25–33.

94. Petsche H, Stumpf C, Gogolak G. The significance of the rabbit's septum as a relay station between the midbrain and the hippocampus. The control of hippocampus arousal activity by septum cells. *Electroencephalography and Clinical Neurophysiology* 1962;**14**:202–211.

95. Alonso A, Garcia-Austt E. Neuronal sources of theta rhythm in the entorhinal cortex of the rat. I. Laminar distribution of theta field potentials. *Experimental Brain Research* 1987;**67**:493–501.

96. Mitchell SJ, Ranck JB, Jr. Generation of theta rhythm in medial entorhinal cortex of freely moving rats. *Brain Research* 1980; **189**:49–66.

97. Boeijinga PH, Lopes da Silva FH. Differential distribution of beta and theta EEG activity in the entorhinal cortex of the cat. *Brain Research* 1988;**448**:272–286.

98. Buzsaki G, Czopf J, Kondakor I, Kellenyi L. Laminar distribution of hippocampal rhythmic slow activity (RSA) in the behaving rat: current-source density analysis, effects of urethane and atropine. *Brain Research* 1986;**365**:125–137.

99. Soltesz I, Deschenes M. Low- and high-frequency membrane potential oscillations during theta activity in CA1 and CA3 pyramidal neurons of the rat hippocampus under ketamine-xylazine anesthesia. *Journal of Neurophysiology* 1993;**70**:97–116.

100. Bland BH, Anderson P, Ganes T. Two generators of hippocampal theta activity in rabbits. *Brain Research* 1975;**94**:199–218.

101. Green JD, Maxwell DS, Schindler WJ, Stumpf C. Rabbit EEG "theta" rhythm: its anatomical source and relation to activity in single neurons. *Journal of Neurophysiology* 1960;**23**:403–420.

102. Winson J. Patterns of hippocampal theta rhythm in the freely moving rat. *Electroencephalography and Clinical Neurophysiology* 1974;**36**:291–301.

103. Fujita Y, Sato T. Intracellular records from hippocampal pyramidal cells in rabbit during theta rhythm activity. *Journal of Neurophysiology* 1964;**27**:1012–1025.

104. Nunez A, Garcia-Austt E, Buno W, Jr. Intracellular theta-rhythm generation in identified hippocampal pyramids. *Brain Research* 1987;**416**:289–300.

105. Niedermeyer E. The normal EEG of the waking adult. In Niedermeyer E, Lopes da Silva FH, eds. *Electroencephalography: Basic Principles, Clinical Applications, and Related Fields*. Baltimore: Lippincott, Williams & Wilkins; 2005, pp. 167–192.

106. Andersen P, Andersson SA. *Physiological Basis of the Alpha Rhythm*. New York: Appleton-Century-Crofts; 1968.

107. Creutzfeld O, Grünvald G, Simonova O, Schmitz H. Changes of the basic rhythms of the EEG during the performance of mental and visuomotor tasks. In Evans CR, Mulholland TB, eds. *Attention in Neurophysiology*. London: Butterworth; 1969, pp. 148–168.

108. Ray WJ, Cole HW. EEG alpha activity reflects attentional demands, and beta activity reflects emotional and cognitive processes. *Science* 1985;**228**:750–752.

109. Lopes da Silva FH, Van Lierop THMT, Schrijer CFM, Storm Van Leeuwen W. Organization of thalamic and cortical alpha rhythm: spectra and coherences. *Electroencephalography and Clinical Neurophysiology* 1973;**35**:627–639.

110. Lopes da Silva FH, Storm Van Leeuwen W. The cortical alpha rhythm in dog: depth and surface profile of phase. In Brazier MAB, Petsche H, eds. *Architecture of the Cerebral Cortex, IBRO Monograph Series, Vol. 3*. New York: New York; 1978, pp. 319–333.

111. Lopes da Silva FH, Vos JE, Mooibroek J, Van Rotterdam A. Relative contributions of intracortical and thalamo-cortical processes in the generation of alpha rhythms, revealed by partial coherence analysis. *Electroencephalography and Clinical Neurophysiology* 1980;**50**:449–456.

112. Morison RS, Bassett DL. Electrical activity of the thalamus and basal ganglia in decorticate cats. *Journal of Neurophysiology* 1945;**8**:309–314.

113. Steriade M, Llinas RR. The functional states of the thalamus and the associated neuronal interplay. *Physiological Review* 1988;**68**:649–742.

114. Steriade M. Cellular substrates of brain rhythms. In Niedermeyer E, Lopes da Silva FH, eds. *Electroencephalography: Basic Principles, Clinical Applications and Related Fields, 5th edn*. Baltimore: Lippincott Williams & Wilkins; 2005, pp. 31–84.

115. Jones EG. *The Thalamus*. New York: Plenum; 1985.

116. Domich L, Oakson G, Deschenes M, Steriade M. Thalamic and cortical spindles during early ontogenesis in kittens. *Brain Research* 1987;**428**:140–142.

117. Steriade M, Deschenes M, Domich L, Mulle C. Abolition of spindle oscillations in thalamic neurons disconnected from nucleus reticularis thalami. *Journal of Neurophysiology* 1985;**54**:1473–1497.

118. Leung LW, Borst JG. Electrical activity of the cingulate cortex. I. Generating mechanisms and relations to behavior. *Brain Research* 1987;**407**:68–80.

119. Steriade M, Domich L, Oakson G, Deschenes M. The deafferented reticular thalamic nucleus generates spindle rhythmicity. *Journal of Neurophysiology* 1987;**57**:260–273.

120. Contreras D, Steriade M. Spindle oscillation in cats: the role of corticothalamic feedback in a thalamically generated rhythm. *Journal of Physiology* 1996;**490 (Pt 1)**:159–179.

121. Contreras D, Destexhe A, Sejnowski TJ, Steriade M. Control of spatiotemporal coherence of a thalamic oscillation by corticothalamic feedback. *Science* 1996; **274**:771–774.

122. Contreras D, Destexhe A, Sejnowski TJ, Steriade M. Spatiotemporal patterns of spindle oscillations in cortex and thalamus. *Journal of Neuroscience* 1997; **17**:1179–1196.

123. Finelli LA, Borbely AA, Achermann P. Functional topography of the human non REM sleep electroencephalogram. *European Journal of Neuroscience* 2001;**13**: 2282–2290.

124. Sanford AJ. A periodic basis for perception and action. In Colquhoun WP, ed. *Biological Rhythms and Human Perception.* New York: Academic Press; 1971, pp. 179–209.

125. Moruzzi G, Magoun HW. Brain stem reticular formation and activation of the EEG. *Electroencephalography and Clinical Neurophysiology* 1949;**1**:455–473.

126. Hu B, Steriade M, Deschenes M. The cellular mechanism of thalamic ponto-geniculo-occipital waves. *Neuroscience* 1989;**31**:25–35.

127. McCormick DA, Prince DA. Acetylcholine induces burst firing in thalamic reticular neurones by activating a potassium conductance. *Nature* 1986;**319**:402–405.

128. McCormick DA, Wang Z. Serotonin and noradrenaline excite GABAergic neurones of the guinea-pig and cat nucleus reticularis thalami. *Journal of Physiology* 1991;**442**:235–255.

129. McCormick DA, Pape HC. Noradrenergic and serotonergic modulation of a hyperpolarization-activated cation current in thalamic relay neurones. *Journal of Physiology* 1990;**431**:319–342.

130. Steriade M, Amzica F, Nunez A. Cholinergic and noradrenergic modulation of the slow (approximately 0.3 Hz) oscillation in neocortical cells. *Journal of Neurophysiology* 1993;**70**:1385–1400.

131. Buzsaki G, Bickford RG, Ponomareff G *et al.* Nucleus basalis and thalamic control of neocortical activity in the freely moving rat. *Journal of Neuroscience* 1988;**8**:4007–4026.

132. Bremer F, Stoupel N, Van Reeth PC. Nouvelles recherches sur la facilitation et l'inhibition des potentiels évoqués corticaux dans l'éveil réticulaire. *Archives Italiennes de Biologie* 1960;**98**:229–247.

133. Lopes da Silva FH, van Rotterdam A, Storm van Leeuwen W, Tielen AM. Dynamic characteristics of visual evoked potentials in the dog. II. Beta frequency selectivity in evoked potentials and background activity. *Electroencephalography and Clinical Neurophysiology* 1970;**29**:260–268.

134. Freeman WJ, van Dijk BW. Spatial patterns of visual cortical fast EEG during conditioned reflex in a rhesus monkey. *Brain Research* 1987;**422**:267–276.

135. Murthy VN, Fetz EE. Coherent 25- to 35-Hz oscillations in the sensorimotor cortex of awake behaving monkeys. *Proceedings of the National Academy of Science USA* 1992;**89**:5670–5674.

136. Bouyer JJ, Montaron MF, Vahnee JM, Albert MP, Rougeul A. Anatomical localization of cortical beta rhythms in cat. *Neuroscience* 1987;**22**:863–869.

137. Freeman WJ. *Mass Action in the Nervous System.* New York: Academic Press; 1975.

138. Eckhorn R, Bauer R, Jordan W *et al.* Coherent oscillations: a mechanism of feature linking in the visual cortex? Multiple electrode and correlation analyses in the cat. *Biological Cybernetics* 1988;**60**:121–130.

139. Engel AK, Konig P, Gray CM, Singer W. Stimulus-dependent neuronal oscillations in cat visual cortex: inter-columnar interaction as determined by cross-correlation analysis. *European Journal of Neuroscience* 1990;**2**:588–606.

140. Gray CM, Konig P, Engel AK, Singer W. Oscillatory responses in cat visual cortex exhibit inter-columnar synchronization which reflects global stimulus properties. *Nature* 1989;**338**:334–337.

141. Gray CM, Engel AK, Konig P, Singer W. Stimulus-dependent neuronal oscillations in cat visual cortex: receptive field properties and feature dependence. *European Journal of Neuroscience* 1990; **2**:607–619.

142. Gray CM, Singer W. Stimulus-specific neuronal oscillations in orientation columns of cat visual cortex. *Proceedings of the National Academy of Sciences USA* 1989;**86**:1698–1702.

143. von der Malsburg C, Schneider W. A neural cocktail-party processor. *Biological Cybernetics* 1986;**54**:29–40.

144. Steriade M, Contreras D, Amzica F, Timofeev I. Synchronization of fast

(30–40 Hz) spontaneous oscillations in intrathalamic and thalamocortical networks. *Journal of Neuroscience* 1996; **16**:2788–2808.

145. Yuval-Greenberg S, Tomer O, Keren AS, Nelken I, Deouell LY. Transient induced gamma-band response in EEG as a manifestation of miniature saccades. *Neuron* 2008;**58**:429–441.

146. Llinas RR, Grace AA, Yarom Y. In vitro neurons in mammalian cortical layer 4 exhibit intrinsic oscillatory activity in the 10- to 50-Hz frequency range. *Proceedings of the National Academy of Sciences USA* 1991;**88**:897–901.

147. Nunez A, Amzica F, Steriade M. Voltage-dependent fast (20–40 Hz) oscillations in long-axoned neocortical neurons. *Neuroscience* 1992;**51**:7–10.

148. Steriade M, Dossi RC, Pare D, Oakson G. Fast oscillations (20–40 Hz) in thalamocortical systems and their potentiation by mesopontine cholinergic nuclei in the cat. *Proceedings of the National Academy of Sciences USA* 1991; **88**:4396–4400.

149. Cunningham ET, Jr., Levay S. Laminar and synaptic organization of the projection from the thalamic nucleus centralis to primary visual cortex in the cat. *Journal of Comparative Neurology* 1986;**254**:66–77.

150. Chagnac-Amitai Y, Connors BW. Synchronized excitation and inhibition driven by intrinsically bursting neurons in neocortex. *Journal of Neurophysiology* 1989;**62**:1149–1162.

151. Steriade M, Amzica F. Intracortical and corticothalamic coherency of fast spontaneous oscillations. *Proceedings of the National Academy of Sciences USA* 1996;**93**:2533–2538.

152. Llinás RR. Intrinsic electrical properties of mammalian neurons and CNS function. *Fidia Research Foundation Neuroscience Award Lectures.* New York: Raven Press; 1990, pp. 175–194.

153. Seigneur J, Kroeger D, Nita DA, Amzica F. Cholinergic action on cortical glial cells in vivo. *Cerebral Cortex* 2006;**16**:655–668.

# Chapter 2

# Scalp field maps and their characterization

Thomas Koenig and Lorena R.R. Gianotti

The present chapter gives a comprehensive introduction into the display and quantitative characterization of scalp field data. After introducing the construction of scalp field maps, different interpolation methods, the effect of the recording reference and the computation of spatial derivatives are discussed. The arguments raised in this first part have important implications for resolving a potential ambiguity in the interpretation of differences of scalp field data.

In the second part of the chapter different approaches for comparing scalp field data are described. All of these comparisons can be interpreted in terms of differences of intracerebral sources either in strength, or in location and orientation in a nonambiguous way.

In the present chapter we only refer to scalp field potentials, but mapping also can be used to display other features, such as power or statistical values. However, the rules for comparing and interpreting scalp field potentials might not apply to such data.

## Generic form of scalp field data

Electroencephalogram (EEG) and event-related potential (ERP) recordings consist of one value for each sample in time and for each electrode. The recorded EEG and ERP data thus represent a two-dimensional array, with one dimension corresponding to the variable "time" and the other dimension corresponding to the variable "space" or electrode. Table 2.1 shows ERP measurements over a brief time period. The ERP data (averaged over a group of healthy subjects) were recorded with 19 electrodes during a visual paradigm. The parietal midline Pz electrode has been used as the reference electrode. Because by definition the reference is zero, the values at Pz in the Table 2.1 are all zero. The measurements at the other electrodes are voltage differences against this reference. The reference issue will be discussed in detail later in this chapter.

The time course of the measured EEG data is easily inferred from the values in Table 2.1 because adjacent time points are shown in subsequent columns of the table. Thus electrode-wise line plots of the values over time visualize the time course of the measured EEG data (Figure 2.1A). An alternative view to the electrode-wise line plots is shown in Figure 2.1B, where voltage differences against a given reference are expressed in terms of different colors (red denotes in our case a positive voltage difference and blue a negative voltage difference) and different color intensity (the greater the color intensity, the larger the voltage difference). On the other hand, it is not possible to represent the scalp location of the electrodes in Table 2.1. The aim of the next section is to explain how to construct a so-called "scalp field map."

*Electrical Neuroimaging*, ed. Christoph M. Michel, Thomas Koenig, Daniel Brandeis, Lorena R.R. Gianotti and Jiří Wackermann. Published by Cambridge University Press. © Cambridge University Press 2009.

**Table 2.1** Event-related potential voltage measurements (in microvolt) recorded during a visual paradigm with the placed according to the International 10–20 System[25]. The columns show samples adjacent in time. The bold numbers indicate electrodes Pz (left panel) or Cz (right panel) as reference electrode. The table rows represent the 19 electrodes that were the sample at 100 ms that will be further investigated.

|      |      | 84 ms | 92 ms | 100 ms | 108 ms | 116 ms |
|------|------|-------|-------|--------|--------|--------|
| Fp1  | ...  | 0.90  | 1.00  | **0.35**  | −0.40  | −0.80  |
| Fp2  | ...  | 0.90  | 1.00  | **0.40**  | −0.25  | −0.75  |
| F7   | ...  | 1.10  | 1.20  | **0.75**  | 0.05   | −0.55  |
| F3   | ...  | 0.65  | 0.50  | **−0.05** | −0.70  | −1.00  |
| Fz   | ...  | 0.55  | 0.35  | **−0.30** | −0.90  | −1.25  |
| F4   | ...  | 0.55  | 0.45  | **−0.15** | −0.65  | −0.90  |
| F8   | ...  | 1.05  | 1.15  | **0.70**  | 0.05   | −0.55  |
| T3   | ...  | 1.45  | 1.70  | **1.45**  | 0.75   | −0.15  |
| C3   | ...  | 0.40  | 0.35  | **0.00**  | −0.45  | −1.00  |
| Cz   | ...  | −0.15 | −0.35 | **−0.65** | −1.10  | −1.50  |
| C4   | ...  | 0.20  | 0.20  | **−0.05** | −0.50  | −0.95  |
| T4   | ...  | 1.20  | 1.50  | **1.30**  | 0.75   | −0.05  |
| T5   | ...  | 3.00  | 3.95  | **4.05**  | 2.95   | 1.15   |
| P3   | ...  | 0.80  | 1.10  | **1.00**  | 0.45   | −0.25  |
| Pz   | ...  | 0.00  | 0.00  | **0.00**  | 0.00   | 0.00   |
| P4   | ...  | 0.80  | 1.05  | **1.00**  | 0.50   | −0.35  |
| T6   | ...  | 2.80  | 3.75  | **3.85**  | 2.75   | 0.70   |
| O1   | ...  | 3.40  | 4.65  | **4.85**  | 3.25   | 0.80   |
| O2   | ...  | 3.65  | 4.60  | **4.35**  | 2.35   | −0.65  |

## Display of a scalp field map

In order to capture the spatial information, the data needs to be graphically arranged such that the position of the electrodes on the scalp and the distances between the electrodes are adequately represented. In Figure 2.2A, a two-dimensional scheme of the electrode positions on the scalp is drawn. The three-dimensional positions of the electrodes have been warped on a two-dimensional plane with Cz as center. Electrodes were shifted away from the center based on their distance to Cz. Note that warping a sphere-like shape, as for instance the scalp surface, to a two-dimensional plane implies some distortions, similar to, for example, two-dimensional representations of the earth's surface in geographic maps. The method employed here allows the display of all the electrodes in one scheme, but overemphasizes areas at the lower boundary of the electrode array. Alternatively, one could make several schemes showing the electrode positions on the scalp seen from different angles.

Having constructed an electrode scheme, the voltage values shown in Table 2.1 are assigned to their positions, for each sample in time. This procedure is illustrated in Figure 2.2B using the values at time point 100 ms. Looking carefully at Figure 2.2B, it becomes apparent that there is a considerable order in the data: the differences between values at neighboring electrodes are often smaller than the differences between values at remote electrodes. Furthermore, in the given example, the positive and negative values form two spatially distinct groups: most negative values are found at centro-frontal electrodes, while the most

**Table 2.1** (cont.)

| | ... | 84 ms | 92 ms | 100 ms | 108 ms | 116 ms |
|---|---|---|---|---|---|---|
| Fp1 | ... | 1.05 | 1.35 | **1.00** | 0.70 | 0.70 |
| Fp2 | ... | 1.05 | 1.35 | **1.05** | 0.85 | 0.75 |
| F7 | ... | 1.25 | 1.55 | **1.40** | 1.15 | 0.95 |
| F3 | ... | 0.80 | 0.85 | **0.60** | 0.40 | 0.50 |
| Fz | ... | 0.70 | 0.70 | **0.35** | 0.20 | 0.25 |
| F4 | ... | 0.70 | 0.80 | **0.50** | 0.45 | 0.60 |
| F8 | ... | 1.20 | 1.50 | **1.35** | 1.15 | 0.95 |
| T3 | ... | 1.60 | 2.05 | **2.10** | 1.85 | 1.35 |
| C3 | ... | 0.55 | 0.70 | **0.65** | 0.65 | 0.50 |
| Cz | ... | 0.00 | 0.00 | **0.00** | 0.00 | 0.00 |
| C4 | ... | 0.35 | 0.55 | **0.60** | 0.60 | 0.55 |
| T4 | ... | 1.35 | 1.85 | **1.95** | 1.85 | 1.45 |
| T5 | ... | 3.15 | 4.30 | **4.70** | 4.05 | 2.65 |
| P3 | ... | 0.95 | 1.45 | **1.65** | 1.55 | 1.25 |
| Pz | ... | 0.15 | 0.35 | **0.65** | 1.10 | 1.50 |
| P4 | ... | 0.95 | 1.40 | **1.65** | 1.60 | 1.15 |
| T6 | ... | 2.95 | 4.10 | **4.50** | 3.85 | 2.20 |
| O1 | ... | 3.55 | 5.00 | **5.50** | 4.35 | 2.30 |
| O2 | ... | 3.80 | 4.95 | **5.00** | 3.45 | 0.85 |

positive values are found at occipital and temporal electrodes. A first impression of the spatial structure of the data is thus already achieved.

In a next step, one can connect with a line all electrode locations with a given measurement, let us say +1 microvolt (µV), and all points in between with, in this case, an interpolated value of 1 µV (see below for the interpolation issue). Such lines are called isopotential lines, and are analogous for instance to the isobar lines that are used in meteorology to indicate points in our atmosphere that are measuring the same atmospheric pressure, or the contour lines that are used in geographic cartography to indicate height. If isopotential lines are drawn for different voltage values, the obtained picture can be read out in the same way as a geographic map, with "valleys" representing areas of the scalp where lower potential values have been recorded and "mountains" where higher potential values have been recorded. These pictures are called scalp field maps.

In Figure 2.2C, isopotential lines have been drawn for values that correspond to the voltages −1, 0, 1, 2, 3 and 4 µV; the bold line corresponds to 0 µV. The isopotential lines visualize something that was not evident before: the lines appear most densely at the posterior part of the scalp, indicating that the differences between adjacent electrodes are largest there. It is important to note that the density of the field lines does not only depend on the potentials that are being displayed, but also on the projection used to map the scalp positions of

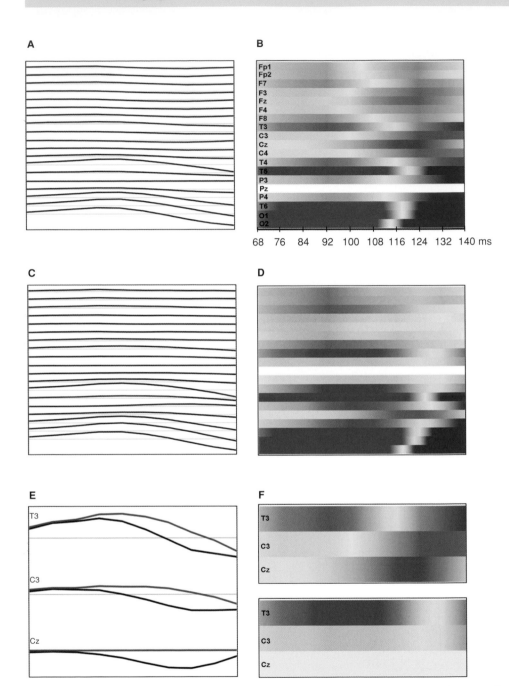

**Figure 2.1** Electrode-wise line plots and intensity plots of the data described in Table 2.1. A. Line plot against Pz. B. Intensity plot against Pz. C. Line plot against Cz. D. Intensity plot against Cz. In E, the line plots of the three electrodes T3, C3 and Cz were magnified; in black line plots computed against Pz, in red line plots computed against Cz. In F, the line plots of the three electrodes T3, C3 and Cz were magnified; upper panel shows the data computed against Pz, lower panel shows the data computed against Cz. The red color used in the intensity plots represents a positive voltage difference compared with the reference electrode, whereas the blue color represents a negative voltage difference compared with the reference electrode. The greater the intensity of the colors, the larger the differences measured compared with the reference electrode.

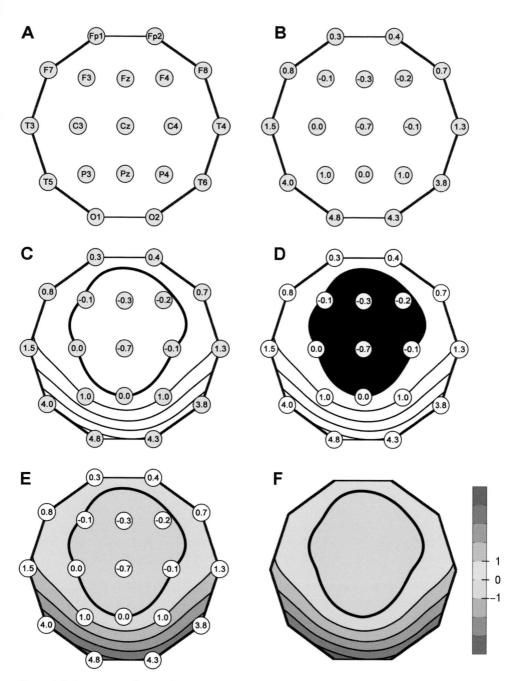

**Figure 2.2** Construction of a scalp field map. A. Scheme of the electrode positions projected on a two-dimensional plane. The head is seen from above, nose up. B. Scheme of the electrode positions with the values (in microvolts) at time point 100 ms. C. Values with isopotential lines at −1, 0 (bold line), 1, 2, 3 and 4 microvolts. D. Same as C, but negative areas are shown in black. E. Same as D, but with blue areas indicating negative, and red areas indicating positive values. The color intensity is proportional to the voltage differences from zero. F. Same as E, but with an additional color scale and the numbers removed.

the electrodes on a plane. Depending on the distortion of the electrode distances introduced by the projection, the density of the field lines may also appear distorted.

A further improvement in the visualization of the scalp field map is achieved by adding visual codes for specific values. One way to reach this goal is shown in Figure 2.2D, where all negative scalp areas are shown in black with white isopotential lines, and all positive scalp areas are shown in white with black isopotential lines. The introduction of colors further facilitates the visualization of the scalp field map (Figure 2.2E): negative scalp areas are now drawn in a particular color (typically blue) and positive scalp areas are drawn in another color (typically red). Moreover, different color intensities code different voltages, i.e. color intensity increases (or decreases) with increasing voltage differences from zero. Finally, by adding a color scale, the numbers shown in the figures can be removed, still maintaining an unequivocal display (Figure 2.2F). Note that scalp field maps starting from Panel C onward represent only visualization enhancements.

## Interpolation

The interpolation of scalp potentials serves several purposes:

(1) For the visualization of scalp field maps, a sufficient number of points between the electrode positions need to be estimated.

(2) If for technical reasons the data recorded at an electrode are not useable, it may be convenient to interpolate those data based on the other electrodes. Whether or not to interpolate "bad" data from one or many electrodes is a question of the signal-to-noise ratio. Initially, data recorded at these electrodes have a bad signal-to-noise ratio. Excluding the electrodes from the analysis eliminates both signal and noise, whereas the interpolation of the electrodes by neighboring electrodes introduces a signal, but also noise coming both from the neighboring electrodes and from uncertainties in the interpolation. Which one of these possibilities produces an optimal signal-to-noise ratio cannot be answered in general and needs to be considered in each particular situation. In general, the interpolation requires that neighboring channels have a good signal-to-noise ratio and that the electrodes to be interpolated are not at the edge of the electrode array.

(3) If the data have been recorded with a dense electrode array and the variance of the electrode positions across subjects is large in relation to the inter-electrode distances, it may be useful to normalize the electrode positions across subjects before averaging, to remove noise in the spatial sampling of the data (see also Chapter 4).

There are several procedures for the interpolation of two-dimensional data structures. In general, the problem of interpolation consists of computing a value at a location that was not measured, based on other measured values at other locations. A method suitable for our purpose should produce interpolated values that are as similar as possible to the values that would have been obtained by measuring at the location where the value has been interpolated.

Most of the interpolation routines used for EEG scalp potentials belong to the family of spline interpolations. Using spline interpolations, values at new locations are obtained based on some weighted average of the existing measurements in the neighborhood. The weights are determined by fitting polynomials of some degree to the measured data.

Spline interpolations can be linear (based on a polynomial of first degree), which means that the potentials between neighboring electrodes change in a strictly linear way. This has

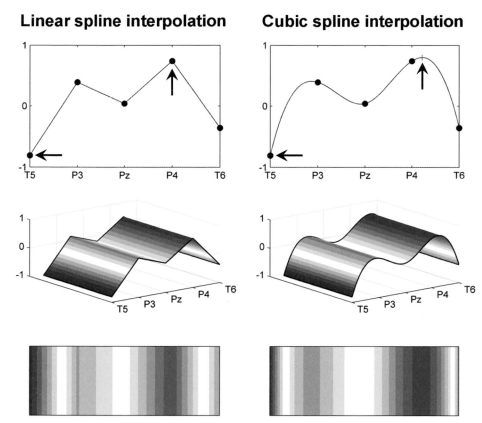

**Figure 2.3** The linear and the cubic spline interpolation. The dots in the upper graphs show the potentials of an ERP at one moment in time at five temporal-parietal electrodes, going from left to right. The lines correspond to the potential values interpolated between electrodes. Horizontal (vertical) arrows indicate the location of the minima (maxima). Note that in the case of the linear interpolation, the extreme values coincide with the electrode positions. This is not necessarily the case with the spline interpolated data. The central panels show a color-coded 3D profile from left to right, and the lower panels show the color-coded potential values across the five electrodes. While the linear spline interpolation shows sharp edges, the cubic spline interpolation produces a smooth surface.

also been called nearest neighbor interpolation[1], but to avoid confusion, we will not use this term, because it commonly refers to setting the value of the point to be interpolated to the value of the nearest known point. Consequently, linear spline interpolation limits the location of the minima and maxima of the scalp potential field (see below) to the electrode positions where measured data are available. On the other hand, it produces edges at the lines that connect neighboring electrodes, which is unlikely to occur in reality. Higher order (cubic, quadratic or higher) spline interpolation produces interpolated values that change smoothly across the scalp, minimizing spatial frequencies, but the minima and maxima of the field can be localized between electrode positions, where no measured data are available. Figure 2.3 shows EEG data recorded from five electrodes with interpolated values obtained by linear (first degree) or cubic (third degree) spline interpolation.

In order to evaluate the appropriateness of different interpolation methods, one can make theoretical considerations and/or empirical tests. From a theoretical point of view, we know from the properties of the lead-field (see Chapter 3) that intracerebral generators produce smooth spatial fields. We therefore know that the edges introduced by the linear interpolation are an artifact. To the contrary, the putative scalp field minima and maxima localized between electrodes that might arise from the spline interpolation are not necessarily an artifact: although there is no evidence that they are correctly interpolated, there is also no reason to assume that they were actually located at electrode positions.

The different interpolation algorithms have been tested based on real data, using cross-validation tests. These tests consist of removing part of the electrodes and interpolating these missing values. The difference between the interpolated values and the actual measures is then used as an index for the appropriateness of the chosen interpolation method. In general, it was concluded that higher order spline interpolations perform reasonably well in sufficiently dense electrode arrays[1,2].

The estimation of potentials is less reliable when the potentials are located outside of the electrode array and not between some electrodes. Extrapolating potentials beyond the electrode array should thus be avoided. This also implies that the interpolation of electrodes at the border of the electrode array is more prone to artifacts. The electrode array should therefore be chosen such that the fields produced by the events of interest are well covered and that no extrapolation is needed to capture their essential features.

## The reference electrode

In the example of Table 2.1, the electrode Pz is the reference against which all data shown so far were computed. What would happen if the data were recorded against another reference? The values are actually differences with regard to the reference electrode. The value at the reference electrode is thus by definition zero. Computationally, if another reference is chosen, the new values at each electrode correspond to the voltage difference between the electrode and the new reference. Note that if the new reference is a single electrode, the measurement at that electrode is also subtracted from itself, thus the new value at that electrode is always zero. The recomputation of references is easy if all measurements are against the same reference. Recording setups that do not employ the same reference for all electrodes (bipolar or differential montages) may even make it impossible to recompute the data against a reference of choice.

The procedure of recomputation of references is exemplified in Table 2.1: the previous data that used the electrode Pz as reference (left panel), are recomputed against Cz (right panel). As described above, for each sample in time the measurement of the new reference (Cz) needs to be subtracted from each electrode. In Figure 2.1C, the time course of the ERP data displayed in the right panel of Table 2.1 is line-plotted separately for each electrode (see Figure 2.1D for the intensity plot). It is important to note that since the value we have subtracted from each electrode varies from sample point to sample point, the wave shapes have changed, too (see Figures 2.1E and F).

What happens to the scalp map topography after recalculation of the data against the new reference? Figures 2.4A and B displays the two scalp map topographies before and after recomputation of the new reference. Since the topography of the mapped brain electric field reflects the relative potential differences between the recording sites, it is not affected by the location of the reference. As described above, recalculating the data against a new reference means that for all electrodes, the same value is being subtracted from the original measurements for each sample in time. The potential differences between electrodes therefore remain unchanged. Changing the site of the recording reference will only influence the decision as to which one of the field lines (isopotential lines) is to be called the zero potential line. Thus,

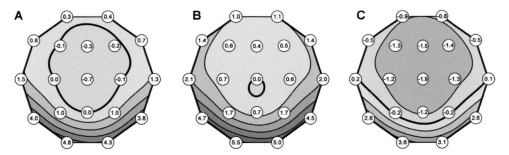

**Figure 2.4** Scalp field map with potential values computed (A) against Pz; (B) against Cz; and (C) against the average reference (see below).

**Figure 2.5** Midline section of the scalp field map of Figure 2.4 crossing electrodes Fz, Cz and Pz, shown as relief. The reference defines the zero level. Positive (negative) amplitudes are drawn in red (blue). The color intensity is proportional to the amplitude difference from the zero level. Obviously changing the zero level changes the color labeling, but not the shape of the landscape.

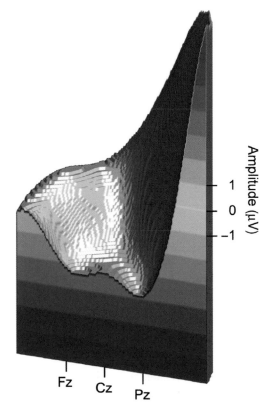

the spatial configuration of the field distribution, its "landscape," with the characteristic gradients, mountain peaks and valley troughs, remains invariant; only the labeling of the field lines changes. Using again the comparison with geographic maps: the topographical features remain identical when the electrical landscape is viewed from different points (references), similar to the constant relief of a geographical map where sea level is arbitrarily defined as zero (Figure 2.5). It is thus crucial to observe here that the topographic distribution of scalp fields (in terms of differences) does not depend on the reference.

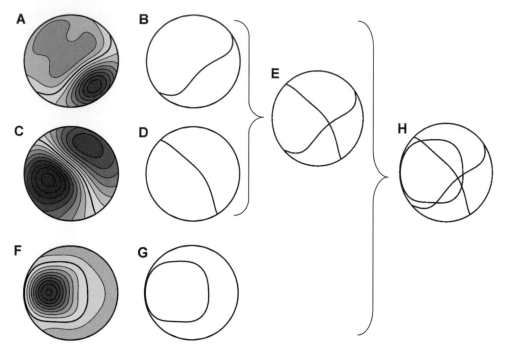

**Figure 2.6** No electrically inactive point on the scalp. A. Forward solution of a dipole located in the right parietal cortex. B. Zero line corresponding to the dipole in A. C. Forward solution of a second dipole located in the middle frontal cortex. D. Zero line corresponding to the dipole in C. E. Zero lines corresponding to the dipoles in A and C. F. Forward solution of a third dipole located in the left frontal cortex. G. Zero line corresponding to the dipole in F. H. Zero lines corresponding to the dipoles in A, C and F.

For analyses to be reference independent, it is thus sufficient, but essential that the extracted features can still be attributed to differences in scalp potentials. These differences can either be dealt with in a global manner (all electrodes against all electrodes) or, if a feature is extracted based on the difference between two electrodes, it has to be considered that both electrodes may have been active, and that the difference thus depends on the activity of both electrodes. The assumption that a measured potential represents the activity at only one position, while the other is always zero, is in general false, and results based on such assumptions remain ambiguous, because they change with the reference. This is namely the case for power maps (see Chapter 7).

The problem of reference-dependent results has produced a considerable amount of confusion in the field and seriously limited the interpretability of results reported. By using methods that consider the distribution of the scalp field rather than the raw scalp potential values, the results and interpretation of the data do not depend on the reference chosen. In the remainder of the book, we will take care that the procedures proposed are formulated in a reference independent way.

Is there a point on the scalp that is electrically always inactive and that would therefore constitute an appropriate location for placing the reference? The general answer to this question is no. Let us assume that at a certain sample in time there is only one single dipole active in the whole head. The dipole is located in the right parietal cortex and the forward solution produces a scalp map topography that is shown in Figure 2.6A. The ensemble of points that would be a correct reference location for this single source is located on the zero line that runs around the scalp (Figure 2.6B). Let us now assume that another single source is active: there would be another, different zero line around the scalp that would be suitable as the reference location for this other source (Figures 2.6C and D). If we now assume that the two sources are simultaneously active, the location that would be suitable as the reference is the intersection of the two zero-lines (usually two points, see Figure 2.6E). When a third source is added (Figures 2.6F and G), there is usually no single point on the scalp where all three zero-lines intersect (Figure 2.6H). This is even the case if the electrode is placed remotely from the brain, i.e. on the earlobes, nose or anywhere else on the body. References that electrically link different locations on the head (like linked earlobes) may even change the electric properties of the head and therefore introduce artificial distortions in the data.

In the general case of an unknown number of generators it is thus not possible to prove the electric inactivity of any location on the scalp. Even for the case of a single source, it would be necessary to know the location of the source for the proper placement of a reference electrode. But if the location of the source is already known, there is usually little need to measure it.

However, the properties of the EEG forward solution are such that for any source, the voltage integral across the entire head surface is zero[3]. If we could cover the entire head with a sufficient number of equally spaced electrodes, we could thus approximate this voltage integral by the sum of the measurements at all electrodes. Accordingly, we could assume that the sum of the potential differences from all recorded electrodes would be equal to zero. The sum of the potential differences would thus approximate a "correct" zero-reference. Mathematically, this is achieved by using as a reference the average of the measurements at all electrodes. This reference is called the "average reference" (Figure 2.4C).

The validity of the assumptions upon which the average reference is justified depends on the goodness of coverage of the entire head by the electrode array. This coverage is however limited, because it is impossible to cover the entire volume, especially the lower part of the brain.

The arguments raised above apply to the case of initially unknown generators in the brain. Sometimes, we have previously characterized a generator of interest and would only like to measure its activity in some conditions. We can then optimize the location of a recording and of the reference electrode such that the signal of that generator is maximized. Typically, this is achieved by placing the recording and reference electrode on the positive and negative maximum of the field produced by that generator.

# Spatial derivatives: gradients, current source density and spatial deblurring

Some topographic features seen in scalp field maps can be enhanced or removed using spatial transformations[4]. Spatial transformations are the computation of the first and second spatial derivatives of the data and yield physically meaningful reference-independent quantities within a subspace of the electrode array[5].

The first spatial derivative is usually called a gradient. Gradients are vectors that vary in strength and direction. Although they have rarely been used in spatial analysis, they are related to the localization of sources. The use of bipolar derivations that is common and useful in the visual inspection of clinical EEG corresponds to the computation of gradients.

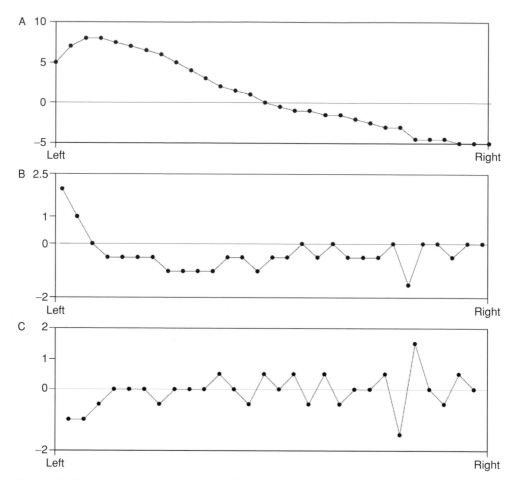

**Figure 2.7** First and second spatial derivatives. A. Thirty electrodes (corresponding to the 30 dots) of a potential map are shown. Horizontal axis: electrode position on the x-axis (from left to right); vertical axis: potential values. B. First spatial derivative (i.e. gradient) of the 30 electrodes. C. Second spatial derivative (i.e. current source density) of the 30 electrodes.

Current source density approximates the second spatial derivative of the field[6] and corresponds to the application of a spatial high-pass filter, as for instance the Laplacian operator to the data. Current source density is sometimes computed to enhance and separate focal activity and remove low spatial frequency assumed to originate from deeper sources. For the construction of the spatial high-pass filter, a series of models has been proposed, based on spline interpolation[7] or spherical harmonics[8].

The enhancement and isolation of focal activity by spatial filtering has been further developed taking into account realistic head geometry and finite element volume conductor models of the skull and scalp. These methods have been referred to as deblurring methods[9,10].

In Figure 2.7, we describe how first and second spatial derivative maps are constructed from a given potential map. In order to simplify the procedure we have drawn a series of 30 electrodes, corresponding to the 30 dots shown in Figure 2.7A. Let us assume that the

**Figure 2.8** Scalp field map of an ERP 260 ms after a visual stimulus presentation in a mental rotation task[11] and its spatial derivatives. A. Scalp field map. Ba. Same data as in A, recomputed into gradients (first spatial derivative of the potential distribution). Within the electrode array, for each square formed by four electrodes the gradient was computed and entered as an arrow which points in the direction of the resultant gradient. The origin of the arrow is at the center of the four-electrode square. The length shows the relative magnitude of the gradient. Bb. Magnitude of local gradients of Ba mapped with equigradient lines in steps of 0.5 µV cm$^{-1}$, linearly interpolated between gradient locations of Ba. Orientation is omitted. C. Same data as in A, recomputed into current source density values (second spatial derivative), using the potential values of the four surrounding electrodes for each current source density computation.

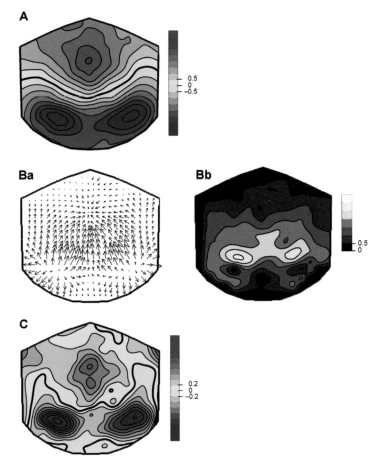

horizontal axis represents the electrode position on the x-axis (left to right) of a potential map and the vertical axis represents the recorded potential values in a given moment. The first electrode, the second electrode and the third electrode (starting from the left) measured a potential difference (to the recording reference) of +5 µV, +7 µV and +8 µV respectively. The first spatial derivative (gradient, see Figure 2.7B) corresponds to the difference between two adjacent electrodes. If we proceed from left to right the gradient between electrodes 1 and 2 is +2 µV and the gradient between electrodes 2 and 3 is +1 µV (respectively −1 µV and −2 µV if we proceed from right to left.) Please note that the position on the horizontal axis of the gradients is set between the corresponding electrodes in the top panel. The same rationale is applied for the computation of the second spatial derivative (current source density, see Figure 2.7C). We note that the direction of the computation (i.e. whether we start from the left or from the right) plays a crucial role for the first derivative (i.e. it reversed the values) but not for the second derivative. In a two-dimensional array, which is usually used to represent potential maps, we additionally have to take into account the electrode position on the anterior–posterior axis. In Figure 2.8 the potential map and the first two spatial derivatives maps of ERP data recorded in a mental rotation task with 123 electrodes[11] are illustrated.

## Map descriptors

Mapping implies no data reduction. It actually increases the amount of data through interpolation. Mapping is "just" another way to interpolate and display the recorded EEG signals. For the description and interpretation of these maps, it can be useful to extract features that reflect specific properties of these maps.

The spatial configuration of the brain's electric field on the scalp reflects the activities of neuronal populations (see Chapter 1). A change of the spatial configuration must have been caused by a change of the distribution of intracranial sources, i.e. some sources have become active or inactive, or have become proportionally more or less active than other sources[12,13]. Conversely, however, similar spatial configurations may or may not have been generated by the same intracranial sources. When the relative distribution of active sources is stable and the amount of activity of all sources changed in a proportional way, the topography of the brain electric field will remain unchanged and only the strength of the field will change. More specifically, when the activity of the intracranial sources is scaled by a common factor, all measured potential values will be scaled by the same factor. By looking at changes of potential values at isolated electrodes, it is thus impossible to infer whether these changes were caused by a global change of source strength, or by a change of source distribution, i.e. local changes of source strength.

Since the interpretation of global change of source strength and changes of source distribution can be quite different, it is often helpful to have on the one hand map descriptors which are sensitive to changes in the spatial distribution, but insensitive to global strength, and on the other hand, map descriptors which are sensitive to changes in the global strength, but insensitive to spatial distribution.

## Map descriptors of the spatial distribution of scalp fields: extreme potential values, centroids, electric gravity center

### Extreme potential values

Simple descriptors of the scalp field distribution can already be obtained by assessing the location of the maximal and minimal scalp field potential values[14]. The positive extreme is the location of the electrode where the most positive voltage has been recorded; the negative extreme is the location of the electrode where the most negative voltage has been recorded (see Figure 2.9A). The choice of the reference electrode does not affect the locations of these two spatial descriptors because the most positive/negative voltage is a relative statement and does not depend on absolute values. Note that unless one uses spline interpolated data, extremes are confined to electrode positions. The measure thus becomes increasingly sparse with decreasing number of electrodes. Figure 2.9A shows the location of the extremes mapped on the anterior–posterior, on the left–right and on the superior–inferior axes over time[15]. Thus, in our example, the extremes describe the topography of a map by three location parameters each. The location of the extremes is driven by the projection of the poles of the active elements; they are therefore sensitive to the orientation of these elements. If one or both extremes are located at the border of the electrode array, it is unclear whether the real extreme would have been outside the electrode array. The usage of extremes therefore requires that the electrode array covers a maximally large area of the scalp with sufficient density.

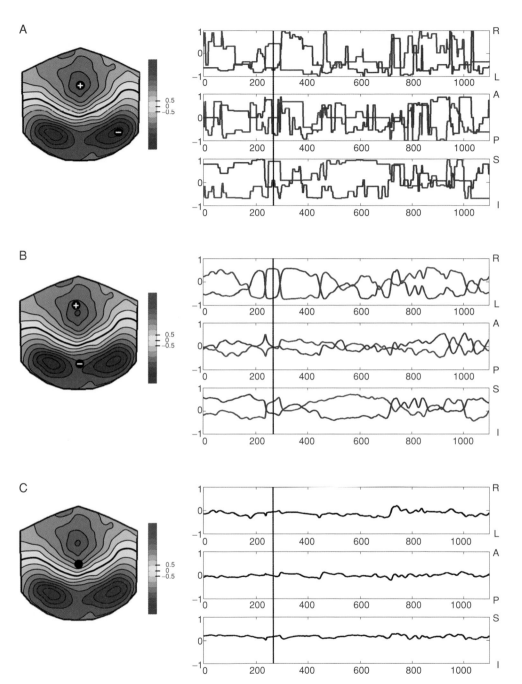

**Figure 2.9** Map descriptors of the spatial distribution of scalp field maps after a visual stimulus presentation in a mental rotation task[11]. Trajectory of the locations of the (A) extreme positive (red line) and negative (blue line) potential values, (B) positive (red line) and negative (blue line) centroids and (C) gravity center (black line) over time (x-axis) along the right–left (y-axis, upper graphs), anterior–posterior (y-axis, middle graphs), and superior–inferior (y-axis, lower graphs) axes. The ERP scalp field map at 260 ms (black vertical line in the right panels) and the location of the map descriptors are shown on the left.

## Centroids of positive and negative potential areas

The description obtained with extreme values maps only the tips of the dipolar source configurations. It depends on only those two electrodes where the maximally positive and negative potential values were recorded. For a similar description of the location of the positive and negative poles of a map using all electrodes, the position of the centroids[16] of the positive and negative map areas (against average reference) can be computed. The position of the positive centroid on the x-axis is defined as

$$C_x = \sum_{i=1}^{N_{pos}} u_i x_i \bigg/ \sum_{i=1}^{N_{pos}} u_i \tag{1}$$

where $u_i$ is the voltage of the map $u$ at the positive electrode $i$, $x_i$ is the location of the electrode $i$ on the x-axis, and $N_{pos}$ is the total number of positive electrodes of the map $u$.

"Centroid" has the same meaning as "center of gravity," but in order to distinguish the measure from the global measure defined below, this terminology was chosen. Figure 2.9B shows the location of the centroids mapped on the anterior–posterior, on the left–right and on the superior–inferior axes. Different from the case of the extremes, centroids can be located anywhere within the mapped electrode array, i.e. they are not restricted to the electrode positions since they use the information of all electrodes[5,16]. Compared with the extreme locations, centroid locations have a tendency to be nearer to the center of the field and are less likely to occur near the borders of the electrode array.

## Electric gravity center

When the location of the positive and the negative centroids are averaged for each axis separately, the electric gravity center is obtained[17].

The position of the gravity center on the x-axis is defined as

$$G_x = \sum_{i=1}^{N} |u_i| x_i \bigg/ \sum_{i=1}^{N} |u_i| \tag{2}$$

where $u_i$ is the voltage of the map $u$ at the electrode $i$, $x_i$ is the location of the electrode $i$ on the x-axis and $N$ is the total number of electrodes of the map $u$.

The center of gravity is insensitive to the orientation of sources and tends to move in parallel with the center of gravity of the intracerebral active neural elements[18]. Figure 2.9C shows the location of the gravity center mapped on the anterior–posterior, on the left–right and on the superior–inferior axes. Besides using electric gravity centers as outlined above, there is also a series of studies that fitted a single dipole to scalp potential maps with potentially many sources. The location and amplitude of this single dipole were not regarded as evidence for activity at the location of the dipole, but as mere descriptors representing the center of gravity and strength of the intracerebral activity[19,20].

## Advantages and limitations of map descriptors

Spatial descriptors achieve a massive data reduction and drastically reduce the amount of data to be analyzed. They are therefore an alternative to de-correlation techniques such as PCA or ICA. Extracting map features as described above provides simple and comprehensive descriptors of map topographies. However, it implies certain assumptions about the number of features in the data, and imposes limitations when these assumptions are violated. The data presented in Figure 2.9 showed two bilateral posterior negative peaks. The "dipolar" representation with one descriptor for the positive pole and one descriptor for the negative pole does not represent such a field well: the negative centroid is located somewhere in the middle between the two posterior peaks, where the potentials are low, and the location of the maximum will only represent either one of the peaks, while the other one is ignored, falsely suggesting a very lateralized topography.

## Map descriptor of the global strength of scalp fields: Global Field Power

In order to quantify the strength of a scalp potential field, all electrodes have to be considered equally. For the measure to be reference independent, it should be based on potential differences between electrodes. The simplest approach is to construct a measure that includes the differences between all possible electrode pairs. If the measure is defined by the sum of all squared potential differences, it can be shown that it is equivalent to the computation of the standard deviation of the potentials. This measure was introduced by Lehmann and Skrandies in 1980[21] and was later called "Global Field Power" (typically abbreviated as GFP[22]) and is defined as

$$GFP = \sqrt{\left. \sum_{i=1}^{N} (u_i - \bar{u})^2 \middle/ N \right.}$$

(3)

where $u_i$ is the voltage of the map $u$ at the electrode $i$, $\bar{u}$ is the average voltage of all electrodes of the map $u$ and $N$ is the number of electrodes of the map $u$.

Global Field Power is closely related and sometimes confused with the root mean square (RMS). The difference between GFP and RMS is that in the computation of GFP, the mean potential of all electrodes is subtracted from each potential before the square-sum is computed. Global Field Power therefore implicitly contains the average reference, but can be considered reference independent with the initial definition as mean potential difference between all possible pairs of electrodes. This does not apply to RMS, where no mean potential is subtracted; RMS is thus a reference-dependent measure.

Scalp potential fields with steep gradients and pronounced peaks and troughs, i.e. very "hilly" maps, will result in high GFP, while GFP is low in electrical fields with only shallow gradients that have a "flat" appearance (Figure 2.10). Maps at times of maximal GFP imply an optimal signal-to-noise ratio. High GFP is typically associated with stable landscape configuration, while low GFP is associated with changes in the landscape configurations. When a time-series of maps is to be analyzed, GFP is computed separately for each map of the series. This results in a single value at each sample in time that can be plotted as a function of time (Figure 2.10).

The GFP has a simple geometrical representation: in Figure 2.11, two electrodes (C3 and P3) are shown against the common average reference, at a certain time point. The potential value of the first electrode has been mapped onto the horizontal axis; the potential value of the second electrode has been mapped onto the vertical axis. In this graph, the combined potentials of these two electrodes are thus represented as a single point. This type of display is called a state space representation and will be discussed in more detail in Chapter 9. The Euclidean distance $u$ of this point from the origin (i.e. the reference) is the root of the *sum* of the squared potentials of both electrodes, or in more technical terms,

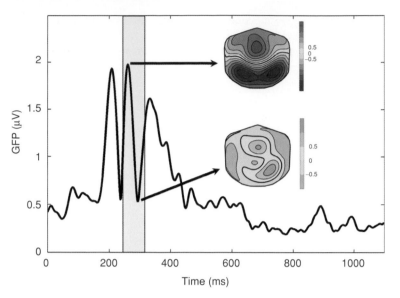

**Figure 2.10** Map descriptor of the global strength of scalp fields. Curve of the Global Field Power (GFP, y-axis, µV) over time (x-axis, ms) for the ERP data[11]. The scalp field maps corresponding to the highest (260 ms) and lowest (292 ms) GFP points in the gray area are shown.

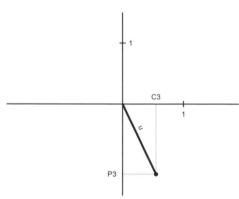

**Figure 2.11** Potentials of two electrodes represented in a state-space diagram. The potential value of C3 (P3) at a certain time point is mapped onto the x-axis (y-axis).

their L2 norm. The GFP has been defined as the root of the *mean* of the squared potentials. The only difference between $u$ and GFP is thus a constant factor $\sqrt{N}$, by which the GFP is smaller than $u$ For the present example only two electrodes are used: if $N$ electrodes were used, the state-space display would change from two-dimensional to $N$-dimensional. The computation of $u$ would still be defined as the root of the sum of all squared potentials of the $N$ electrodes, and remain proportional to the GFP by a factor $\sqrt{N}$. Note that it is also possible to use the L1 norm (the mean or sum of absolute values, or "hilliness") or the maximal absolute potential difference between electrodes (range) as global measures of map strength[21,22].

## Difference maps, amplitude normalization and dissimilarity
### Difference maps and pre-stimulus baseline
In Chapter 1, it has been shown that the scalp field map produced by a set of intracerebral sources is the sum of the scalp field maps produced by each of these sources. This implies

that if we have two conditions where different sources are active, the difference map between the scalp field maps of the two conditions is equivalent to the scalp field map produced by those sources that differ between the two conditions and therefore represents location and orientation of these sources.

The computation of difference maps is a standard procedure for many paradigms; it is employed when a pre-stimulus baseline correction is being computed, or when the effect of interest is defined as difference between two conditions. Typical examples for such effects are the "mismatch negativity" that is defined as the difference between potentials evoked by standard and deviant tones, or the "N400" that is defined as the difference between potentials evoked by semantically expected and unexpected words. Comparing difference maps across observations implies that the relevant parts of generators have a consistent orientation. There is good reason to assume that this is the case[23] and the same assumption is made whenever an average evoked potential is being computed.

Computing inverse solutions of difference maps between two conditions may yield different results than computing differences of inverse solutions of the two conditions, because some assumptions differ in the two procedures. The difference map contains information about the localization and orientation of the generators that accounts for the differences, whereas the orientation is typically ignored in inverse solutions. Average difference maps across subjects thus represent generators that differ between conditions and that have a common location and orientation over subjects. Differences of inverse solutions represent generators that differ between conditions and have a common location, whereas orientation is irrelevant.

Difference maps are also obtained when an ERP is computed against a pre-stimulus baseline: the obtained ERP maps are then the difference between the post-stimulus ERP maps and the mean map of the chosen pre-stimulus period. The implication made is that the ERP adds onto a pre-stimulus state that remains constant throughout the post-stimulus period, and that is constant across the conditions that are compared. The validity of this assumption varies. The activity of those generators that have shown significant activation in the pre-stimulus period is likely to be present in the early post-stimulus period, but is also likely to decay with time. Across conditions, the pre-stimulus state depends on the subjects' possibilities to recruit preparatory neural resources for the processing of the expected stimulus. These possibilities depend on the experimental task and setup, and on the subjects' state. While one can expect that preparatory processes are similar if the different experimental conditions cannot be predicted by the subject, the capacity of subjects to prepare may vary consistently, especially if different patient groups are studied. Pre-stimulus baseline correction may therefore significantly alter the hypotheses that are actually being tested when comparing post-stimulus ERPs. Care should therefore be taken to ensure that these hypotheses correspond to the research questions, and that the results are interpreted in these terms. Namely, if a pre-stimulus baseline correction is applied, one should ensure that (a) the subject groups compared do not differ in regard to the recruitment of preparatory neural resources (which can be tested by comparing the pre-stimulus period between groups); (b) the occurrence of the stimuli to be compared is not predictable for the subject and thus does not allow a differential recruitment of resources; and (c) the pre-stimulus processes are likely to be still active during those time periods where an effect is observed. The effects of a pre-stimulus baseline correction on a sample ERP channel are shown in Figure 2.12.

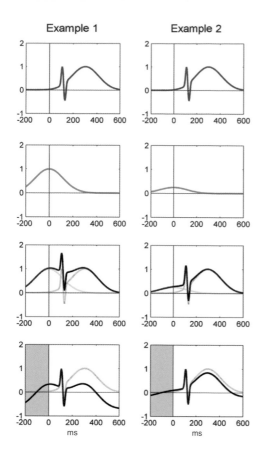

Example 1     Example 2

**Figure 2.12** Effects of pre-stimulus baseline correction on a sample ERP channel. Two examples are shown. For both examples the same ERP trace (first row, red lines) with early, fast (100–150 ms) and late, slow (150–600 ms) potentials is used. The baseline activity (second row, green lines) shows potentials related to preparatory processes that decay after stimulus onset. This potential is strong in Example 1 and weak in Example 2. In a between-subject design, this difference in the preparatory processes might be the case for groups with different attentional resources, whereas in a within-subject design this could be the case if the two stimulus categories to be compared are predictable for the subject and thus do allow a differential recruitment of resources. In the third row, the resulting potential sums (black lines) without baseline correction are shown. The peak amplitudes of the early ERP potentials are strongly affected by the amount of preparatory potentials, while the late ERP potentials are rather unaffected. The lower row shows the same data after pre-stimulus (−200 to 0 ms) baseline correction. While there is little effect of preparatory activity on the peaks in the early ERP potentials, the baseline correction strongly affected the peaks of the late ERP potentials.

## Normalization and map dissimilarity

Following the distinction between changes in total map amplitude and amplitude-independent changes in spatial distribution, we can distinguish two cases:

(a) A given difference map is observed because all active sources changed their strength in a proportional manner.

(b) A given difference map is observed because some sources changed their strength in a manner that was disproportional to the strength of the other sources.

In case (a), the maps of the two conditions would differ only by a global scaling factor. If this scaling factor is eliminated, the potentials of the difference map should be zero at all electrodes. Note that in the real case, when noise is present, this will however only approximately be the case. The hypothesis that there is zero difference plus noise can be tested with statistics (see Chapter 8).

In case (b), map differences exist although possible differences in scaling have been eliminated by map normalization. The map normalization is achieved by dividing the potential values at each electrode of a given map by its GFP. This procedure is somewhat similar to the computation of relative power, where the power spectrum is normalized by the total power.

Similar to the GFP (as discussed earlier), difference maps and map normalization have a simple geometrical equivalent in the state space representation (see Chapter 9): in

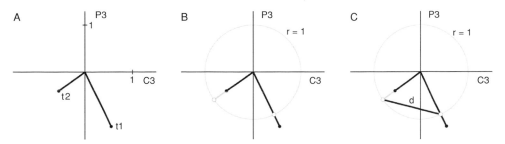

**Figure 2.13** Potentials of two electrodes at two different time points and their dissimilarity represented in a state-space diagram. A. The potential values of the two electrodes C3 and P3 at two different time points (t1 and t2) are mapped onto the x- and y-axis, respectively, forming two vectors. The origin of the diagram represents the reference. B. The vectors' lengths are normalized by a projection on a unity circle. C. Global map dissimilarity (GMD) is defined as the distance d between the endpoints of the two normalized vectors. For maps with n channels, the computation is done in an n-dimensional space (see also Chapter 9).

Figure 2.11, it has been shown how two electrodes of one map (at time t1) are mapped onto a point of a plane of the state space representation. In Figure 2.13A, a second map (at time t2) is added. The map occupies another point of the state space diagram. The maps differ in GFP, because they have different distances to the reference. Normalizing the maps by their GFP makes them equidistant to the reference and thus projects them onto a circle (Figure 2.13B).

If the two maps differed only in their total strength, i.e. in GFP, but not in their topography, the normalization would project them to the same point on the circle. Their difference could thus be fully explained by a GFP difference, which would correspond to case (a) described above. In the current example, this is not the case, and normalization projects the two maps onto different points on the sphere: the difference between the two maps cannot be explained by GFP alone, but there is an additional topographical difference.

The distance $d$ between the two projections on the sphere is an amplitude-independent measure of map difference and corresponds to the GFP of the difference of the normalized maps (Figure 2.13C). This measure has been introduced as global map dissimilarity (GMD[21]) and is defined as

$$GMD = \sqrt{\frac{1}{N}\sum_{i=1}^{N}\left\{\frac{u_i - \bar{u}}{\sqrt{\sum_{i=1}^{N}\frac{(u_i-\bar{u})^2}{N}}} - \frac{v_i - \bar{v}}{\sqrt{\sum_{i=1}^{N}\frac{(v_i-\bar{v})^2}{N}}}\right\}^2} \tag{4}$$

where $u_i$ is the voltage of map $u$ at the electrode $i$, $v_i$ is the voltage of map $v$ at the electrode $i$, $\bar{u}$ is the average voltage of all electrodes of map $u$, $\bar{v}$ is the average voltage of all electrodes of map $v$ and $N$ is the total number of electrodes.

From Figure 2.13C, it becomes apparent that GMD is 0 when two maps are equal, and that GMD maximally reaches 2 for the case where the two maps point in the opposite direction, i.e. have the same topography with reversed polarity. Global map dissimilarity can also be computed using the Pearson's product-moment correlation coefficient between the potentials of the two maps to be compared[24].

# References

1. Fletcher EM, Kussmaul CL, Mangun GR. Estimation of interpolation errors in scalp topographic mapping. *Electroencephalography and Clinical Neurophysiology* 1996;**98**:422–434.

2. Perrin F, Pernier J, Bertrand O, Echallier JF. Spherical splines for scalp potential and current density mapping. *Electroencephalography and Clinical Neurophysiology* 1989;**72**:184–187.

3. Bertrand O, Perrin F, Pernier J. A theoretical justification of the average reference in topographic evoked potential studies. *Electroencephalography and Clinical Neurophysiology* 1985;**62**:462–464.

4. Brandeis D, Lehmann D, Michel CM, Mingrone W. Mapping event-related brain potential microstates to sentence endings. *Brain Topography* 1995;**8**:145–159.

5. Lehmann D. Principles of spatial analysis. In Gevins A, Remond A, eds. *Handbook of Electroencephalography and Clinical Neurophysiology: Methods of Analysis of Brain Electrical and Magnetic Signals.* Amsterdam: Elsevier; 1987, pp. 309–354.

6. Hjorth B. An on-line transformation of EEG scalp potentials into orthogonal source derivations. *Electroencephalography and Clinical Neurophysiology* 1975;**39**:526–530.

7. Babiloni F, Babiloni C, Carducci F et al. Spline Laplacian estimate of EEG potentials over a realistic magnetic resonance-constructed scalp surface model. *Electroencephalography and Clinical Neurophysiology* 1996;**98**:363–373.

8. Pascual-Marqui RD, Gonzalez-Andino SL, Valdes-Sosa PA, Biscay-Lirio R. Current source density estimation and interpolation based on the spherical harmonic Fourier expansion. *International Journal of Neuroscience* 1988;**43**:237–249.

9. Cincotti F, Babiloni C, Miniussi C et al. EEG deblurring techniques in a clinical context. *Methods Inf Med.* 2004;**43**:114–117.

10. Gevins A, Le J, Brickett P, Reutter B, Desmond J. Seeing through the skull: advanced EEGs use MRIs to accurately measure cortical activity from the scalp. *Brain Topography* 1991;**4**:125–131.

11. Arzy S, Thut G, Mohr C, Michel CM, Blanke O. Neural basis of embodiment: distinct contributions of temporoparietal junction and extrastriate body area. *Journal of Neuroscience* 2006;**26**:8074–8081.

12. McCarthy G, Wood CC. Scalp distributions of event-related potentials: an ambiguity associated with analysis of variance models. *Electroencephalography and Clinical Neurophysiology* 1985;**62**:203–208.

13. Vaughan HG, Jr. The neural origins of human event-related potentials. *Annals of the New York Academy of Sciences* 1982;**388**: 125–138.

14. Lehmann D. Multichannel topography of human alpha EEG fields. *Electroencephalography and Clinical Neurophysiology* 1971;**31**:439–449.

15. Brandeis D, Vitacco D, Steinhausen HC. Mapping brain electric micro-states in dyslexic children during reading. *Acta Paedopsychiatrica* 1994;**56**:239–247.

16. Wackermann J, Lehmann D, Michel CM, Strik WK. Adaptive segmentation of spontaneous EEG map series into spatially defined microstates. *International Journal of Psychophysiology* 1993;**14**:269–283.

17. Kinoshita T, Strik WK, Michel CM et al. Microstate segmentation of spontaneous multichannel EEG map series under diazepam and sulpiride. *Pharmacopsychiatry* 1995;**28**:51–55.

18. Pizzagalli D, Lehmann D, Koenig T, Regard M, Pascual-Marqui RD. Face-elicited ERPs and affective attitude: brain electric microstate and tomography analyses. *Clinical Neurophysiology* 2000;**111**:521–531.

19. Dierks T, Ihl R, Frolich L, Maurer K. Dementia of the Alzheimer type: effects on the spontaneous EEG described by dipole sources. *Psychiatry Research* 1993;**50**:151–162.

20. Lehmann D, Michel CM. Intracerebral dipole source localization for FFT power maps. *Electroencephalography and Clinical Neurophysiology* 1990;**76**:271–276.

21. Lehmann D, Skrandies W. Reference-free identification of components of checkerboard-evoked multichannel potential fields. *Electroencephalography and Clinical Neurophysiology* 1980;**48**:609–621.

22. Lehmann D, Skrandies W. Spatial analysis of evoked potentials in man – a review. *Progress in Neurobiology* 1984;**23**:227–250.

23. Koenig T, Melie-García L, Stein M, Strik W, Lehmann C. Establishing correlations of scalp field maps with other experimental variables using covariance analysis and resampling methods. *Clinical Neurophysiology* 2008;**119**:1262.

24. Brandeis D, Naylor H, Halliday R, Callaway E, Yano L. Scopolamine effects on visual information processing, attention, and event-related potential map latencies. *Psychophysiology* 1992;**29**:315–336.

25. Jasper HA. The ten-twenty system of the international federation. *Electroencephalography and Clinical Neurophysiology* 1958;**10**:371–375.

# Chapter 3

# Imaging the electric neuronal generators of EEG/MEG

Roberto D. Pascual-Marqui, Kensuke Sekihara, Daniel Brandeis and Christoph M. Michel

## Introduction

In order to try to understand "how the brain works," one must make measurements of brain function. And ideally, the measurements should be as noninvasive as possible, i.e. the brain should be disturbed as little as possible during the measurement of its functions. One of the first types of noninvasive measurements reported in the literature, by Hans Berger[1], that directly tapped brain function was the human electroencephalogram (EEG), consisting of scalp electric potential differences as a function of time. In fact, Berger saw the EEG as a "window into the brain." One of Berger's first observations that showed compelling evidence of having tapped brain function was the alpha rhythm. This oscillatory activity, at around 10–12 Hz, is optimally recorded from a posterior electrode with an anterior reference. The activity is very pronounced when the human subject is with eyes closed, awake, alert, resting. By simply being instructed to perform a mental task such as overtly subtracting the number seven serially, starting at 500, the alpha activity disorganizes and almost disappears.

The main subject matter addressed in this chapter is the use of noninvasive extracranial measurements, i.e. the EEG and the magnetoencephalogram (MEG), for the estimation of the distribution in the brain of their electric neuronal generators. This can be seen as an extension of Berger's initial efforts towards developing a window into the brain. This chapter is also partly motivated by the rapidly advancing technologies of invasive and noninvasive functional imaging of the human brain, such as functional magnetic resonance imaging (fMRI), positron emission tomography (PET) and near infrared spectroscopy (NIRS) imaging, to name just a few.

Noninvasive EEG/MEG neuroimaging offers two unique attractions: high time resolution in the millisecond range, and direct access to neuronal signaling rather than the indirect metabolic signals picked up by fMRI, PET and NIRS.

However, one must emphasize from the outset that there are seemingly severe limitations to an EEG/MEG tomography. As early as 1853, Helmholtz showed that this type of inverse problem does not have a unique solution, i.e. there exist many different current density distributions in 3D space that are consistent with the electric potential distribution on a surface enclosing the volume. This implies that EEG/MEG measurements (even with an infinite number of electrodes/sensors) can be explained by many different distributions of generators.

*Electrical Neuroimaging*, ed. Christoph M. Michel, Thomas Koenig, Daniel Brandeis, Lorena R.R. Gianotti and Jiří Wackermann. Published by Cambridge University Press. © Cambridge University Press 2009.

The general conditions under which Helmholtz's result applies can be stated informally as follows: Let there be a finite volume enclosed by a surface. Electric potential differences and magnetic fields are known on the surface. If the current density in the volume is totally unrestricted, i.e. "anything goes," then the surface measurements have insufficient information to determine the current density.

If these conditions were applicable to the case of EEG/MEG measurements from a human brain, then it would certainly render hopeless the task of developing an EEG/MEG tomography. Fortunately, this is not the case, as will be argued further on. Indeed, the EEG and the MEG are not due to capricious distributions of electrical events. Rather, electric neuronal activity obeys certain electrophysiological and neuroanatomical constraints, that when plugged into the laws of electrodynamics, offer at least an approximate solution to the inverse problem.

In particular, it is known that EEG/MEG is not generated unrestrictedly in the brain, but it is confined to cortical gray matter. This information narrows significantly the non-uniqueness of the inverse solution. Moreover, it is known that non-negligible EEG/MEG measurements are possible only if large clusters of cortical pyramidal neurons undergo highly synchronous postsynaptic potentials. This additional information narrows even further the possible inverse solutions.

## Origin of scalp electric potential differences

Excluding artifacts such as eye movements or muscle movements, the generators of the EEG are thought to be the postsynaptic potentials that take place on the pyramidal cortical neurons[2].

For instance, Figure 3.1 represents schematically a particular case, in which the cortical pyramidal neuron denoted by the letter "B" is undergoing an excitatory postsynaptic

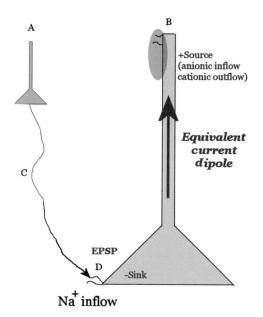

**Figure 3.1** Schematic representation of the generators of EEG/MEG. "B" corresponds to a cortical pyramidal neuron undergoing an excitatory postsynaptic potential (EPSP) at its basal dendrites ("D"). The distant presynaptic neuron "A," with axon "C," has its axonal termination at "D." The EPSP event induces specific channels to open in the postsynaptic neuron "B," allowing an inflow of $Na^+$, and producing an active sink of current. Due to electrical neutrality conservation, an active source of current is produced at the apical regions of "B" (by way of anionic inflow and cationic outflow) shown as a transparent blue ellipse (containing apical dendrites). The final consequence is that the neuron behaves as a simple physical entity known as a current dipole, shown as the blue arrow.

potential (EPSP) at its basal dendrites (denoted by the letter "D"). Note that the distant presynaptic neuron denoted by the letter "A" has its axonal (denoted by letter "C") termination at "D." Such an event induces specific channels to open in the postsynaptic neuron "B," and typically an inflow of $Na^+$ takes place, producing an active sink of current. Electrical neutrality prevails, and an active source of current is produced at the apical regions of "B" (by way of anionic inflow and cationic outflow), shown in the transparent blue ellipse. The final consequence is that the neuron behaves as a simple physical entity known as a current dipole, shown as the solid blue arrow.

The current dipole consists of two active, energy-consuming "poles": the source and the sink. These induce, by means of volume conduction, passive flows of Ohmic currents, which eventually pass through the skull and reach the scalp, thus producing scalp electric potentials. These same current dipoles are also responsible for the magnetic fields measured in the MEG.

However, a single active neuron is not enough to produce measurable scalp electric potential differences or extracranial magnetic fields. There are two additional mandatory prerequisites: relatively large spatial clusters of cortical pyramidal cells must be geometrically arranged parallel to each other, and the neurons in a cluster must simultaneously undergo the same type of postsynaptic potential (synchronization). A violation of any of these conditions will result in a total summed activity that is too weak to produce non-negligible extracranial fields.

According to calculations reviewed in Hämäläinen et al.[3], a typical cluster size must cover at least 40–200 mm$^2$ of cortical surface for the production of non-negligible extracranial fields.

Mitzdorf[4] presents ample experimental evidence on the neuronal postsynaptic potential source/sink configuration as the basis for the generation of the EEG. Mitzdorf's results justify the use of "current dipoles" as the basic entity for the representation of cortical activity as seen from extracranial electrodes/sensors, since the distance between source and sink is in the order of a few hundreds of microns, at most.

All these facts are discussed in detail in Chapter 1 of this book. They are also reviewed in general[2,5,6]. In addition, independent experimental evidence demonstrating high synchronization of neighboring neurons can be found[7,8,9]. The basic underlying physics can be studied[10].

The electrophysiological and neuroanatomical constraints described here for the generation of EEG/MEG can be taken into account when setting up the inverse problem for the estimation of electric neuronal activity. In addition, the implicit fact that the generators are limited to gray matter narrows even more the inverse solution. It is in this sense that the Helmholtz non-uniqueness of the unconstrained inverse problem does not apply to the EEG/MEG case.

To conclude this section, an important clarification is in order. One must distinguish the "*electrical*" phenomena underlying the EEG/MEG, as explained above, from the "*physiological*" mechanisms originating the EEG/MEG. For instance, the "*electrical*" generators (in the sense explained above) of the alpha rhythm are thought to be located in occipital/parietal cortices. But this activity is thought to be due (i.e. the "*physiological*" mechanism) to a thalamo-cortical feedback loop. The EEG/MEG measurements only "see" the electrically active neurons, as explained above, regardless of the physiological mechanism by which the neurons became active (see also Chapter 1).

# Some first steps in estimating cortical activity: from single waves to scalp topography to intracranial dipoles

At the time of Hans Berger's measurements of the EEG, it was already quite fascinating to tap brain function by the observation of changes in the temporal characteristics of a time-varying EEG signal. The example referred to above was the appearance and disappearance of 8–12 Hz oscillations (alpha rhythm). At that time, it was thought that the observed signal was due to the cortex just below the electrode. However, this assumption is in general incorrect, i.e. it is not generally true that an electrode picks up activity of the underlying cortex. In the general case, a scalp electric potential difference (which involves two electrodes, not one electrode) is determined by the strength and orientation of all cortical pyramidal neurons.

Seemingly, it took 20 years after Berger's publication for the proposal of the current dipole to appear in the literature. Brazier[11] considered the electric field at the surface of a conductor (the "scalp topography") due to a current dipole within it. She indicated that electric field theory can be employed to deduce the location and orientation of the current dipole from the pattern of potentials it creates at the surface. This was perhaps the origin of what was later popularized as "dipole fitting."

At about the same time, two papers appeared with the equations that related electric potential differences on the surface of a homogeneous conduction sphere (which had been used as the head model), due to a current dipole within it[12,13]. Ten years later, an improved, more realistic head model considered the different conductivities of neural tissue, skull and scalp[14]. Use was made of these early techniques by Lehmann *et al.*[15] to locate the generator of a visual evoked potential.

The basic assumption/constraint in the single current dipole model is that at a given moment in time, brain activity is due to a single, small area of active cortex. If one considers that the total number of cortical pyramidal neurons is very large, and that they are all quite active, this model seems very simplistic and nonrealistic. Even for the multiple dipole model, where two or a few more dipoles are allowed to wander (variable locations), wiggle (variable orientations), and grow or shrink (variable strengths) in the brain all at the same time, the basic assumption remains not too realistic in general.

Quite astonishingly, the dipole model does produce reasonable results under some particular conditions. This was shown very clearly by Henderson *et al.*[16], both in an experimentally simulated head (a head "phantom") and with real human EEG recordings.

The conditions under which a dipole model makes sense are limited to cases where electric neuronal activity is dominated by a small brain area. Two examples where the model performs very well are in some epileptic spike events, and in the description of the early components of the brain-stem auditory evoked potential (see Scherg & von Cramon[17]).

However, it would seem that the localization of higher cognitive functions cannot be reliably modeled by dipole fitting.

At this point, the basic dipole equation will be introduced. Consider first the simplest case of a current dipole in an infinite homogeneous medium with conductivity $\sigma$. The scalp electric potential $\phi_{e,v}$ at an electrode located at position vector $\mathbf{r}_e \in \mathbb{R}^{3\times1}$, due to a dipole located at position vector $\mathbf{r}_v \in \mathbb{R}^{3\times1}$, with dipole moment $\mathbf{j}_v \in \mathbb{R}^{3\times1}$, is:

$$\phi_{e,v} = \mathbf{j}_v^T \mathbf{k}_{e,v} + c \tag{1}$$

where "$c$" is an arbitrary constant, the superscript "$T$" denotes vector/matrix transpose, and $\mathbf{k}_{e,v} \in \mathbb{R}^{3 \times 1}$ denotes the lead field, given by:

$$\mathbf{k}_{e,v} = \frac{1}{4\pi\sigma} \frac{(\mathbf{r}_e - \mathbf{r}_v)}{\|\mathbf{r}_e - \mathbf{r}_v\|^3} \tag{2}$$

The arbitrary constant appearing in Eqn 1 is a consequence of the physical nature of electric potentials, which are determined up to an arbitrary constant. Measurements are necessarily based on the difference between two electrodes, thus eliminating the arbitrary constant. The moment $\mathbf{j}_v$ contains information on the orientation and strength of the dipole. The lead field is a vector with three components corresponding to the coordinate axes $XYZ$. The $X$-component of the lead field is the electric potential at electrode "$e$" due to a unit strength current dipole at "$v$" that is oriented along the $X$-axis. Similar definitions hold for the $Y$- and $Z$-components.

A more complicated, but slightly more realistic model corresponds to a homogeneous conducting sphere in air, where the lead field is:

$$\mathbf{k}_{e,v} = \frac{1}{4\pi\sigma}\left[ 2\frac{(\mathbf{r}_e - \mathbf{r}_v)}{\|\mathbf{r}_e - \mathbf{r}_v\|^3} + \frac{\mathbf{r}_e\|\mathbf{r}_e - \mathbf{r}_v\| + (\mathbf{r}_e - \mathbf{r}_v)\|\mathbf{r}_e\|}{\|\mathbf{r}_e\|\|\mathbf{r}_e - \mathbf{r}_v\|\left[\|\mathbf{r}_e\|\|\mathbf{r}_e - \mathbf{r}_v\| + \mathbf{r}_e^T(\mathbf{r}_e - \mathbf{r}_v)\right]} \right] \tag{3}$$

In Eqn 3, the notation:

$$\|\mathbf{X}\|^2 = tr\left(\mathbf{X}^T\mathbf{X}\right) = tr\left(\mathbf{X}\mathbf{X}^T\right) \tag{4}$$

is used, where $tr$ denotes the trace, and $\mathbf{X}$ is any matrix or vector. If $\mathbf{X}$ is a vector, then this is the squared Euclidean $L_2$ norm; if $\mathbf{X}$ is a matrix, then this is the squared Frobenius norm.

If one takes into account all aspects of a real human head, considering its shape (which is not a sphere) and different tissues with different conductivities, then numerical methods need to be used in order to calculate the lead field (see[18] and[19]). This is discussed in some more detail in the last paragraph of this chapter.

Regardless of the actual head model used, the basic equation giving the scalp electric potential due to a dipole has the simple form of Eqn 1, where:

(1) The lead field depends on the locations of the electrode and the dipole.

(2) The lead field is the collection of electric potentials at an electrode due to unit strength dipoles, each one oriented along the coordinate axes.

In practice, the dipole location and moment form a set of six unknown parameters, typically found by using a non-linear least squares fit. Informally, this means that, given a set of measured scalp electric potential differences, the dipole parameters are changed (location and moment), using some algorithm, until the model extracranial fields (given by Eqn 1) match as closely as possible the measured instantaneous EEG scalp map.

Note that the scalp potential due to two dipoles denoted $v1$ and $v2$ is simply a linear superposition:

$$\phi_e = \mathbf{j}_{v1}^T \mathbf{k}_{e,v1} + \mathbf{j}_{v2}^T \mathbf{k}_{e,v2} + c \tag{5}$$

This can be extended straightforwardly to any number of dipoles.

There are two major problems in dipole fitting procedures. First, as soon as two or more dipoles are considered, the best-fitting dipole parameters are almost impossible to find, because there are multiple "best fits." This means that there are several different configurations of the dipole parameters that reproduce almost identically well the measured EEG/MEG. The second problem is estimating or defining the number of dipoles to be fitted. Typically, completely different localization results are obtained by sequentially fitting (in the least squared sense) more and more dipoles. This means that if one fits two dipoles, and then separately one starts all over again and now fits three dipoles, the results are likely to be totally disparate, with no commonality between them. These problems are also discussed in Baillet et al.[6].

A noteworthy improvement in dipole localization was introduced by Scherg and von Cramon[17]: the spatio-temporal dipole model. This technique is applied to time varying recordings, and it assumes, as before, that the dipole positions are unknown, but fixed throughout time. This spatio-temporal constraint provides stability to the results, and has been very successful in modeling the first stages of the auditory pathway. The actual number of dipoles to be fitted remains an unsolved problem.

## Imaging the electric neuronal generators with discrete, 3D distributed, linear tomographies

This family of techniques has a very simple structure that leads to a linear system of equations. The "known" part of the system of equations consists of the measurements, i.e. the instantaneous scalp electric potential differences or magnetic fields. The "unknowns" consist of the current density vector sampled at points throughout the cortical gray matter. The collection of points in the brain where the current density vector is to be determined is often called the "solution space." It can be defined, for instance, by constructing a regular cubic grid through the whole brain volume, and retaining only those points that correspond to the cortical gray matter (see last paragraph). At these points, a current density vector, i.e. a dipole, is placed. If the exact cortical geometry is known, then the orientation of the dipole is known, otherwise all three components are considered unknown. Finally, the coefficients of the linear system of equations correspond to the lead fields, which embody the laws of electrodynamics relating an extracranial measurement and a source.

Without loss of generality, the system of equations for scalp electric potential differences will be considered:

$$\boldsymbol{\Phi} = \mathbf{K}\mathbf{J} + c\mathbf{1} \tag{6}$$

In Eqn 6, $\boldsymbol{\Phi} \in \mathbb{R}^{N_E \times 1}$, with $\boldsymbol{\Phi} = (\phi_1, \phi_2, \ldots, \phi_{N_E})^T$, contains the measurements at $N_E$ electrodes, all using the same reference (which can be one of the measurement electrodes or not). The parameter "$c$," which is common to all electrodes, accounts for the physical nature of electric potentials, which are determined up to an arbitrary constant. $\mathbf{1} \in \mathbb{R}^{N_E \times 1}$ is a vector of ones. $\mathbf{J} \in \mathbb{R}^{(3N_V) \times 1}$ contains the current density vector defined on a total of $N_V$ points throughout the cortical gray matter. Note that the case considered here corresponds to an unknown cortical geometry, and therefore, at any point in the solution space, the current density vector has three unknown components, i.e. the dipole moment $\mathbf{j}_v \in \mathbb{R}^{3 \times 1}$, for $v = 1 \ldots N_V$. The lead field matrix $\mathbf{K} \in \mathbb{R}^{N_E \times (3N_V)}$ embodies the laws of electrodynamics that related scalp potentials and current densities. The coefficients in $\mathbf{K}$ are determined by all the properties of the head, i.e. geometry and conductivity profile. The detailed structure of the lead field matrix is:

$$\mathbf{K} = \begin{pmatrix} \mathbf{k}_{1,1}^T & \mathbf{k}_{1,2}^T & \cdots & \mathbf{k}_{1,N_V}^T \\ \mathbf{k}_{2,1}^T & \mathbf{k}_{2,2}^T & \cdots & \mathbf{k}_{2,N_V}^T \\ \cdots & & & \\ \mathbf{k}_{N_E,1}^T & \mathbf{k}_{N_E,2}^T & \cdots & \mathbf{k}_{N_E,N_V}^T \end{pmatrix} \tag{7}$$

where $\mathbf{k}_{e,v} \in \mathbb{R}^{3\times1}$ is the lead field vector with three components corresponding to the coordinate axes $XYZ$. As explained above, the $X$-component of the lead field is the electric potential at electrode "$e$" due to a unit strength current dipole at "$v$" that is oriented along the $X$-axis. Similar definitions hold for the $Y$- and $Z$-components.

The basic system of equations expressed in Eqn 6 above is written in matrix notation. This might be obscure to non-mathematicians. A completely equivalent and perhaps less obscure way of stating the system is:

$$\phi_e = \mathbf{j}_1^T \mathbf{k}_{e,1} + \mathbf{j}_2^T \mathbf{k}_{e,2} + \mathbf{j}_3^T \mathbf{k}_{e,3} + \cdots + \mathbf{j}_{N_V}^T \mathbf{k}_{e,N_V} + c \tag{8}$$

This means that, up to an arbitrary constant, the potential at electrode "$e$" is due to the linear combination of contributions from all possible sources. Each source contributes to the potential at electrode "$e$" according to the lead field, which will in turn depend on the distance between the source and the electrode, but in general it depends on the detailed head model (geometry and conductivity profile).

All that is needed now is to solve the system of equations in Eqn 6 for the unknown current density. This should produce a 3D image of electric neuronal activity throughout the cortex.

It is enlightening to note the similarity between this problem and the dipole fitting techniques described above. In fact, one way to interpret this linear distributed setup summarized in Eqn 6 is that there are $N_V$ dipoles, with known and fixed locations, but with unknown moments. However, the similarity goes no deeper. The essential difference is that while dipole fitting assumes that there are only a few active locations in the brain at any one moment in time, the distributed tomography in Eqn 6 allows for the whole cortex to be active in any general way, including the particular case of a few "hot spots." Another important difference is that in the distributed tomography there is no need to specify beforehand the "number of sources," since the very concept of "source" is now that of a distribution, allowing for any activity pattern on the cortex.

The problem presented here in Eqn 6 has the same structure and form of a much earlier tomography: the x-ray based computerized axial tomography (CAT) scan[20,21]. This was one of the first tomographies in the medical sciences, and it has had a tremendously beneficial impact on health. In many of its implementations, a CAT scan can be described as a discrete, 3D distributed, linear inverse solution[22]. However, it so happens that the CAT scan inverse problem has a unique solution, whereas the EEG/MEG problem does not[23].

In general, in order to obtain a particular solution, the current density must satisfy at least two conditions:

(1) It must respect the measurements, i.e. the current density should produce EEG/MEG values that in some sense must be as close as possible to the actual measurements.

(2) It should satisfy some property, i.e. the current density should deviate minimally from a predefined property.

Informally, this may be expressed as follows: find the current density $\mathbf{J}$ and the nuisance parameter $c$ that minimizes the functional $F$:

$$F = G\{d_1[\mathbf{\Phi}, (\mathbf{KJ} + c\mathbf{1})], d_2[\mathbf{J}, P]\} \tag{9}$$

In Eqn 9, $G$ is a monotonic increasing function of both arguments, i.e. $G$ increases with increasing $d_1$ or $d_2$. The function $d_1$ measures "distance" between its two arguments, i.e. small values correspond to a current density that is faithful to the measurements. The function $d_2$ measures deviation of the current density from an a-priori defined property denoted by $P$.

Equation 9 is an informal representation of almost all approaches that attempt to fit a model to some data, and at the same time demands that the model has certain properties. Some common approaches include the functional analysis formulation[24], the penalized likelihood formulation[25] and the Bayesian framework[26].

Within this context, the particular solution to Eqn 6 introduced by Hämäläinen[27], is the one that not only tries to satisfy the measurements, but also has the smallest possible value for $(\mathbf{J}^T\mathbf{J})$, i.e. it is the minimum norm solution. The formal problem statement is:

$$\min_{\mathbf{J},c} F \tag{10}$$

with:

$$F = \|\mathbf{\Phi} - \mathbf{KJ} - c\mathbf{1}\|^2 + \alpha\mathbf{J}^T\mathbf{J} \tag{11}$$

In Eqn 11, the parameter $\alpha > 0$ controls the relative importance between the two terms on the right-hand side: a penalty for being unfaithful to the measurements and a penalty for a large current density norm. This parameter is known as the Tikhonov regularization parameter[24]. The solution is:

$$\hat{\mathbf{J}} = \mathbf{T}\mathbf{\Phi} \tag{12}$$

with:

$$\mathbf{T} = \mathbf{K}^T\mathbf{H}\left(\mathbf{HKK}^T\mathbf{H} + \alpha\mathbf{H}\right)^+ \tag{13}$$

$$\mathbf{H} = \mathbf{I} - \frac{1}{N_E}\mathbf{1}\mathbf{1}^T \tag{14}$$

where $\mathbf{I}$ is the identity matrix of dimension $N_E \times N_E$, and $\mathbf{1}$ is a vector of $N_E$ ones. The superscript "$+$" denotes the Moore–Penrose generalized inverse[28]. The matrix $\mathbf{H}$ in Eqn 14 is the average reference operator. The matrix $\mathbf{T}$ in Eqn 13 is known as a pseudoinverse matrix. In this presentation the nuisance parameter "$c$" is estimated and plugged into the final equations to eliminate it. The effect is that the final solution is reference electrode invariant, due to the natural appearance of the average reference operator. It is important to emphasize this reference independency of EEG inverse solutions. The choice of the recording reference does not in any way influence the result of source localization algorithms, as it does not influence the topography of the scalp electric field (see Chapter 2).

Note that when considering the MEG case, all equations in this section are valid with the following substitutions:

(1) The arbitrary constant "$c$" is set to zero for MEG.

(2) The matrix $\mathbf{H}$ (average reference operator) is set to the identity matrix $\mathbf{I}$ for MEG.

The original minimum norm method[27] was applied to MEG data. The main property of the method was illustrated by showing that it localized test point sources correctly, albeit with low spatial resolution. Informally speaking, the method was accepted by the nascent neuroimaging community because it was linear, and it was capable of correct, but blurred localization of point sources. The actual simulation tests were carried out with MEG sensors distributed on a plane, and with the cortex represented as a square grid of points on a plane, parallel and just below the sensor plane. The test point source (a dipole) was placed somewhere on the cortical grid, and the theoretical MEG measurements were computed, which were then used as input in Eqn 12 to obtain the estimated minimum norm current density, showing maximum activity at the correct location, but with some blurring (dispersion) in the neighboring cortex. These first results were very encouraging. But there was one essential fact that was not emphasized, even to this day: the method does not localize deep sources. If the actual source is deep, the method misplaces it to the outermost cortex. The reason for this behavior was rigorously explained (including theoretical proof) in Pascual-Marqui[29], where it was noted that the EEG/MEG minimum norm solution is a harmonic function[30] that can attain extreme values (maximum activation) only at the boundary of the solution space, i.e. the outermost cortex.

In trying to correct for depth localization error, one school of thought has been to give more importance (more weight) to deep cortical areas. This method has been termed "depth-weighting," and a recent version of it can be found in Lin et al.[31]. The general inverse problem of this type is known as the diagonally weighted minimum norm, given by:

$$\min_{\mathbf{J}, c} F_D \tag{15}$$

with:

$$F_D = \|\boldsymbol{\Phi} - \mathbf{KJ} - c\mathbf{1}\|^2 + \alpha \mathbf{J}^T \mathbf{DJ} \tag{16}$$

The diagonal matrix $\mathbf{D}$ contains the weights. The solution is:

$$\hat{\mathbf{J}}_D = \mathbf{T}_D \boldsymbol{\Phi} \tag{17}$$

with pseudoinverse:

$$\mathbf{T}_D = \mathbf{D}^{-1} \mathbf{K}^T \mathbf{H} \left( \mathbf{HKD}^{-1} \mathbf{K}^T \mathbf{H} + \alpha \mathbf{H} \right)^+ \tag{18}$$

The diagonal elements of $\mathbf{D}^{-1}$ should be large for deep sources as compared with shallow sources, as shown in Lin et al.[31]. That study showed that with proper depth-weighting, the average depth localization error was reduced from 12 mm to 7 mm.

Several other weighting strategies have been proposed, such as the PROMS method by Greenblatt et al.[32] where the covariance data matrix is used to construct a weighting function in the source space, the regularized location-wise normalization proposed in the FOCUSS algorithm[33], the iterative change of the weights according to the previous solution[34], or the radially weighted minimum norm solution[35].

Another discrete, 3D distributed, linear imaging method is LORETA: low resolution electromagnetic tomography[36]. The development of this method was profoundly influenced by the minimum norm solution[27]. Informally, the basic property of the solution is that the current density at any given point on the cortex must be as close as possible to the average current density of its closest neighbors. This local property (activity at a cortical point and in its immediate neighborhood) is applied globally to the whole cortex, and is known as "smoothing"[37,38].

The "smoothness" property that defined LORETA actually constitutes an approximation to the electrophysiological constraint under which EEG/MEG is generated: relatively large spatial clusters of cortical pyramidal cells must simultaneously and synchronously undergo the same type of postsynaptic potentials. It is of course evident that the scale and the neuroanatomical boundaries of this synchronization are not supposed to be adequately modeled by the general "unbounded" smoothness constraint.

The general inverse problem that includes LORETA as a particular case is stated as:

$$\min_{\mathbf{J},c} F_W \tag{19}$$

with:

$$F_W = \|\mathbf{\Phi} - \mathbf{KJ} - c\mathbf{1}\|^2 + \alpha \mathbf{J}^T \mathbf{WJ} \tag{20}$$

The solution is:

$$\hat{\mathbf{J}}_W = \mathbf{T}_W \mathbf{\Phi} \tag{21}$$

with the pseudoinverse given by:

$$\mathbf{T}_W = \mathbf{W}^{-1} \mathbf{K}^T \mathbf{H} \left( \mathbf{HKW}^{-1} \mathbf{K}^T \mathbf{H} + \alpha \mathbf{H} \right)^+ \tag{22}$$

The weight matrix $\mathbf{W}$ appearing in Eqn 19 to Eqn 22 is not restricted to be diagonal.

Informally, in the case of LORETA, the weights are constructed in such a way that the second term on the right hand side of Eqn 20 has the form:

$$\mathbf{J}^T \mathbf{WJ} = \sum_v \|\mathbf{j}_v - AveNeighb(\mathbf{j}_v)\|^2 \tag{23}$$

where $AveNeighb(\mathbf{j}_v)$ is an informal notation indicating "average of current densities in the immediate neighborhood of point $v$, excluding point $v$." By keeping this penalty term as small as possible, a current density is achieved that produces localization errors much smaller than the minimum norm solution. Note that for the sake of simplicity, lead field normalization (i.e. depth-weighting described above) was not mentioned in this description, although it is also part of the weight matrix used in LORETA[29,36].

Also based on the idea of dependency between neighbored solution points, Grave de Peralta Menendez et al.[39] proposed to incorporate the fact that the strength of the source regresses with distance according to electromagnetic laws. These laws are integrated as a constraint in terms of a local autoregressive average with homogeneous regression coefficients depending on the distance between solution points. This inverse solution method has been abbreviated as LAURA (Local Autoregressive Average). It should be emphasized that the LAURA method suffers from the same problem as the LORETA method, in that both model inadequately the actual physiological dependency, because the local dependency constraint is applied to inter-voxel distances that are extremely large as compared with the neuronal dependency scale.

In keeping with the formulations given above, the LAURA method corresponds to the constraint:

$$\mathbf{J}^T \mathbf{W}_{Laura} \mathbf{J} = \sum_v \|\mathbf{j}_v - WeightedAveNeighb(\mathbf{j}_v)\|^2 \tag{24}$$

where the weight matrix $W_{Laura}$ implements the spatial autoregressive model, which informally corresponds to a "distance-weighted average of current densities in the immediate neighborhood of voxel $v$."

Other prominent variants of the minimum-norm solution proposed to incorporate a-priori information by statistical Bayesian formulations[40-42], by weighted resolution optimization (WROP method[43]), or by estimating the source-current covariance in a Wiener formulation[44].

As can be seen, because of the non-uniqueness of the inverse problem formulated in Eqn 9, different "discrete, 3D distributed, linear" solutions have been proposed with incorporation of different a-priori constraints. This chapter does not intend to give an overview of all proposals that have been made and does not make any judgment with respect to the goodness of the different proposals. Comprehensive reviews on inverse solutions have been provided[29,33,35,45-49].

In a simulation study, Michel et al.[49] compared the dipole localization error of some of the distributed linear inverse solutions in dependency of the number of recording electrodes (see also Figure 4.3). The mean localization error of LORETA and LAURA was, on average, three times smaller than the minimum norm, independent of the number of electrodes.

Over the years, distributed linear inverse solutions have been extensively applied to experimental and clinical data and the solutions have been validated with intracranial recordings, clinical outcome or other imaging methods.

An important application of EEG source imaging concerns the localization of epileptic foci. Because of their high temporal resolution EEG and MEG allow the distinguishing of activity of the primary focus from propagated activity. Besides the clinical value these studies also offer a means of validating the localization capabilities of the different inverse solution methods. Intracranial recordings in these patients as well as seizure-freedom after surgical resection of the focus provide excellent validation possibilities (for a comprehensive review see[50]). Such studies have repeatedly shown the high spatial precision of the distributed linear inverse solutions, both for mesial temporal as well as for extratemporal lobe epilepsy[33,45,51-57], particularly when high density EEG systems (up to 256 channels) were used[58-62].

Figure 3.2 shows the result of different distributed linear inverse solutions (weighted minimum norm, LORETA and LAURA) for two cases with intractable epilepsy, the first due to a non-lesional mesial temporal lobe epilepsy, the second due to a lesion in the right frontal lobe. The solution space was constrained to the individual MRI using the SMAC-transformed head model[63] (discussed in the final section of this chapter). The same lead fields were used for all inverse solutions. In the first patient, validation is provided by intracranial subdural recordings of the spikes. In the second patient, validation is given by the successful resection of the epileptogenic zone and comparison with the postoperative MRI. Figure 3.2 illustrates the highly similar results of LORETA, developed in 1994[36], and LAURA, that was proposed several years later[64]. Both solutions provide precise and correct localization of the focus. The weighted minimum norm solution, however, is imprecise and slightly outside of the focus region in both cases.

A second possible validation is the comparison with other imaging modalities. Still in the case of epilepsy, such cross-modal comparison has been made with PET and SPECT by Sperli et al.[57]. While correspondence between modalities was very high, electric source imaging was superior to the other two imaging modalities with respect to correct focus localization

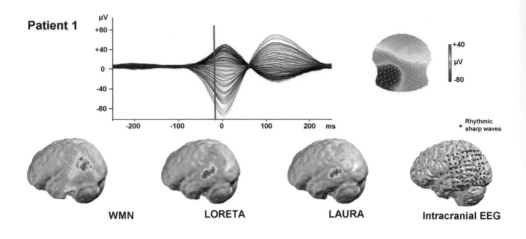

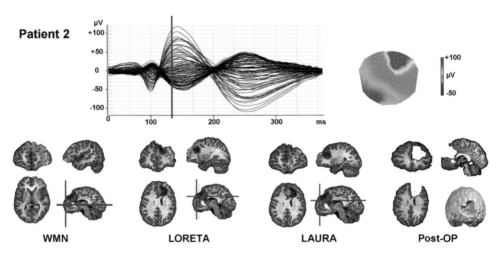

**Figure 3.2** Example of electric source imaging in epilepsy with two types of validation: intracranial subdural recordings in Patient 1, and postoperative MRI after successful resection of the epileptogenic focus in Patient 2. Three different inverse solutions were applied to the same data point (50% rising phase of the average spike). A spherical head model with anatomical constraints (SMAC) based on the individual MRI was used in both cases. Around 4000 solution points were equally distributed in the gray matter of the individual brain. The same lead field and the same regularization parameters were used for all inverse solutions. The first patient was recorded with 128 electrodes, the second with 256 electrodes using the EGI geodesic sensor nets (Electrical Geodesics, Inc., Eugene). The analysis was performed with the free academic software CARTOOL programmed by D. Brunet at the Functional Brain Mapping Laboratory in Geneva (http://brainmapping.unige.ch/).

(SPECT: 70%, PET: 82%, source imaging: 90%). Comparison with fMRI was performed with one epileptic case[65], where LORETA allowed the assignation of initiation and propagation to the different fMRI spots. More direct comparisons between LORETA and fMRI have been performed in cognitive studies[66,67]. In a recent study, Schulz *et al.*[68] compared fMRI with LORETA and LAURA evoked potentials in dyslexic children during sentence reading. Very high correspondence between fMRI and both inverse solutions was found. Differences between LAURA and LORETA were again minimal and mainly found with respect to the susceptibility to individual variation. Cross-modal imaging using EEG source localization and other imaging modalities is discussed in detail in Chapter 10.

## Statistical standardization

Up to this point, the tomographies described correspond to methods that estimate the electric neuronal activity directly as current density. Another approach, still within the realm of "discrete, 3D distributed, linear imaging methods" is to estimate activity as the statistically standardized current density.

This approach was introduced by Dale *et al.* in 2000[5], and is referred to as dynamic statistical parametric maps (dSPM) or noise-normalized current density. In their derivations, the first step consists of using the ordinary minimum norm solution for estimating the current density (Eqns 12 and 13). The second step consists of computing the standard deviation of the minimum norm current density, assuming that its variability is exclusively due to noise in the measured extracranial fields (i.e. EEG/MEG noise).

If $\mathbf{S}_{\Phi}^{Noise} \in \mathbb{R}^{N_E \times N_E}$ denotes the EEG/MEG noise covariance matrix, then the corresponding current density covariance is:

$$\mathbf{S}_{\hat{\jmath}}^{Noise} = \mathbf{T}\mathbf{S}_{\Phi}^{Noise}\mathbf{T}^{T} \qquad (25)$$

with $\mathbf{T}$ given by Eqn 13. This result is based on the quadratic nature of the covariance in Eqn 25, as derived from the linear transform in Eqn 12 (see Mardia *et al.*[69]). From Eqn 25, let $[\mathbf{S}_{\hat{\jmath}}^{Noise}]_v \in \mathbb{R}^{3\times 3}$ denote the covariance matrix at voxel $v$. Note that this is the $3 \times 3$ diagonal block matrix in $\mathbf{S}_{\hat{\jmath}}^{Noise}$, and it contains current density noise covariance information for all three components of the dipole moment. Finally, the noise-normalized imaging method of Dale *et al.*[5] gives:

$$\mathbf{q}_v = \frac{\hat{\mathbf{\jmath}}_v}{\sqrt{tr\left[\mathbf{S}_{\hat{\jmath}}^{Noise}\right]_v}} \qquad (26)$$

with $\hat{\mathbf{\jmath}}_v$ being the minimum norm current density at voxel $v$. The squared norm of $\mathbf{q}_v$, i.e.:

$$\mathbf{q}_v^t\mathbf{q}_v = \frac{\hat{\mathbf{\jmath}}_v^T\hat{\mathbf{\jmath}}_v}{tr\left[\mathbf{S}_{\hat{\jmath}}^{Noise}\right]_v} \qquad (27)$$

is an *F*-distributed statistic.

Note that the noise-normalized minimum norm in Eqn 26 is a linear imaging method when it uses an estimated EEG/MEG noise covariance matrix based on a set of measurements that are thought to contain no signal of interest (only noise), and that are independent from the measurements whose generators are sought.

Pascual-Marqui *et al.*[70] and Sekihara *et al.*[71] showed that this method has significant non-zero localization error, even under quasi-ideal conditions of negligible measurement noise.

Another member of the family of discrete, 3D distributed, linear statistical imaging methods is sLORETA: standardized low resolution brain electromagnetic tomography[70]. In sLORETA, it is assumed that the current density variance receives contributions from possible noise in the EEG/MEG measurements, but more importantly, from biological variance, i.e. variance in the actual electric neuronal activity. In its simplest form, the biological variance is assumed to be due to electric neuronal activity that is independent and identically distributed all over the cortex. This means that all neurons are equally likely to be active. Under this hypothesis, sLORETA produces a linear imaging method that has exact, zero-error localization under ideal conditions, as shown empirically in Pascual-Marqui et al.[70] and as proven by Sekihara et al.[71] and by Greenblatt et al.[32].

Under the sLORETA assumptions, the covariance matrix for the EEG/MEG measurements is:

$$\mathbf{S_\Phi} = \mathbf{K S_J K}^T + \mathbf{S_\Phi}^{Noise} \tag{28}$$

where $\mathbf{S_\Phi}^{Noise}$ represents noise in the measurements, and where $\mathbf{S_J}$ is the biological source of variability, i.e. the covariance for the actual current density. When $\mathbf{S_J}$ is set to the identity matrix, it is equivalent to allowing equal contribution of all cortical neurons to the biological noise. Typically, the covariance of the noise in the measurements $\mathbf{S_\Phi}^{Noise}$ is assumed to be proportional to the identity matrix (or to the equivalent average reference operator matrix). Under these conditions, the EEG/MEG covariance in Eqn 28 produces an estimated current density covariance given by:

$$\mathbf{S_{\hat{j}}} = \mathbf{T S_\Phi T}^T = \mathbf{T}\left(\mathbf{K S_J K}^T + \mathbf{S_\Phi}^{Noise}\right)\mathbf{T}^T = \mathbf{T}(\mathbf{KK}^T + \alpha\mathbf{H})\mathbf{T}^T$$
$$= \mathbf{K}^T(\mathbf{KK}^T + \alpha\mathbf{H})\mathbf{K} \tag{29}$$

Finally, the sLORETA linear imaging method is:

$$\boldsymbol{\sigma}_v = \left[\mathbf{S_{\hat{j}}}\right]_v^{-1/2}\hat{\mathbf{j}}_v \tag{30}$$

where $[\mathbf{S_{\hat{j}}}]_v \in \mathbb{R}^{3\times3}$ denotes the $3 \times 3$ diagonal block matrix in $\mathbf{S_{\hat{j}}}$ (Eqn 29), containing the current density covariance information for all three components of the dipole moment; and $[\mathbf{S_{\hat{j}}}]_v^{-1/2}$ denotes the symmetric square root inverse (as in the Mahalanobis transform[69]). The squared norm of $\boldsymbol{\sigma}_v$, i.e.:

$$\boldsymbol{\sigma}_v^T\boldsymbol{\sigma}_v = \hat{\mathbf{j}}_v^T\left[\mathbf{S_{\hat{j}}}\right]_v^{-1}\hat{\mathbf{j}}_v \tag{31}$$

can be viewed as a pseudo-statistic with the form of an $F$-distribution.

As a practical example, Figure 3.3 shows a 3D sLORETA map ($F$-pseudo-statistic in Eqn 31), corresponding to a visual evoked potential to pictures of flowers. The free academic sLORETA-KEY software and the data can be downloaded from the appropriate links at the homepage of the KEY Institute for Brain-Mind Research, University of Zurich (http://www.keyinst.uzh.ch). Maximum sLORETA global field power occurs at about 170 ms latency after stimulus onset (shown in panel D). Standardized electric neuronal activity is color coded, with maximum values represented in bright yellow. Maximum activation is found in Brodmann area 18 (panel B). Panel A shows three orthogonal slices through the point of maximum activity. Panel C shows a 3D rendering of the posterior cortex.

In general, statistical parametric or nonparametric mapping methods can be applied to distributed inverse solutions in exactly the same way as to other functional imaging data. Thereby, the inverse solution is calculated for each subject, each experimental condition and each time point (or selected time windows). Voxel-wise comparison between conditions can then be performed using randomization tests or simple paired or unpaired t-tests. This strategy has been successfully applied to localize the onset of interictal epileptic activity with LORETA[56] and with weighted minimum norm[57] algorithms. The method is described and illustrated in detail in Chapter 6. Statistical parametric or nonparametric mapping in

**Figure 3.3**
Three-dimensional sLORETA map consisting of the F-pseudo-statistic (Eqn 31 in the text), corresponding to a visual evoked potential to pictures of flowers. Maximum sLORETA global field power occurs at about 170 ms latency after stimulus onset (shown in panel D). Standardized electric neuronal activity is color coded, with maximum values represented in bright yellow. Maximum activation is found in Brodmann area 18 (panel B). Panel A shows three orthogonal slices through the point of maximum activity. Panel C shows a 3D rendering of the posterior cortex.

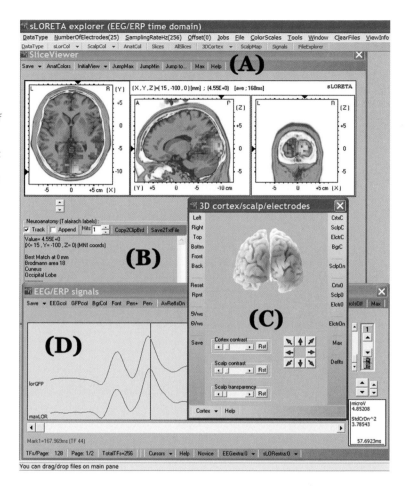

the inverse space has also been used in several recent experimental studies to localize those voxels in the brain that significantly differ between two experimental conditions[72–76].

# The regularization parameter

In all the discrete, 3D, linear tomographies previously described, there appeared the regularization parameter $\alpha$ as part of the solution. But, what is the role of this parameter? Is it important? What effect does it have on the solution? How can it be determined?

Some very brief answers to these essential questions follow.

An inverse solution will smooth out gradually as Tikhonov's regularization parameter increases in value. This means that the images will look more blurred as $\alpha$ increases. The reason for this is that the parameter controls the spatial frequency components of the inverse solution: the higher the value of $\alpha$, the lower the low-pass spatial frequency (i.e. large $\alpha$ cuts off higher spatial frequencies, small $\alpha$ lets through higher spatial frequencies).

Seen from this point of view, using a correct value for $\alpha$ is just as important as correctly filtering the time-varying EEG/MEG recordings. Typically, noisy measurements produce, due to the principle of "garbage in, garbage out," very noisy tomographic images. One way to fit the inverse solution to the signal rather than to the noise is to increase appropriately the value of $\alpha$.

Informally speaking, if the signal-to-noise ratio (SNR) of the EEG/MEG measurements is known, then a good "guesstimate" can be found in Lin et al.[31]. The use of the SNR value for determining $\alpha$ will not change the fact that all the tomographies reviewed above remain linear and independent of the actual data being analyzed. This procedure is an option that has been implemented in the free academic sLORETA-KEY software.

Another approach to determine the regularization parameter $\alpha$ is to use cross-validation. The concept behind cross-validation is to select the value of the regularization parameter that produces the best genuine and objective prediction of the measurements. For instance, in the case of EEG measurements, suppose there are $N_E$ electrodes. Select a particular inverse solution, and set the value of the regularization parameter to any initial value. Select one electrode and form a new data set without it, i.e. with only $N_E - 1$. Next, estimate the current density, and compute the scalp electric potential at the eliminated electrode. Next, compare the predicted value with the actual measurement (squared difference). Repeat this prescription, one electrode at a time, and compute the total prediction error, i.e. the cross-validation error $CVE(Inverse\ method, \alpha)$. Note that in this notation it has been emphasized that the cross-validation error depends on the actual inverse method used, and on the regularization parameter. The best method and the best parameter are the ones that minimize this predictive error. Details of this technique can be found in Pascual-Marqui[77]. If the regularization parameter is determined by this technique, then the tomography is data dependent, or adaptive, and it is not linear.

## Adaptive spatial filter for bioelectromagnetic source imaging

This family of techniques has appeared in the literature under several names, such as beamformers and adaptive spatial filters. These techniques have been widely used in MEG. In common with spatio-temporal dipoles, they make use of time-varying recordings, and they use such temporal information to achieve improved localization results.

This section provides an overview on the adaptive spatial filter technique used for electromagnetic source imaging. We describe basic principles, underlying assumptions, and the extension to incorporate the estimation of the source orientation. In what follows, the MEG case will be treated, bearing in mind that without any loss of generality they apply as well to the EEG case.

## Definitions

Let us define the time-varying magnetic field measured by the $e$-th sensor at time $t$ as $b_{e,t}$, and a column vector:

$$\mathbf{b}_t = (b_{1,t}\ \ b_{2,t}\ \ \ldots \ \ b_{N_E,t})^T \tag{32}$$

as a set of measured data where $N_E$ is the total number of sensors. Let us define the measurement covariance matrix $\mathbf{C}$ as:

$$\mathbf{C} = \frac{1}{N_T} \sum_{t=1}^{N_T} \mathbf{b}_t \mathbf{b}_t^T \tag{33}$$

where $N_T$ denotes the number of discrete time samples in the recorded time window of interest. Extending our previous notation, let $\mathbf{j}_{v,t} \in \mathbb{R}^{3\times 1}$ denote the time-varying dipole moment vector at time $t$, at position $\mathbf{r}_v \in \mathbb{R}^{3 \times 1}$. Note that the source $\mathbf{j}_{v,t}$ can be equivalently written as:

$$\mathbf{j}_{v,t} = j_{v,t} \boldsymbol{\eta}_v \tag{34}$$

where $j_{v,t}$ denotes the source magnitude, and $\boldsymbol{\eta}_v \in \mathbb{R}^{3 \times 1}$ denotes its orientation. Note that it is assumed that the source orientation is time independent.

Let $\mathbf{l}_{e,v} \in \mathbb{R}^{3 \times 1}$ denote the lead field for the magnetic field case. As before, for the EEG case, the magnetic lead field is a vector with three components corresponding to the coordinate axes $XYZ$. The $X$-component of the lead field is the magnetic field at sensor "$e$" due to a unit strength current dipole at "$v$" that is oriented along the $X$-axis. Similar definitions hold for the $Y$- and $Z$-components. Particular examples of magnetic lead fields for spherical head models can be found, for example, in Sarvas[10].

In analogy with the EEG case, the forward equation for MEG is:

$$b_{e,t} = \sum_{v=1}^{N_V} \mathbf{l}_{e,v}^T \mathbf{j}_{v,t} \tag{35}$$

where $N_V$ is the number of sources. In the presence of additive measurement noise, Eqn 35 generalizes to:

$$b_{e,t} = \sum_{v=1}^{N_V} \mathbf{l}_{e,v}^T \mathbf{j}_{v,t} + n_{e,t} \tag{36}$$

Note that Eqn 36 can be written in vector/matrix notation as:

$$\mathbf{b}_t = \sum_v \mathbf{L}_v \mathbf{j}_{v,t} + \mathbf{n}_t = \mathbf{L}\mathbf{J}_t + \mathbf{n}_t \tag{37}$$

where $\mathbf{b}_t \in \mathbb{R}^{N_E \times 1}$ is given by Eqn 32; $\mathbf{L}_v \in \mathbb{R}^{N_E \times 3}$ contains in each row (sensor) the corresponding transposed lead field; $\mathbf{n}_t \in \mathbb{R}^{N_E \times 1}$ is the time varying noise vector; $\mathbf{L} \in \mathbb{R}^{N_E \times (3N_V)}$ is the lead field matrix for all sensors and sources; and $\mathbf{J}_t \in \mathbb{R}^{(3N_V) \times 1}$ is the current density vector for all sources.

Note that the summations in Eqn 35 and Eqn 36, and the matrix multiplication in Eqn 37 correspond, equivalently and formally, to integration over the source space, in the case of continuously distributed sources.

In the case of known orientation $\boldsymbol{\eta}_v$ for the sources, and by making use of Eqn 34, the previous equations can be written as:

$$b_{e,t} = \sum_{v=1}^{N_V} l_{e,v} j_{v,t} + n_{e,t} \tag{38}$$

and:

$$\mathbf{b}_t = \sum_v L_v j_{v,t} + \mathbf{n}_t \tag{39}$$

with:

$$l_{e,v} = \mathbf{l}_{e,v}^T \boldsymbol{\eta}_v \tag{40}$$

$$L_v = \mathbf{L}_v \boldsymbol{\eta}_v \tag{41}$$

where, as before, the scalar $j_{v,t}$ denotes the source magnitude.

# Source reconstruction using spatial filter

From the measurements $\mathbf{b}_t$, the spatial filter reconstructs the source magnitude $j_{v,t}$ as:

$$\hat{j}_{v,t} = \mathbf{w}_v^T \mathbf{b}_t \tag{42}$$

where $\hat{j}_{v,t}$ is the estimated or reconstructed source magnitude at location $v$ and time $t$ (see Van Veen & Buckley[78]). Using Eqn 42, the power of the spatial filter outputs is given by:

$$\frac{1}{N_T} \sum_{t=1}^{N_T} \hat{j}_{v,t}^2 = \mathbf{w}_v^T \left( \frac{1}{N_T} \sum_{t=1}^{N_T} \mathbf{b}_t \mathbf{b}_t^T \right) \mathbf{w}_v = \mathbf{w}_v^T \mathbf{C} \mathbf{w}_v \tag{43}$$

In Eqn 42 and Eqn 43, $\mathbf{w}_v$ is the weight vector, which characterizes the properties of the spatial filter. There are two types of spatial filters. One is the nonadaptive spatial filter in which the weight vector depends solely on the lead field of the sensor array. The other is the adaptive spatial filter in which the weight vector depends on the measured data as well as the lead field of the sensor array.

Because a biomagnetic source is the electric current density, which is a 3D vector quantity, we need to know the source orientation $\boldsymbol{\eta}_v$ when deriving the weight vector $\mathbf{w}_v$. The information on the source orientation may be predetermined if an accurate 3D MRI of the subject provides information on the orientation. In most cases, however, the source orientation $\boldsymbol{\eta}_v$ should be estimated also from the data.

When $\boldsymbol{\eta}_v$ is unknown, we first derive the weight $\mathbf{w}_{v,\eta}$ that depends on both the location $\mathbf{r}_v$ and orientation $\boldsymbol{\eta}_v$, and using $\mathbf{w}_{v,\eta}$, the source estimate $\hat{j}_{v,t,\eta}$ is obtained as:

$$\hat{j}_{v,t,\eta} = \mathbf{w}_{v,\eta}^T \mathbf{b}_t \tag{44}$$

The source orientation at $\mathbf{r}_v$ is estimated by maximizing the power of $\hat{j}_{v,t,\eta}$ with respect to $\boldsymbol{\eta}_v$. That is, the optimum source orientation $\boldsymbol{\eta}_{opt,v}$ is obtained from:

$$\boldsymbol{\eta}_{opt,v} = \arg \max_{\eta} \frac{1}{N_T} \sum_{t=1}^{N_T} \hat{j}_{v,t,\eta}^2 = \arg \max_{\eta} \mathbf{w}_{v,\eta}^T \mathbf{C} \mathbf{w}_{v,\eta} \tag{45}$$

Then, the weight vector $\mathbf{w}_v$ is redefined as the weight associated with this optimum orientation $\boldsymbol{\eta}_{opt,v}$, i.e.:

$$\mathbf{w}_v = \mathbf{w}_{v,\eta_{opt,v}} \tag{46}$$

We use this $\mathbf{w}_v$ to reconstruct the source intensity at location $\mathbf{r}_v$ such that:

$$\hat{j}_{v,t} = \mathbf{w}_v^T \mathbf{b}_t \tag{47}$$

The spatial filter that reconstructs 3D source vectors in this manner is called the scalar spatial filter. (Although there is a vector formulation of spatial filters, we do not describe it due to the space limitation. In practice the scalar and vector formulations give very similar results.)

# Nonadaptive spatial filter

Many tomographic reconstruction methods can be interpreted as nonadaptive spatial filters. For example, the well-known minimum-norm method[27] described above can be formulated as a nonadaptive spatial filter, of which weight is expressed as (see Sekihara et al.[71]):

$$\mathbf{w}_v = \mathbf{G}^{-1} \mathbf{L}_v \tag{48}$$

where $\mathbf{G} \in \mathbb{R}^{N_E \times N_E}$ is often referred to as the gram matrix, given by:

$$\mathbf{G} = \mathbf{L}\mathbf{L}^T \tag{49}$$

The sLORETA method introduced above[70] can also be reformulated as a nonadaptive spatial filter, of which weight is expressed as[71]:

$$\mathbf{w}_v = \frac{\mathbf{G}^{-1} L_v}{\sqrt{L_v^T \mathbf{G}^{-1} L_v}} \tag{50}$$

According to the Rayleigh–Ritz formula[79], the optimum orientation $\eta_{opt,v}$ for the minimum-norm filter is obtained as:

$$\eta_{opt,v} = \boldsymbol{v}_{\max} \left\{ L_v^T \mathbf{G}^{-1} \mathbf{C} \mathbf{G}^{-1} L_v \right\} \tag{51}$$

For sLORETA, it is obtained as:

$$\eta_{opt,v} = \boldsymbol{v}_{\max} \left\{ L_v^T \mathbf{G}^{-1} \mathbf{C} \mathbf{G}^{-1} L_v, \, L_v^T \mathbf{G}^{-1} L_v \right\} \tag{52}$$

In the above equations, the eigenvector corresponding to the maximum eigenvalues of a matrix $\mathbf{A}$ is denoted $\boldsymbol{v}_{\max}\{\mathbf{A}\}$ and the eigenvector corresponding to the maximum generalized eigenvalue of a matrix $\mathbf{A}$ with a metric $\mathbf{B}$ as $\boldsymbol{v}_{\max}\{\mathbf{A}, \mathbf{B}\}$. For later use, we denote the minimum generalized eigenvalue of a matrix $\mathbf{A}$ with a metric $\mathbf{B}$ as $\varepsilon_{\min}\{\mathbf{A}, \mathbf{B}\}$ and the corresponding eigenvector as $\boldsymbol{v}_{\min}\{\mathbf{A}, \mathbf{B}\}$.

## Adaptive spatial filter
## Minimum-variance spatial filter with the unit-gain constraint
Let us derive the weight of the minimum-variance spatial filter, which is the best-known adaptive spatial filter[80]. The weight vector of the minimum-variance spatial filter $\mathbf{w}_v$ is derived as the one which minimizes the output power $\mathbf{w}_v^T \mathbf{C} \mathbf{w}_v$ under the constraint of $\mathbf{w}_v^T L_v = 1$, i.e.:

$$\mathbf{w}_v = \arg \min_{\mathbf{w}_v} \mathbf{w}_v^T \mathbf{C} \mathbf{w}_v \text{ subject to } \mathbf{w}_v^T L_v = 1 \tag{53}$$

The inner product $\mathbf{w}_v^T L_v$ represents the spatial filter outputs from a unit magnitude source located at $v$. Therefore, setting $\mathbf{w}_v^T L_v$ equal to 1 guarantees that the spatial filter passes the signal from $v$ with a gain equal to 1 (unit gain). The output power of the spatial filter $\mathbf{w}_v^T \mathbf{C} \mathbf{w}_v$ generally contains not only the noise contributions but also unwanted contributions such as the influences of sources located at other than $v$. Therefore, by minimizing the output power with this unit gain constraint, we can derive a weight that minimizes such unwanted influence without affecting the signal coming from $v$, the pointing location of the spatial filter.

By solving the minimization problem in Eqn 53, the explicit form of the weight vector is given by:

$$\mathbf{w}_v = \frac{\mathbf{C}^{-1} L_v}{L_v^T \mathbf{C}^{-1} L_v} \tag{54}$$

It is easy to see that, using Eqn 43, the output power of this spatial filter is expressed as:

$$\frac{1}{N_T} \sum_{t=1}^{N_T} \hat{j}_{v,t}^2 = \mathbf{w}_v^T \mathbf{C} \mathbf{w}_v = \frac{1}{L_v^T \mathbf{C}^{-1} L_v} \tag{55}$$

The adaptive spatial filter in Eqn 54, which is obtained with the unit-gain constraint, is often called the minimum-variance distortionless spatial filter.

## Minimum-variance spatial filter with the array gain constraint

The constraint $\mathbf{w}_v^T L_v = 1$ is given in a somewhat arbitrary manner, and there should be other possibilities, depending on the characteristics of the problem to be solved. For the bio-electromagnetic source imaging, the norm of the lead field vector $\|L_v\|$ has a spatial dependence. Particularly when the spherical homogeneous conductor model is used for calculating the lead field, $\|L_v\|$ becomes zero at the center of the sphere for the MEG case (not for the EEG case). This causes a false intensity increase around the center of the sphere in the source reconstruction obtained using the minimum-variance distortionless filter, because the weight becomes infinity at the center.

When $\|L_v\|$ has a spatial dependence, it should be more reasonable to use the constraint of $\mathbf{w}_v^T L_v = \|L_v\|$, instead of using $\mathbf{w}_v^T L_v = 1$. Because $\|L_v\|$ is the gain of the sensor array, we derive, by using $\mathbf{w}_v^T L_v = \|L_v\|$, the spatial filter whose gain exactly matches the gain of the sensor array. The weight vector in this case, is obtained as:

$$\mathbf{w}_v = \frac{\mathbf{C}^{-1} \tilde{L}_v}{\tilde{L}_v^T \mathbf{C}^{-1} \tilde{L}_v} \tag{56}$$

Where $\tilde{L}_v$ is the normalized lead field vector defined as $\tilde{L}_v = L_v / \|L_v\|$. The output power from this spatial filter is given by:

$$\frac{1}{N_T} \sum_{t=1}^{N_T} \hat{j}_{v,t}^2 = \frac{1}{\tilde{L}_v^T \mathbf{C}^{-1} \tilde{L}_v} = \frac{L_v^T L_v}{L_v^T \mathbf{C}^{-1} L_v} \tag{57}$$

The output power obtained in Eqn 57 is sometimes called the neural activity index[81]. In Eqns 56 and 57, we can see that the weight is independent from the norm of the lead field, and we can avoid the artifacts caused due to the nonuniformity $\|L_v\|$.

## Prerequisite for the adaptive spatial filter formulation

As described in the preceding sections, the weight vectors of the adaptive spatial filters are obtained by minimizing the output power $\mathbf{w}_v^T \mathbf{C} \mathbf{w}_v$ with a constraint. Let us look at this minimization process in detail. We assume that total $N_V$ sources are located at $\mathbf{r}_1, \mathbf{r}_2, \ldots, \mathbf{r}_{N_V}$, and that their time courses are denoted $j_{1,t}, j_{2,t}, \ldots, j_{N_V,t}$. Ignoring the noise term, and assuming that the spatial filter is pointing at $\mathbf{r}_p$, the location of the $p$-th source, the output power of the spatial filter is given by:

$$\mathbf{w}_p^T \mathbf{C} \mathbf{w}_p = \frac{1}{N_T} \sum_{t=1}^{N_T} \left[ \mathbf{w}_p^T \sum_{v=1}^{N_V} j_{v,t} L_v \right] \left[ \mathbf{w}_p^T \sum_{v=1}^{N_V} j_{v,t} L_v \right]^T \tag{58}$$

Considering the unit gain constraint $\mathbf{w}_v^T L_v = 1$, we have:

$$\mathbf{w}_p^T \mathbf{C} \mathbf{w}_p = \frac{1}{N_T} \sum_{t=1}^{N_T} j_{p,t}^2 + \sum_{\substack{v=1 \\ v \neq p}}^{N_V} \left[ \frac{1}{N_T} \sum_{t=1}^{N_T} j_{v,t}^2 \right] \left\| \mathbf{w}_p^T L_v \right\|^2$$
$$+ \sum_{v=1}^{N_V} \sum_{\substack{u=1 \\ u \neq v}}^{N_V} \left[ \frac{1}{N_T} \sum_{t=1}^{N_T} j_{v,t} j_{u,t} \right] \mathbf{w}_p^T L_v L_u^T \mathbf{w}_p \tag{59}$$

We assume that source activities are uncorrelated with each other, i.e.:

$$\frac{1}{N_T} \sum_{t=1}^{N_T} j_{p_1,t} j_{p_2,t} = 0, \quad \text{for } p_1 \neq p_2 \tag{60}$$

Then, the third term in the right-hand side of Eqn 59 becomes equal to zero, and we have:

$$\mathbf{w}_p^T \mathbf{C} \mathbf{w}_p = \frac{1}{N_T} \sum_{t=1}^{N_T} j_{p,t}^2 + \sum_{\substack{v=1 \\ v \neq p}}^{N_V} \left[ \frac{1}{N_T} \sum_{t=1}^{N_T} j_{v,t}^2 \right] \left\| \mathbf{w}_p^T L_v \right\|^2 \tag{61}$$

Therefore, the weight vector that minimizes the output power $\mathbf{w}_p^T \mathbf{C} \mathbf{w}_p$ satisfies the relationship $\mathbf{w}_p^T L_q = 0$, for $p \neq q$. Using such weight vectors, we have:

$$\mathbf{w}_p^T \mathbf{C} \mathbf{w}_p = \frac{1}{N_T} \sum_{t=1}^{N_T} j_{p,t}^2 \tag{62}$$

In summary, the weight vector obtained by minimizing the output power with the unit gain constraint has the property:

$$\mathbf{w}_p^T L_q = \delta_{pq} \tag{63}$$

where $\delta_{pq}$ is the Kronecker delta, i.e. $\delta_{pq} = 1$ when $p = q$ and $\delta_{pq} = 0$ when $p \neq q$. Equation 63 indicates that the weight vector passes a signal from a source at the pointing location but does not pass signals from other sources. The weight vector of the adaptive spatial filter attains such performance without being explicitly informed about the locations of other sources. This is because the covariance matrix R contains this information, and adaptive spatial filters automatically utilize it. It is obvious that the arguments in this section hold for the array-gain constraint minimum-variance filter, except that the weight property is expressed as:

$$\mathbf{w}_p^T L_q = \delta_{pq} \| L_q \| \tag{64}$$

## Scalar minimum-variance spatial filter

The source orientation can be determined in the following manner for the minimum-variance spatial filter. In this subsection, the minimum-variance spatial filter indicates the minimum-variance spatial filter obtained with the array-gain-constraint. The weight vector that depends both on the location and the source orientation is obtained using:

$$\mathbf{w}_{v,\eta} = \arg \min_{\mathbf{w}_{v,\eta}} \mathbf{w}_{v,\eta}^T \mathbf{C} \mathbf{w}_{v,\eta} \text{ subject to } \mathbf{w}_{v,\eta}^T L_v \boldsymbol{\eta}_v = \| L_v \boldsymbol{\eta}_v \| \tag{65}$$

The resulting weight vector is given by:

$$\mathbf{w}_{v,\eta} = \|\mathbf{L}_v\boldsymbol{\eta}_v\| \frac{\mathbf{C}^{-1}\mathbf{L}_v\boldsymbol{\eta}_v}{\boldsymbol{\eta}_v^T\mathbf{L}_v^T\mathbf{C}^{-1}\mathbf{L}_v\boldsymbol{\eta}_v} \tag{66}$$

and the output power is given by:

$$\frac{1}{N_T}\sum_{t=1}^{N_T}\hat{j}_{v,t,\eta} = \frac{\boldsymbol{\eta}_v^T\mathbf{L}_v^T\mathbf{L}_v\boldsymbol{\eta}_v}{\boldsymbol{\eta}_v^T\mathbf{L}_v^T\mathbf{C}^{-1}\mathbf{L}_v\boldsymbol{\eta}_v} \tag{67}$$

Therefore, the orientation $\boldsymbol{\eta}_{opt,v}$ that gives the maximum spatial filter outputs is obtained as[82,83]:

$$\boldsymbol{\eta}_{opt,v} = \arg\max_{\eta} \frac{\boldsymbol{\eta}_v^T\mathbf{L}_v^T\mathbf{L}_v\boldsymbol{\eta}_v}{\boldsymbol{\eta}_v^T\mathbf{L}_v^T\mathbf{C}^{-1}\mathbf{L}_v\boldsymbol{\eta}_v} \tag{68}$$

According to the Rayleigh–Ritz formula[79], the optimum orientation $\boldsymbol{\eta}_{opt,v}$ is given by:

$$\boldsymbol{\eta}_{opt,v} = \boldsymbol{v}_{\min}\left\{\mathbf{L}_v^T\mathbf{C}^{-1}\mathbf{L}_v, \mathbf{L}_v^T\mathbf{L}_v\right\} \tag{69}$$

The output power of this spatial filter is given by:

$$\frac{1}{N_T}\sum_{t=1}^{N_T}\hat{j}_{v,t,\eta} = \frac{1}{\boldsymbol{\varepsilon}_{\min}\left\{\mathbf{L}_v^T\mathbf{C}^{-1}\mathbf{L}_v, \mathbf{L}_v^T\mathbf{L}_v\right\}} \tag{70}$$

The minimum-variance spatial filter can be extended to the eigenspace-projection minimum-variance filter, which is known to be tolerant of errors in the forward modeling or in the estimation of the data covariance matrix[84]. The extension is attained by projecting the weight vector onto the signal subspace of the measurement covariance matrix. That is, redefining the weight vector as $\mathbf{w}_{MV,v}$, the weight vector for the eigenspace-projection beamformer is obtained using:

$$\mathbf{w}_v = \mathbf{E}_s\mathbf{E}_s^T\mathbf{w}_{MV,v} \tag{71}$$

where $\mathbf{E}_s$ is a matrix whose columns consist of the signal-level eigenvectors of $\mathbf{C}$, and $\mathbf{E}_s\mathbf{E}_s^T$ is the projection matrix that projects a vector onto the signal subspace of $\mathbf{C}$.

## Examples of the source reconstruction

The somatosensory response was recorded using a 160-channel whole-head sensor array (MEGVISION, Yokogawa Electric Corp, Tokyo, Japan) with an electric stimulus delivered to the right median nerve at the subject's wrist with a 1 s interstimulus interval. An epoch of 300 ms duration (100 ms pre- and 200 ms post-stimulus) was digitized at 1 kHz sampling frequency and a total of 400 epochs were averaged. The averaged magnetic recordings are shown in the lower panel of the right-hand side of Figure 3.4.

We applied the minimum-variance spatial filter to this somatosensory response. The weight vector of the minimum-variance filter was computed using Eqns 66, 69 and 71, and used for spatial filtering. The sample covariance matrix was calculated using a time window between 15 and 65 ms. The reconstructed results are shown in Figure 3.4. The MRI overlay shows that the reconstructed results demonstrate a clear localized activation at the subject's SI cortex. The upper panel in the right-hand side shows the reconstructed source time course at

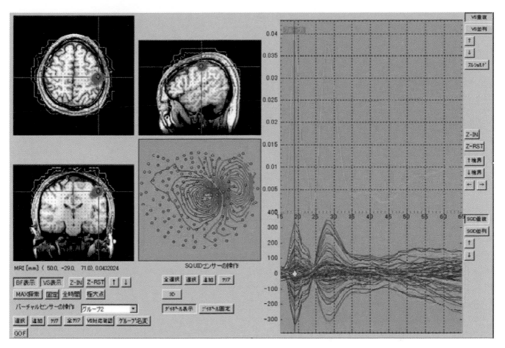

**Figure 3.4** Three panels (two upper panels and bottom-left panel) in the left-hand side show the results of MRI overlay in which the source reconstruction at 20 ms (the latency at the N20 peak) is overlaid onto the subject MRI. The bottom-right panel in the left-hand side shows the iso-contour map of the magnetic field at 20 ms of latency. The upper panel in the right-hand side shows the reconstructed source time course at the position that has the maximum source intensity. (This position is indicated by the diamond-like marks on the MRI.) The lower panel of the right-hand side shows the 160-channel magnetic recordings averaged over 400 epochs.

the SI cortex. These results clearly demonstrate the high-resolution reconstruction capability of adaptive spatial filtering.

# Head volume conductor model and solution space

Source localization consists of a source model and a volume conductor model. The different source models have been explained in detail above. They can in principle be applied to any head volume conductor model. The head model (geometry and conductive characteristics) defines the transfer matrix or lead field matrix. Equation 2 above describes the lead field matrix for the simplest head volume conductor model, the sphere. Different conductivity properties can be attributed to the different tissues of the head represented as homogeneous shells (Eqn 3). This approach has been used in most of the source localization studies, particularly when using equivalent dipole models. Most of these studies use the conductivity parameters of the different compartments as defined 40 years ago by Rush & Driscoll[85]. They proposed that the skull resistivity is 80 times higher than the resistivity of the scalp and the brain. These values are most probably wrong and the conductivity ratio between skull and brain is only about 20:1 or even lower, leading to much higher spatial resolution of the EEG[86]. This issue will be discussed in detail in Chapter 4, because it crucially influences the question of the number of electrodes that are needed for electric source imaging.

Spherical head models with uniform conductivity properties allow an analytical solution of the inverse problem and are thus fast and easy to calculate. However, they are not realistic. The brain is neither spherical, nor are the conductivity values homogeneous over the whole head. Therefore, more sophisticated realistic head volume conductor models based on the structural high resolution MRI of the individual subject are required. The realistic geometry can be implemented by numerical methods such as the finite element model (FEM[87]) or the boundary element method (BEM[88]). The FEM model allows a tessellation of the whole volume (typically restricted to the gray matter) and therefore allows the consideration of different conductivity values for each element. In addition, different orientation of the current dipole can be predetermined for each element based on the local cortical folding (for a review see Fuchs et al.[89]). While such realistic head models will certainly soon replace the simple spherical head models, this is not the case yet, because of the complexity, instability and computer demands of the FEM algorithms.

In an attempt to combine the computational efficiency of the spherical head model with a more accurate description of the head shape, Spinelli et al.[63] proposed a Spherical head Model with Anatomical Constraints (SMAC). It consists in calculating a best-fitting sphere for the individual head surface derived from the structural MRI. The brain is then transformed to this best-fitting sphere using homogeneous transformation operators. A multishell spherical model can then be used to calculate the inverse problem analytically, but the solutions are directly calculated for this (though slightly deformed) MRI.

The realistic head models (including the SMAC model) allow a restriction of the solution space, i.e. the space in which electrical activity can be generated, to the gray matter of the cortex. This drastically reduces the number of unknowns, and it allows the exclusion of cavities and lesions from the potential source space. For dipolar models, the search space is restricted to this individual source space. For distributed source models, the solution points are only distributed in this anatomically defined source space. While most of the experimental studies with healthy subjects tend to use one and the same realistic head model for all subjects (as offered for example in the LORETA software), clinical studies generally use the individual MRI of the patient and define an individual solution space in the gray matter of the patient[57,60].

## Conclusion

This chapter provides an overview of the different algorithms that are proposed to solve the electromagnetic inverse problem. We have focused on distributed source models that do not require a-priori assumptions on the number of sources, and we focused on those algorithms that are currently most widely used in the EEG and MEG community. We tried to make clear that the EEG/MEG inverse problem can be solved by incorporating physically and physiologically meaningful constraints and we tried to illustrate the capacity of these methods to noninvasively determine the distribution of electrically active neuronal populations at each moment in time in the healthy as well as in the pathological brain. The very high temporal resolution of the EEG and MEG make these methods unique to study the spatio-temporal dynamics of large-scale neuronal networks in the human brain. Recording systems with a high number of sensors combined with sophisticated source models and powerful realistic head volume conductor models make the EEG and MEG a reliable functional imaging method that can answer many scientific and clinical questions on how the human brain works.

# References

1. Berger H. Über das Elektroenkephalogramm des Menschen. *Archiv für Psychiatrie und Nervenkrankheiten* 1929;**87**:527–570.

2. Martin JH. The collective electrical behavior of cortical neurons: the electroencephalogram and the mechanisms of epilepsy. In Kandel ER, Schwartz JH, Jessell TM, eds. *Principles of Neural Science.* London: Prentice Hall International; 1991, pp. 777–791.

3. Hämäläinen MS, Hari R, Ilmoniemi RJ, Knuutila JE, Lounasmaa OV. Magnetoencephalography – theory, instrumentation, and applications to noninvasive studies of the working human brain. *Review of Modern Physics* 1993;**65**:413–497.

4. Mitzdorf U. Current source-density method and application in cat cerebral cortex: investigation of evoked potentials and EEG phenomena. *Physiology Review* 1985;**65**:37–100.

5. Dale AM, Liu AK, Fischl BR *et al.* Dynamic statistical parametric mapping: combining fMRI and MEG for high-resolution imaging of cortical activity. *Neuron* 2000;**26**:55–67.

6. Baillet S, Mosher JC, Leahy RM. Electromagnetic brain mapping. *IEEE Signal Processing Magazine* 2001;**18**:14–30.

7. Llinas RR. The intrinsic electrophysiological properties of mammalian neurons: insights into central nervous system function. *Science* 1988;**242**:1654–1664.

8. Haalman I, Vaadia E. Dynamics of neuronal interactions: relation to behavior, firing rates, and distance between neurons. *Human Brain Mapping* 1997;**5**:249–253.

9. Sukov W, Barth DS. Three-dimensional analysis of spontaneous and thalamically evoked gamma oscillations in auditory cortex. *Journal of Neurophysiology* 1998;**79**:2875–2884.

10. Sarvas J. Basic mathematical and electromagnetic concepts of the biomagnetic inverse problem. *Physics in Medicine and Biology* 1987;**32**:11–22.

11. Brazier MAB. A study of the electrical fields at the surface of the head. *Electroencephalography and Clinical Neurophysiology Supplement* 1949;**2**:38–52.

12. Wilson FN, Bayley RH. The electric field of an eccentric dipole in a homogeneous spherical conducting medium. *Circulation* 1950;**1**:84–92.

13. Frank E. Electric potential produced by 2 point current sources in a homogeneous conducting sphere. *Journal of Applied Physics* 1952;**23**:1225–1228.

14. Geisler CD, Gerstein GL. The surface EEG in relation to its sources. *Electroencephalography and Clinical Neurophysiology* 1961;**13**:927–934.

15. Lehmann D, Kavanagh RH, Fender DH. Field studies of averaged visually evoked EEG potentials in a patient with a split chiasm. *Electroencephalography and Clinical Neurophysiology* 1969;**26**:193–199.

16. Henderson CJ, Butler SR, Glass A. The localization of equivalent dipoles of EEG sources by the application of electrical field theory. *Electroencephalography and Clinical Neurophysiology* 1975;**39**:117–130.

17. Scherg M, von Cramon D. A new interpretation of the generators of BAEP waves I-V: Results of a spatio-temporal dipole model. *Electroencephalography and Clinical Neurophysiology* 1985;**62**:290–299.

18. Mosher JC, Leahy RM, Lewis PS. EEG and MEG: forward solutions for inverse methods. *IEEE Transactions on Biomedical Engineering* 1999;**46**:245–259.

19. Wolters CH, Anwander A, Tricoche X *et al.* Influence of tissue conductivity anisotropy on EEG/MEG field and return current computation in a realistic head model: a simulation and visualization study using high-resolution finite element modeling. *Neuroimage* 2006;**30**:813–826.

20. Cormack AM. Representation of a function by its line integrals with some radiological applications. *Journal of Applied Physics* 1963;**34**:2722.

21. Hounsfield GN. Computerized transverse axial scanning (tomography). 1. Description of system. *British Journal of Radiology* 1973;**46**:1016–1022.

22. Gordon R, Herman GT. 3-Dimensional reconstruction from projections – review of algorithms. *International Review of*

*Cytology – a Survey of Cell Biology* 1974;**38**:111–151.

23. Helmholtz H. Ueber einige Gesetze der Vertheilung elektrischer Ströme in körperlichen Leitern, mit Anwendung auf die thierisch-elektrischen Versuche. *Annalen der Physikalischen Chemie* 1853;**89**: 211–233; 353–357.

24. Tikhonov A, Arsenin V. *Solutions to Ill-Posed Problems*. Washington, DC: Winston; 1977.

25. Green PJ, Silverman BW. *Nonparametric Regression and Generalized Linear Models: A Roughness Penalty Approach*. London: Chapman and Hall; 1994.

26. Schmidt DM, George JS, Wood CC. Bayesian inference applied to the electromagnetic inverse problem. *Human Brain Mapping* 1999;**7**:195–212.

27. Hämäläinen MS. *Interpreting Measured Magnetic Fields of the Brain: Estimates of Current Distributions*. Tech. Rep. TKK-F-A559. Espoo, Finland: Helsinki University of Technology; 1984.

28. Rao CR, Mitra SK. Theory and application of constrained inverse of matrices. *Siam Journal on Applied Mathematics* 1973;**24**: 473–488.

29. Pascual-Marqui RD. Review of methods for solving the EEG inverse problem. *International Journal of Bioelectromagnetism* 1999;**1**:75–86.

30. Axler S, Bourdon P, Ramey W. *Harmonic Function Theory*. New York: Springer-Verlag; 1992.

31. Lin F-H, Witzel T, Ahlfors SP *et al.* Assessing and improving the spatial accuracy in MEG source localization by depth-weighted minimum-norm estimates. *Neuroimage* 2006;**31**:160–171.

32. Greenblatt RE, Ossadtchi A, Pflieger ME. Local linear estimators for the bioelectromagnetic inverse problem. *IEEE Transactions on Signal Processing* 2005;**53**: 3403–3412.

33. Fuchs M, Wagner M, Köhler T, Wischmann H-A. Linear and nonlinear current density reconstructions. *Journal of Clinical Neurophysiology* 1999;**16**:267–295.

34. Gorodnitsky IF, George JS, Rao BD. Neuromagnetic source imaging with

FOCUSS: a recursive weighted minimum norm algorithm. *Electroencephalography and Clinical Neurophysiology* 1995;**95**:231–251.

35. Grave de Peralta Menendez R, Gonzalez Andino SL. A critical analysis of linear inverse solutions. *IEEE Transactions on Biomedical Engineering* 1998;**45**:440–448.

36. Pascual-Marqui RD, Michel CM, Lehmann D. Low resolution electromagnetic tomography: a new method for localizing electrical activity in the brain. *International Journal of Psychophysiology* 1994;**18**:49–65.

37. Titterington DM. Common structure of smoothing techniques in statistics. *International Statistical Review* 1985;**53**: 141–170.

38. Wahba G. *Spline Models for Observational Data*. Philadelphia, PA: SIAM; 1990.

39. Grave de Peralta Menendez R, Murray MM, Michel CM, Martuzzi R, Gonzalez Andino SL. Electrical neuroimaging based on biophysical constraints. *Neuroimage* 2004;**21**:527–539.

40. Phillips JW, Leahy RM, Mosher JC. MEG-based imaging of focal neuronal current sources. *IEEE Transactions on Medical Imaging* 1997;**16**:338–348.

41. Schmidt DM, George JS, Wood CC. Bayesian inference applied to the electromagnetic inverse problem. *Human Brain Mapping* 1999;**7**:195–212.

42. Baillet S, Garnero L. A Bayesian approach to introducing anatomo-functional priors in the EEG/MEG inverse problem. *IEEE Transactions on Biomedical Engineering* 1997;**44**:374–385.

43. Grave de Peralta Menendez R, Gonzalez Andino SL, Hauk O, Spinelli L, Michel CM. A linear inverse solution with optimal resolution properties: WROP. *Biomedical Engineering (Biomedizinische Technik)* 1997;**42**:53–56.

44. Sekihara K, Scholz B. Average-intensity reconstruction and Wiener reconstruction of bioelectric current distribution based on its estimated covariance matrix. *IEEE Transactions on Biomedical Engineering* 1995;**42**:149–157.

45. Michel CM, Grave de Peralta R, Lantz G *et al.* Spatio-temporal EEG analysis and

distributed source estimation in presurgical epilepsy evaluation. *Journal of Clinical Neurophysiology* 1999;**16**:225–238.

46. Baillet S, Mosher JC, Leahy RM. Electromagnetic brain mapping. *IEEE Signal Processing Magazine* 2001;**18**:14–30.

47. He B, Lian J. High-resolution spatio-temporal functional neuroimaging of brain activity. *Critical Reviews in Biomedical Engineering* 2002;**30**:283–306.

48. He B, Lian J. Electrophysiological neuroimaging: solving the EEG inverse problem. In He B, ed. *Neuronal Engineering*. Norwell, USA: Kluwer Academic Publishers; 2005, pp. 221–261.

49. Michel CM, Murray MM, Lantz G *et al.* EEG source imaging. *Clinical Neurophysiology* 2004;**115**:2195–2222.

50. Plummer C, Harvey AS, Cook M. EEG source localization in focal epilepsy: where are we now? *Epilepsia* 2008;**49**:201–218.

51. Lantz G, Michel CM, Pascual-Marqui RD *et al.* Extracranial localization of intracranial interictal epileptiform activity using LORETA (low resolution electromagnetic tomography). *Electroencephalography and Clinical Neurophysiology* 1997;**102**:414–422.

52. Lantz G, Michel CM, Seeck M *et al.* Frequency domain EEG source localization of ictal epileptiform activity in patients with partial complex epilepsy of temporal lobe origin. *Clinical Neurophysiology* 1999;**110**:176–184.

53. Lantz G, Michel CM, Seeck M *et al.* Space-oriented segmentation and 3-dimensional source reconstruction of ictal EEG patterns. *Clinical Neurophysiology* 2001;**112**:688–697.

54. Zumsteg D, Friedman A, Wennberg RA, Wieser HG. Source localization of mesial temporal interictal epileptiform discharges: correlation with intracranial foramen ovale electrode recordings. *Clinical Neurophysiology* 2005;**116**:2810–2818.

55. Zumsteg D, Andrade DM, Wennberg RA. Source localization of small sharp spikes: low resolution electromagnetic tomography (LORETA) reveals two distinct cortical sources. *Clinical Neurophysiology* 2006;**117**:1380–1387.

56. Zumsteg D, Friedman A, Wieser HG, Wennberg RA. Source localization of interictal epileptiform discharges: comparison of three different techniques to improve signal to noise ratio. *Clinical Neurophysiology* 2006;**117**:562–571.

57. Sperli F, Spinelli L, Seeck M *et al.* EEG source imaging in paediatric epilepsy surgery: a new perspective in presurgical workup. *Epilepsia* 2006;**47**:981–990.

58. Lantz G, Grave de Peralta R, Spinelli L, Seeck M, Michel CM. Epileptic source localization with high density EEG: how many electrodes are needed? *Clinical Neurophysiology* 2003;**114**:63–69.

59. Lantz G, Spinelli L, Seeck M *et al.* Propagation of interictal epileptiform activity can lead to erroneous source localizations: A 128 channel EEG mapping study. *Journal of Clinical Neurophysiology* 2003;**20**:311–319.

60. Michel CM, Lantz G, Spinelli L *et al.* 128-channel EEG source imaging in epilepsy: clinical yield and localization precision. *Journal of Clinical Neurophysiology* 2004;**21**:71–83.

61. Holmes MD, Brown M, Tucker DM. Are "generalized" seizures truly generalized? Evidence of localized mesial frontal and frontopolar discharges in absence. *Epilepsia* 2004;**45**:1568–1579.

62. Holmes MD. Dense array EEG: methodology and new hypothesis on epilepsy syndromes. *Epilepsia* 2008;**49**:3–14.

63. Spinelli L, Andino SG, Lantz G, Seeck M, Michel CM. Electromagnetic inverse solutions in anatomically constrained spherical head models. *Brain Topography* 2000;**13**:115–125.

64. Grave de Peralta R, Gonzalez S, Lantz G, Michel CM, Landis T. Noninvasive localization of electromagnetic epileptic activity. I. Method descriptions and simulations. *Brain Topography* 2001;**14**:131–137.

65. Seeck M, Lazeyras F, Michel CM *et al.* Non invasive epileptic focus localization using

EEG-triggered functional MRI and electromagnetic tomography. *Electroencephalography and Clinical Neurophysiology* 1998;**106**:508–512.

66. Vitacco D, Brandeis D, Pascual-Marqui R, Martin E. Correspondence of event-related potential tomography and functional magnetic resonance imaging during language processing. *Hum Brain Mapping* 2002;**17**:4–12.

67. Mulert C, Jager L, Schmitt R *et al.* Integration of fMRI and simultaneous EEG: towards a comprehensive understanding of localization and time-course of brain activity in target detection. *Neuroimage* 2004;**22**:83–94.

68. Schulz E, Maurer U, Van Der Mark S *et al.* Impaired semantic processing during sentence reading in children with dyslexia: combined fMRI and ERP evidence. *Neuroimage* 2008;**41**:153–168.

69. Mardia KV, Kent JT, Bibby JM. *Multivariate Analysis*. London: Academic Press; 1979.

70. Pascual-Marqui RD. Standardized low-resolution brain electromagnetic tomography (sLORETA): technical details. *Methods and Findings in Experimental and Clinical Pharmacology* 2002:**24 Suppl** C:5–12.

71. Sekihara K, Sahani M, Nagarajan SS. Localization bias and spatial resolution of adaptive and non-adaptive spatial filters for MEG source reconstruction. *Neuroimage* 2005;**25**:1056–1067.

72. Michel CM, Seeck M, Murray MM. The speed of visual cognition. *Supplement in Clinical Neurophysiology* 2004;**57**:617–627.

73. De Santis L, Clarke S, Murray MM. Automatic and intrinsic auditory "what" and "where" processing in humans revealed by electrical neuroimaging. *Cerebral Cortex* 2007;**17**:9–17.

74. Murray MM, Camen C, Gonzalez Andino SL, Bovet P, Clarke S. Rapid brain discrimination of sounds of objects. *Journal of Neuroscience* 2006;**26**:1293–1302.

75. Spierer L, Tardif E, Sperdin H, Murray MM, Clarke S. Learning-induced plasticity in auditory spatial representations revealed by electrical neuroimaging. *Journal of Neuroscience* 2007;**27**:5474–5483.

76. Meylan RV, Murray MM. Auditory-visual multisensory interactions attenuate subsequent visual responses in humans. *Neuroimage* 2007;**35**:244–254.

77. Pascual-Marqui RD. Reply to comments made by R. Grave De Peralta Menendez and S.I. Gozalez Andino; Appendix II. (http://ijbem.k.hosei.ac.jp/2006-/volume1/number2/html/pas-app2.htm). *International Journal of Bioelectromagnetism (online journal)* 1999;**1**.

78. van Veen BD, Buckley KM. Beamforming: a versatile approach to spatial filtering. IEEE ASSP Magazine 1988;**5**:4–24.

79. Lutkepohl H. *Handbook of Matrices*. New York, NY: John Wiley & Sons Ltd.; 1996.

80. Robinson SE, Vrba J. Functional neuroimaging by synthetic aperture magnetometry (SAM). In Yoshimoto T, Kotani M, Kuriki S, Karibe H, Nakasoto N, eds. *Recent Advances in Biomagnetism*. Sendai: Tohoku University Press; 1999, pp. 302–305.

81. van Veen BD, van Drongelen W, Yuchtman M, Suzuki A. Localization of brain electrical activity via linearly constrained minimum variance spatial filtering. *IEEE Transactions on Biomedical Engineering* 1997;**44**:867–880.

82. Sekihara K, Scholz B. Generalized Wiener estimation of three-dimensional current distribution from biomagnetic measurements. *IEEE Transactions on Biomedical Engineering* 1996;**43**:281–291.

83. Sekihara K, Nagarajan SS. Neuromagnetic source reconstruction and inverse modeling. In He B, ed. *Modeling and Imaging of Bioelectric Activity – Principles and Applications*. New York, NY: Kluwer Academic/Plenum Publishers; 2004, pp. 213–250.

84. Sekihara K, Nagarajan SS, Poeppel D, Marantz A, Miyashita Y. Application of an MEG eigenspace beamformer to reconstructing spatio-temporal activities of neural sources. *Human Brain Mapping* 2002;**15**:199–215.

85. Rush S, Driscoll DA. EEG electrode sensitivity – an application of reciprocity. *IEEE Transactions on Biomedical Engineering* 1969;**16**:15–22.

86. Ryynanen OR, Hyttinen JA, Malmivuo JA. Effect of measurement noise and electrode density on the spatial resolution of cortical potential distribution with different resistivity values for the skull. *IEEE Transactions on Biomedical Engineering* 2006;**53**:1851–1858.

87. Bertrand O, Thevenet M, Perrin F. 3D finite element method in brain electrical activity studies. In Nenonen J, Rajala HM, Katila T, eds. *Biomagnetic Localization and 3D Modelling.* Technical Report TKK-F-A689. Helsinki: Helsinki University of Technology; 1991, pp. 154–171.

88. Hämäläinen M, Sarvas J. Realistic conductor geometry model of the human head for interpretation of neuromagnetic data. *IEEE Transactions on Biomedical Engineering* 1989;**36**:165–171.

89. Fuchs M, Wagner M, Kastner J. Development of volume conductor and source models to localize epileptic foci. *Journal of Clinical Neurophysiology* 2007;**24**:101–119.

**Chapter**

# 4 Data acquisition and pre-processing standards for electrical neuroimaging

Christoph M. Michel and Daniel Brandeis

## Introduction

The raw data for electrical neuroimaging is the potential field recorded on the scalp using multichannel EEG systems. Unlike waveform analysis of EEG or evoked potential (EP), electrical neuroimaging is based on the spatial analysis of these potential maps. The quality of these maps determines the goodness of the subsequent analysis steps. It is therefore of crucial importance that these scalp potential fields are recorded and pre-processed in a correct manner. An important issue concerns the number and the distribution of the electrodes on the scalp to provide an adequate spatial sampling of the potential field. Another issue is the measurement of the exact position of each electrode and the spatial normalization of the potential fields when averaging over subjects. Artifact detection and elimination is also an important point, since noise crucially influences source analysis. On the other hand, some factors that pose important problems for the traditional waveform analysis are irrelevant for electric neuroimaging. Obviously the selection of the "correct montage" for EEG analysis, or the "correct electrode" for evoked potential analysis is not relevant when analyzing the potential field. However, most important is that the question of the correct reference is completely obsolete for electrical neuroimaging. This fact was unfortunately often ignored[1-4] and the "reference-problem" has been considered as a major disadvantage of the EEG compared with the MEG[5-8]. It has been explained and illustrated in detail in Chapter 2 that the reference has no effect on the spatial configuration of the potential field and therefore in no way influences spatial EEG analysis[9-13]. This of course also concerns source localization procedures, that are completely reference-independent (see Chapter 3).

Many aspects of EP and EEG data recording are not specifically related to electrical neuroimaging but are standard requirements for all experimental and clinical EEG and EP studies. Such basic requirements (like sampling frequency, hard- and software filters, impedances, etc. are discussed in detail elsewhere[14-16]. Here we only discuss those practical issues that are of particular relevance for electrical neuroimaging (see also Michel *et al.*[12]).

## Spatial sampling

In order to adequately sample the potential field for electrical neuroimaging a large number of electrodes is needed, which is not a great problem any more. Electroencephalogram systems

*Electrical Neuroimaging*, ed. Christoph M. Michel, Thomas Koenig, Daniel Brandeis, Lorena R.R. Gianotti and Jiří Wackermann. Published by Cambridge University Press. © Cambridge University Press 2009.

of up to 256 electrodes are commercially available. Fast application of electrode caps or nets with these large numbers of electrodes is nowadays possible, making even high-density EEG very feasible in clinical routines[17,18].

Intuitively one would assume that more electrodes are always better. However, the issue is complex because the increased spatial resolution depends both on the resistance of the volume layers, particularly the skull, and the spatial smearing induced by these resistances and the measurement noise. The required number of electrodes depends on the spatial frequency of the scalp potential field which has to be correctly sampled to avoid aliasing. Aliasing is a well-known phenomenon for discrete sampling of time series. It appears when the frequency of the measured signal is higher than half of the sampling frequency (Nyquist rate). In this case, higher frequencies are not only poorly characterized; they also distort the energy representation of lower frequencies. This aliasing effect also holds for the sampling in space, since the potential distribution is only sampled at discrete measurement points (electrodes). While the concept of the Nyquist rate does not fully apply to data on the sphere[19,20], spatial frequencies of the potential field that are higher than the spatial sampling frequency (i.e. the distance between electrodes) will distort the map topography[20-24]. This distortion will lead to misinterpretation of maps and mislocalization of the sources.

While temporal aliasing can be diminished by applying pre-sampling low-pass filters, such filtering does not exist for spatial sampling. Therefore, the spatial frequency of the scalp potential fields has to be known. Unfortunately, it can vary for different temporal frequencies in the spontaneous EEG, different components of the evoked potential and different types of pathological activity. It will also vary for different areas of the scalp due to cortical geometry and variations in skull conductivity, the latter of which acts as a "natural" spatial filter. Investigations based on experimental data[25] and simulations[26] proposed that an interelectrode distance of ~2–3 cm is needed. Freeman et al.[27] concluded from spatial spectral density calculations that even less than 1 cm spacing of electrodes is needed. Srinivasan et al.[22] estimated the effective spatial resolution of different electrode montages, using a range from 19–129 electrodes, and concluded that "the smallest topographic feature that can be resolved accurately by a 32-channel array is 7 cm in diameter, or about the size of a lobe of the brain." These authors likewise demonstrated interpretational pitfalls of inadequate spatial sampling on the scalp. Comparison of the scalp topography of the N1 component of the visual evoked potential when recorded with 129 electrodes versus when subsampled to fewer electrodes led to incorrect lateralization of posterior foci and to obfuscation of a fronto-central positive focus with fewer electrodes. One study[28] evaluated the effect of number of recording electrodes on EEG of acute focal ischemic stroke patients. The data were originally recorded from 128 electrodes and then subsampled to 64, 32 and 19 channels. By visually comparing the EEG maps with radiographic images of the patients, it was argued that more than 64 electrodes were needed to avoid mislocalizations of the affected region.

Figure 4.1. illustrates the effect of spatial undersampling with the example of a somatosensory evoked potential after electrical stimulation of the left median nerve. It is a good example of a very focal extreme of the potential field, in this case the negative extreme concentrated on a few electrodes on the superior parietal lobe (the well-known N20 component). A bad spatial sampling of the field could in this case miss the focal minimum and misinterpolate the field. Consequently the estimated source of the N20 component, known to be generated in the primary somatosensory cortex, is not correctly retrieved by the inverse solution algorithm. This example illustrates possible problems of undersampling in the case of a very focal source captured on a few electrodes only.

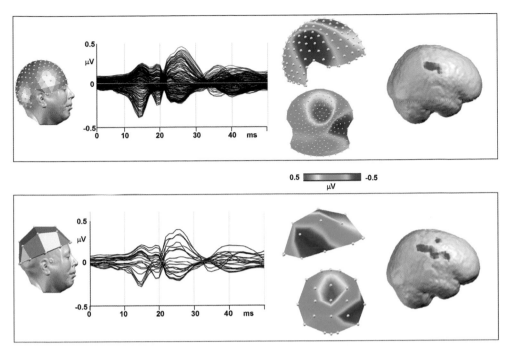

**Figure 4.1** Somatosensory evoked potentials (SSEP) of one subject recorded after electrical stimulation of the left median nerve. The SSEP were recorded from 204 electrodes (top). The overlapped traces are shown with clear components at 15, 20, 25, 38 and 40 ms. The potential map at 20 ms (N20) is shown with the focal negativity on right parietal electrodes. The source localization using a distributed linear inverse solution determines a focal source on the right primary somatosensory cortex of the hand area. The bottom shows the same analysis after subsampling the data to 21 electrodes. The focal minimum is missed in the map and the source localization reveals several activities in the right parieto-frontal region.

A systematic study using this down-sampling strategy was performed by Lantz *et al.*[29] on data from patients with focal partial epilepsy that were originally recorded with 123 electrodes and then subsampled to 63 and 31 channels. The 14 patients were grouped into those with mesial temporal (5), with neocortical (7) and with nonlesional (2) epileptic foci. All but one of the patients were seizure-free after resective surgery, thus the location of the epileptic focus was known. Several interictal spikes were determined from the basis of the 123 channel recordings and were localized using the linear inverse solution EPIFOCUS[30] using a 3-shell spherical head model with anatomical constraints based on the individual MRI (SMAC transformation[31]). The mean distance of the source maximum of the individual spikes to the resected area was determined and statistically compared between the different electrode arrays. Significant smaller localization error was found when using 63 instead of only 31 electrodes. Accuracy still systematically increased from 63 to 123 electrodes, but less significantly (Figure 4.2).

In the same study of Lantz *et al.*[29], as well as in a review by Michel *et al.*[12], simulations were performed with nine different electrode configurations between 25 and 181 electrodes equally distributed over the scalp. For each electrode configuration, the lead field matrix (see Chapter 3) was computed using a 3-shell spherical head model[32] with the resistance values as estimated by Rush and Driscoll[33]. A uniform grid of 1152 solution points was defined in the sphere. At each grid point, the three Cartesian components of a source were used to calculate

81

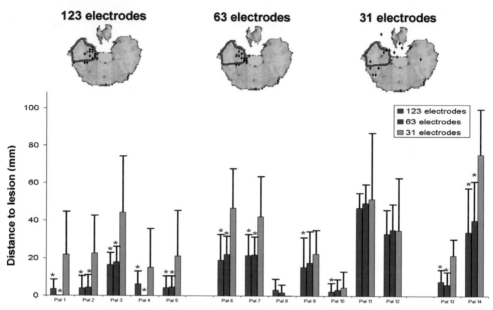

**Figure 4.2** Dependence of the localization precision of interictal spikes on the number of electrodes. Data of 14 patients with seizure-freedom after focus resection were analyzed. In all patients, spikes were recorded with 123 electrodes. Source analysis using the individual head model was performed on the original data and on data subsampled to 63 and 31 electrodes. The linear source localization algorithm EPIFOCUS was used on the individual SMAC-transformed head model and the distance of the maximum to the resection border was determined for all individual spikes and statistically compared between the different recording arrays. The top shows an example of the source maximum of each spike with respect to the resected area delineated in blue. Points appearing outside the brain are lying on another slice. The lower panel shows the mean and standard deviation of distance from source maximum to the lesion. Asterisks indicate significant ($P < 0.05$) better localization. Modified from Lantz et al.[29], Copyright (2003), with permission from the International Federation of Clinical Neurophysiology.

the forward solution, i.e. to produce a scalp potential map. For each electrode configuration, these simulated potentials were subsequently localized, and the averaged localization error was determined. Both studies showed that the localization precision does not increase in a linear fashion, but reaches a plateau at about 100 electrodes for fully distributed inverse solution algorithms (Figure 4.3).

Most of the above-described studies with simulation or with real data estimate that around 100 electrodes are needed for maximal spatial resolution. However, Ryynänen et al.[24] pointed out that this only holds if we assume that the skull resistance is 80 times higher than that of the scalp and the brain, as introduced by Rush & Driscol[33]. The skull resistance has an important effect on the spatial resolution of the EEG by drastically blurring the signals[34]. Several recent studies have shown that the skull resistance is probably considerably lower[35–37]. Ryynänen et al.[23] systematically investigated the gain of the number of electrodes on spatial resolution when lowering the resistance values. They concluded that the usually used high resistance ratio of 80:1 between skull and brain indeed leads to a limited spatial resolution that can be correctly captured with around 64 electrodes. However, when reducing the skull resistance, increasing the number of electrodes clearly increases spatial resolution. With resistances as low as 8, the use of even 512 electrodes would still improve the resolution. The resistance of the skull depends on the skull thickness. In newborns the skull thickness is c. 7–8 times lower than in adults, leading to a ratio of c. 14:1[20,38] between skull

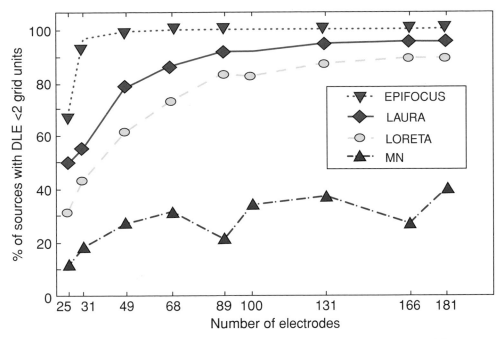

**Figure 4.3** Dependency of source localization precision on the number of electrodes examined by different source localization methods. 181 electrodes were uniformly distributed on a sphere and then down sampled to homogeneously distributed montages ranging from 25 to 166 electrodes. The lead field matrix was computed for each electrode configuration using a 3-shell spherical head model with an equally spaced grid of 1152 solution points. The forward solution was computed for dipolar sources at each of these grid points. These simulated surface potentials were then localized using four different distributed inverse solution algorithms: Minimal Norm (MN), Laplacian weighted Minimum Norm (LORETA), Local Autoregressive Average (LAURA) and EPIFOCUS. The percentage of sources with a dipole localization error of less than 2 grid points are plotted. The localization precision increases nonlinearly with increasing number of electrodes, reaching a plateau at around 100 electrodes. Modified from Michel et al.[12]. Copyright (2004), with permission from the International Federation of Clinical Neurophysiology.

and brain. Ryynänen et al.[24] show that with this ratio, spatial resolution still increases with 256 as compared with 128 electrodes in realistic noise levels. The aspect of number of electrodes in infants has been specifically addressed in the study of Grieve et al.[20]. These authors also concluded that a 256-electrode array is needed to obtain a spatial sampling error of less than 10%.

The conclusion of the above discussion is that with the usually assumed high skull resistance of 80, the blurring caused by volume conductor effects limits the spatial resolution and there would be no great benefit from increasing the number of electrodes much above 64. To the contrary, such large arrays would actually rather aggravate the spatial analysis because they are more influenced by the noise level of the data. As shown by Ryynänen et al.[23,24], the measurement noise (environment and electrode contact) is a critical limiting factor in source localization with high density EEG systems. As the noise increases, the spatial resolution decreases drastically. Thus, in realistic noise levels the use of more than 128 electrodes with the high skull resistance of 80:1 is not a benefit. However, if the resistance is lower, as proposed by several studies, and as is the case in infants, increasing the number of electrodes increases spatial resolution even in a realistic noise environment.

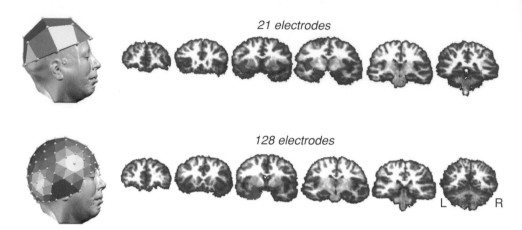

**Figure 4.4** Source analysis of averaged spikes of a patient with mesial temporal lobe epilepsy confirmed by post operative seizure freedom. Top: Localization based on the routine 21-electrode clinical EEG. Bottom: Localization based on the 128-channel recording. Note the shift of the localization maximum to more superior structures with the low resolution recording. Modified from Sperli et al.[40], with permission from John Wiley & Sons, Ltd.

In conclusion, both the intra- and interindividual variability of the resistance values of the skull and the amount of noise need to be more accurately considered in future studies by directly measuring the regional head tissue conductivities through current injection[39].

## Distribution of the electrodes

To correctly interpret the potential field and to adequately estimate the underlying sources, the field has to be sampled as completely as possible. If only one part of the field is captured, interpretation in terms of the generators in the brain is not possible. Ideally, all extremes of the field should lie within the array, so that all positive and negative poles of the dipoles that generated the field are captured. If only one pole is seen, the correct location of the corresponding dipole cannot be estimated. This fact is particularly true for tangential sources, because the maximum and minimum of the generating field do not lie directly above the source. Examples of bad samplings and the corresponding effect on the source estimation are shown in Figure 4.4 with an example of a 128-channel recording of a patient with mesial temporal lobe epilepsy. In this case, the negative extrema of the field is on the inferior temporal lobe. Removing the electrodes that are placed in this area lead to wrong source estimation with a focus proposed on the level of the insula. Since the conventional 10/20 system does not include these inferior electrodes, mesial temporal sources are systematically misplaced, as shown in Sperli et al.[40]. Another example is shown in Figure 4.5 with a visual evoked potential where the bilateral parietal activity of the P300 response evident with 33 electrodes is mistaken as a single posterior midline source when undersampling with only 19 electrodes.

These examples make clear that it is not only the number of electrodes, but also the correct sampling of the field that is essential. If only a low-resolution EEG system is available, it is still better to cover the whole scalp with this sparse electrode array than to put the available electrodes on one region only. Even if a good a-priori hypothesis allows a good estimation of the location of the putative source, the source localization algorithms have major problems if the full potential field is not correctly sampled[12]. This problem is illustrated in Figure 4.6

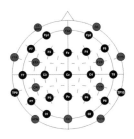

**33 electrodes**

**19 electrodes**

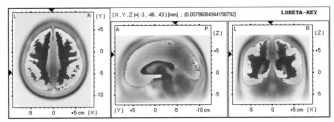

**Figure 4.5** Spatial undersampling can lead to mislocalization of distributed sources. The bilateral parietal activity evident with 33 electrodes (red and black positions) is mistaken ("blurred") as a single posterior midline source when undersampling with only 19 electrodes (black and red positions). LORETA solutions computed for cue P300 data of control children from van Leeuwen *et al.*[65].

with a visual evoked potential recorded from 204 electrodes and then subsampled to lower numbers of electrodes with different distributions.

## Measurement of the electrode positions

Electroencephalogram source localization needs the co-registration of the electrical activity with the anatomical brain space. This co-registration requires knowledge of the 3D position of the electrodes on the scalp. How precise this localization needs to be has not been assessed systematically for different source- and head models. Some studies have evaluated the dipole localization error induced by electrode misplacements. They concluded that the localization error due to electrode misplacement is small and might be negligible compared with the error induced by noise[41–43]. Currently, electrode caps/nets are generally used[44], which leads to a fairly constant electrode placement. In this case, the Cartesian coordinates of the electrodes can be calculated based on the known position of a few landmarks[45,46]. However, even with caps and nets, correct placement is required and the position of at least some of the electrodes should be measured to assure correct placement.

There are different ways to define the position of each electrode (see Koessler *et al.*[47] for a recent review). Manual methods are based on using calipers to measure inter-electrode distances with respect to certain landmarks[45,46]. Electromagnetic digitization utilizes a magnetic field and a transmitter-receiver system to digitize each single electrode[42,46]. Ultrasound

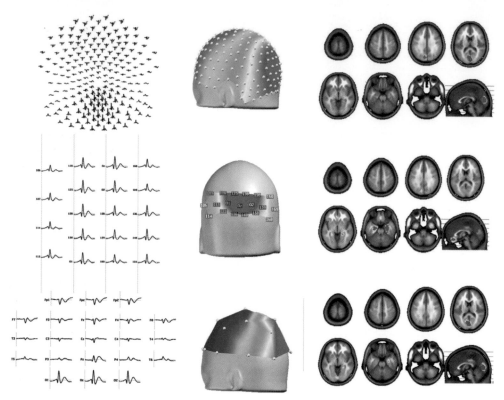

**Figure 4.6** Visual evoked potentials (VEP) of a full-field checkerboard stimulation recorded from 204 electrodes. Top row. VEP of all channels, potential map at 100 ms and source localization using a distributed inverse solution. The maximum is correctly localized in the visual cortex. Second row: Selection of 19 electrodes centered on the occipital "region of interest". Source localization with only these data available incorrectly reveals sources bilaterally in the temporal lobes. Third row: Selection of 19 channels out of the 204 but equally distributed over the scalp: the maximum is again correctly localized in the visual cortex.

digitization measures the time that an ultrasound emitted by a stylus placed on each single electrode needs to travel to a receiver[48]. Because of the considerable time required to digitize each electrode in high-density EEG systems, Russel *et al.*[49] proposed a photogrammetry system, where 11 cameras mounted on the different vertices of a polyhedron-based photogrammetry structure take pictures simultaneously from the head with the electrodes positioned in the middle of this camera array. This allows off-line reconstruction of the electrode positions. All three devices (magnetic, ultrasound, photogrammetry) are commercially available and are widely used. An alternative method consists in marking each (MRI-compatible) electrode with paramagnetic capsules that are localizable on the MRI and making a 3D anatomical T1 scan sequence[50–53]. The electrodes can then directly be determined on the MRI that is used for source imaging without any additional co-registering procedures. The spatial localization in MRI volume data is obviously the most adequate way if the individual MRI is required for the source analysis. While this is usually the case for patients where an MRI is often required for clinical reasons, MRI scans for healthy subjects in pure EEG studies might not always be feasible due to additional financial, organizational and time investment. Since knowledge of 3D electrode position is not only required for source localization, but also for normalization of EEG maps across subjects or within subjects across repeated measures, the measurement options outside the scanner are for the time being more reasonable.

## Spatial normalization and interpolation

Group studies or studies with repeated measures within a subject in different recording sessions require spatial normalization of the electric fields, either on the scalp level, or in the inverse space.

On the scalp level, group analysis requires the normalization of the individual data to a common electrode array[14]. This normalization is evidently only possible if the individual electrode positions have been measured with one of the methods described in the previous paragraph. Interpolation algorithms can then be used to transform the data from the individual electrode space to a general electrode array. Such interpolation algorithms are also needed to remove and replace artifact-contaminated channels or to apply source analysis software that is based on standard electrode arrays[54].

Details of the different interpolation algorithms proposed for EEG maps are given in Chapter 2. Fletcher et al.[55] presented an extended study of interpolation errors in scalp topographic mapping and concluded that spline class algorithms minimize the interpolation errors.

If source analysis is applied to the individual data and group analysis is performed in the inverse space, interpolation of the scalp potential maps is not required any more, but normalization has to be performed on the level of the brain space. There are two levels on which this normalization is performed:

(1) Calculating the lead field (see Chapter 3) for a generic head model, for example based on the averaged brain of the Montreal Neurological Institute (MNI-brain) and a standard distribution of the solution space within the gray matter of this template brain. The individual electrodes are then co-registered on this standard brain and the inverse solution is calculated in this generic brain for all subjects.

(2) Calculating the inverse solution in the individual brain of the subject with the individual gray matter and the solution points distributed within this brain space. These individual 3D functional images can then be normalized to a generic brain in the same way as it is done for individual fMRI data.

## Artifact detection and elimination

In multichannel recordings with hundreds of channels, electrodes with bad contacts cannot be avoided. The logical strategy is to offline detect and eliminate or interpolate bad electrodes. When applying source localization algorithms, the bad electrodes can simply be eliminated when calculating the lead field and the corresponding trace can be erased from the EEG file. Alternatively, the values of bad electrodes can be interpolated from the neighbor electrodes using the above-discussed spline interpolation algorithms. This generally works well as long as the bad electrodes are dispersed and not too much isolated at the border of the electrode array.

While it is relatively easy and not too disastrous to eliminate some bad electrodes from high-density EEG recordings, it is not always trivial to detect them by visual inspection of hundreds of simultaneously recorded EEG channels. While the importance of careful artifact review in high-density recordings has been recognized, algorithms to detect artifacts on

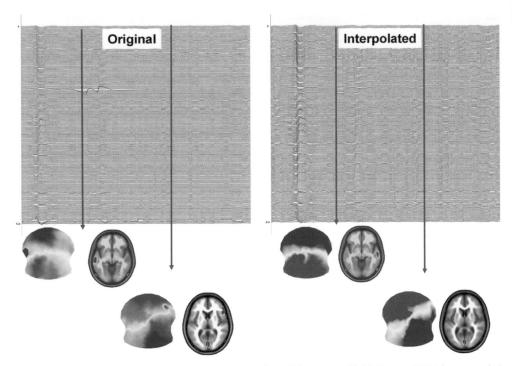

**Figure 4.7** The effect of bad electrodes on the spatial analysis of the potential field. Ongoing EEG is here recorded from 256 electrodes. On the left panel, the original data are shown with maps and inverse solutions at two different time points. The first time point is at the moment of an artifact of a left temporal electrode. The artifact is clearly seen on the traces and on the map as a strong negative potential. Source analysis of this map is completely centered on this artifact. The second time point is selected at a moment where all traces look acceptable. However, the map shows a very focal negativity on a right frontal electrode surrounded by positive potentials. Consequently, the distributed inverse solution places a source below this bad electrode apart from the occipital source. On the right panel, these two electrodes are interpolated and sources are calculated for these corrected maps. The left temporal source at the first time point disappeared and is replaced by a right temporal source. The right frontal source at the second time point completely disappeared and only the occipital source is left.

individual channels automatically are not easy to construct[56]. An important help is provided by the visual inspection of the potential maps. As discussed above, scalp potential maps are by nature spatially smoothed because of the resistance of the skull. Outliers in the topographic arrangement of the potential map are thus easily detected. A single isolated negative value in the middle of an area of positive potentials is most probably an artifact. Such "spatial outliers" can be inconspicuous when inspecting the waveforms, but become readily seen on the maps as "spatial outliers." Such an example is illustrated in Figure 4.7. Even if it is only one out of 256 electrodes that was not recording proper EEG activity, keeping this bad electrode in the subsequent analysis steps, particularly in the source localization calculation, can have drastic effects, as illustrated in Figure 4.7.

Apart from bad electrode contacts, electronic or physiological noise can destroy the electric field. Most important are eye movement artifacts. They can in principle easily be detected by placing electrodes above and below the eye and recording the electrooculogram (EOG). In high-density arrays, eye movement may well be detected from the most frontal channels. The question is whether eye movements inevitably lead to a rejection of the trial, or whether the electric field generated by the eye movement can be detected and subtracted and the non-contaminated EEG can be recovered.

Initial proposals to correct the eye movement artifact were based on simple subtraction of the propagated EOG activity at each channel[57], or by dipole modeling procedures[58]. The currently most popular approach to correct artifacts is based on independent component analysis (ICA)[59]. This technique relies on the hypothesis that brain activity is the result of a superimposition of several independent activities. The activity produced by an eye blink or eye movement is considered to be represented as one such independent component. This interpretation is physiologically well justified and ICA has its undisputed strength in detecting this independent component in the form of a unique map configuration[60,61]. Other types of artifacts have been successfully characterized by ICA, allowing a correction of the EEG[62]. An important use of the ICA correction strategy is in elimination of the cardiac pulse artifact in the EEG recorded in the scanner[63,64], an issue that will be discussed in Chapter 10.

## Conclusions

The basic requirement for electrical neuroimaging is the correct recording of the potential field on the scalp. The quality of the scalp potential map not only depends on technical aspects of the recording apparatus, but also on the number and correct positioning of the electrodes. On the other hand, points that are crucial for waveform analysis, such as the positioning of the reference electrode, are less crucial or even irrelevant for spatial analysis of the potential field. A basic drawback of electrical neuroimaging was for a long time the difficulty of applying a sufficient number of electrodes in a reasonable amount of time. This is not an issue any more with the new commercially available systems. Quickly applied high-density EEG from several hundreds of electrodes with continuous digitization at sampling rates of up to 20 000 Hz per channel are commercially available. Electrical neuroimaging is therefore nowadays possible for any research and clinical laboratory. Efficient and standardized analysis procedures are becoming available, allowing even nonexperienced researchers and clinicians to take advantage of the possibilities that this new functional imaging tool provides.

## References

1. Desmedt JE, Tomberg C, Noel P, Ozaki I. Beware of the average reference in brain mapping. *Electroencephalography and Clinical Neurophysiology Suppl.* 1990; **41**:22–27.

2. Tomberg C, Noel P, Ozaki I, Desmedt JE. Inadequacy of the average reference for the topographic mapping of focal enhancements of brain potentials. *Electroencephalography and Clinical Neurophysiology* 1990;**77**:259–265.

3. Junghofer M, Elbert T, Tucker DM, Braun C. The polar average reference effect: a bias in estimating the head surface integral in EEG recording. *Clinical Neurophysiology* 1999;**110**:1149–1155.

4. Gencer NG, Williamson SJ, Gueziec A, Hummel R. Optimal reference electrode selection for electric source imaging. *Electroencephalography and Clinical Neurophysiology* 1996;**99**:163–173.

5. Williamson SJ, Lu ZL, Karron D, Kaufman L. Advantages and limitations of magnetic source imaging. *Brain Topography* 1991;**4**:169–180.

6. Wikswo JPJ, Gevins A, Williamson SJ. The future of EEG and MEG. *Electroencephalography and Clinical Neurophysiology* 1993;**87**:1–9.

7. Pataraia E, Baumgartner C, Lindinger G, Deecke L. Magnetoencephalography in presurgical epilepsy evaluation. *Neurosurgery Review* 2002;**25**:141–159.

8. Barkley GL. Controversies in neurophysiology. MEG is superior to EEG in localization of interictal epileptiform activity: Pro. *Clinical Neurophysiology* 2004;**115**:1001–1009.

9. Pascual-Marqui RD, Lehmann D. Topographic maps, source localization inference, and the reference electrode: comments on a paper by Desmedt *et al.* *Electroencephalography and Clinical Neurophysiology* 1993;**88**:532–536.

10. Geselowitz DB. The zero of potential. *IEEE Engineering in Medicine and Biology Magazine* 1998;**17**:128–132.

11. Lehmann DSW. Reference-free identification of components of checkerboard-evoked multichannel potential fields. *Electroencephalography and Clinical Neurophysiology* 1980;**48**:609–621.

12. Michel CM, Murray MM, Lantz G *et al.* EEG source imaging. *Clinical Neurophysiology* 2004;**115**:2195–2222.

13. Murray MM, Brunet D, Michel CM. Topographic ERP analyses: a step-by-step tutorial review. *Brain Topography* 2008;**20**:249–264.

14. Picton TW, Bentin S, Berg P *et al.* Guidelines for using human event-related potentials to study cognition: recording standards and publication criteria. *Psychophysiology* 2000;**37**:127–152.

15. Luck SJ. *An Introduction to the Event-Related Potential Technique.* Cambridge, MA: MIT Press; 2005.

16. Nuwer M. Assessment of digital EEG, quantitative EEG, and EEG brain mapping: report of the American Academy of Neurology and the American Clinical Neurophysiology Society. *Neurology* 1997;**49**:277–292.

17. Michel CM, Lantz G, Spinelli L *et al.* 128-channel EEG source imaging in epilepsy: clinical yield and localization precision. *Journal of Clinical Neurophysiology* 2004;**21**:71–83.

18. Holmes MD. Dense array EEG: methodology and new hypothesis on epilepsy syndromes. *Epilepsia* 2008;**49**:3–14.

19. Li T-H, North G. Aliasing effects and sampling theorems of SRFs when sampled on a finite grid. *Annals of the Institute of Statistical Mathematics* 1996;**49**:341–354.

20. Grieve PG, Emerson RG, Isler JR, Stark RI. Quantitative analysis of spatial sampling error in the infant and adult electroencephalogram. *Neuroimage* 2004;**21**:1260–1274.

21. Srinivasan R, Nunez PL, Tucker DM, Silberstein RB, Cadusch PJ. Spatial sampling and filtering of EEG with spline laplacians to estimate cortical potentials. *Brain Topography* 1996;**8**:355–366.

22. Srinivasan R, Tucker DM, Murias M. Estimating the spatial Nyquist of the human EEG. *Behavior Research Methods, Instruments and Computers* 1998;**30**:8–19.

23. Ryynänen OR, Hyttinen JA, Laarne PH, Malmivuo JA. Effect of electrode density and measurement noise on the spatial resolution of cortical potential distribution. *IEEE Transactions on Biomedical Engineering* 2004;**51**:1547–1554.

24. Ryynänen OR, Hyttinen JA, Malmivuo JA. Effect of measurement noise and electrode density on the spatial resolution of cortical potential distribution with different resistivity values for the skull. *IEEE Transactions on Biomedical Engineering* 2006;**53**:1851–1858.

25. Spitzer AR, Cohen LG, Fabrikant J, Hallett M. A method for determining optimal interelectrode spacing for cerebral topographic mapping. *Electroencephalography and Clinical Neurophysiology* 1989;**72**:355–361.

26. Gevins A, Brickett P, Costales B, Le J, Reutter B. Beyond topographic mapping: towards functional-anatomical imaging with 124-channel EEGs and 3-D MRIs. *Brain Topography* 1990;**3**:53–64.

27. Freeman WJ, Holmes MD, Burke BC, Vanhatalo S. Spatial spectra of scalp EEG and EMG from awake humans. *Clinical Neurophysiology* 2003;**114**:1053–1068.

28. Luu P, Tucker DM, Englander R *et al.* Localizing acute stroke-related EEG changes: assessing the effects of spatial undersampling. *Journal of Clinical Neurophysiology* 2001;**18**:302–317.

29. Lantz G, Grave de Peralta R, Spinelli L, Seeck M, Michel CM. Epileptic source localization with high density EEG: how many electrodes are needed? *Clinical Neurophysiology* 2003;**114**:63–69.

30. Grave de Peralta R, Gonzalez S, Lantz G, Michel CM, Landis T. Noninvasive localization of electromagnetic epileptic activity. I. Method descriptions and simulations. *Brain Topography* 2001;**14**: 131–137.

31. Spinelli L, Andino SG, Lantz G, Seeck M, Michel CM. Electromagnetic inverse solutions in anatomically constrained spherical head models. *Brain Topography* 2000;**13**:115–125.

32. Ary JP, Klein SA, Fender DH. Location of sources of evoked scalp potentials: corrections for skull and scalp thicknesses. *IEEE Transactions on Biomedical Engineering* 1981;**128**:447–452.

33. Rush S, Driscoll DA. EEG electrode sensitivity – an application of reciprocity. *IEEE Transactions on Biomedical Engineering* 1969;**16**:15–22.

34. Malmivuo JA, Suihko VE. Effect of skull resistivity on the spatial resolutions of EEG and MEG. *IEEE Transactions on Biomedical Engineering* 2004;**51**:1276–1280.

35. Oostendorp TF, Delbeke J, Stegeman DF. The conductivity of the human skull: results of in vivo and in vitro measurements. *IEEE Transactions on Biomedical Engineering* 2000;**47**:1487–1492.

36. Hoekema R, Wieneke GH, Leijten FS *et al.* Measurement of the conductivity of skull, temporarily removed during epilepsy surgery. *Brain Topography* 2003;**16**:29–38.

37. Lai Y, van Drongelen W, Ding L *et al.* Estimation of in vivo human brain-to-skull conductivity ratio from simultaneous extra- and intra-cranial electrical potential recordings. *Clinical Neurophysiology* 2005;**116**:456–465.

38. Fifer WP, Grieve PG, Grose-Fifer J, Isler JR, Byrd D. High-density electroencephalogram monitoring in the neonate. *Clinical Perinatology* 2006;**33**: 679–691, vii.

39. Ferree TC, Eriksen KJ, Tucker DM. Regional head tissue conductivity estimation for improved EEG analysis. *IEEE Transactions on Biomedical Engineering* 2000;**47**:1584–1592.

40. Sperli F, Spinelli L, Seeck M *et al.* EEG source imaging in paediatric epilepsy surgery: a new perspective in presurgical workup. *Epilepsia* 2006;**47**:981–990.

41. Van Hoey G, De Clercq J, Vanrumste B *et al.* EEG dipole source localization using artificial neural networks. *Physics in Medicine and Biology* 2000;**45**:997–1011.

42. Khosla D, Don M, Kwong B. Spatial mislocalization of EEG electrodes – effects on accuracy of dipole estimation. *Clinical Neurophysiology* 1999;**110**:261–271.

43. Wang Y, Gotman J. The influence of electrode location errors on EEG dipole source localization with a realistic head model. *Clinical Neurophysiology* 2001;**112**: 1777–1780.

44. Tucker DM. Spatial sampling of head electrical fields: the geodesic sensor net. *Electroencephalography and Clinical Neurophysiology* 1993;**87**:154–163.

45. De Munck JC, Vijn PC, Spekreijse H. A practical method for determining electrode positions on the head. *Electroencephalography and Clinical Neurophysiology* 1991;**78**:85–87.

46. Le J, Lu M, Pellouchoud E, Gevins A. A rapid method for determining standard 10/10 electrode positions for high resolution EEG studies. *Electroencephalography and Clinical Neurophysiology* 1998;**106**:554–558.

47. Koessler L, Maillard L, Benhadid A *et al.* Spatial localization of EEG electrodes. *Clinical Neurophysiology* 2007;**37**:97–102.

48. Steddin S, Botzel K. A new device for scalp electrode localization with unrestrained head. *Journal of Neurology* 1995;**242**:65.

49. Russell GS, Jeffrey Eriksen K, Poolman P, Luu P, Tucker DM. Geodesic photogrammetry for localizing sensor positions in dense-array EEG. *Clinical Neurophysiology* 2005;**116**:1130–1140.

50. Brinkmann BH, O'Brien TJ, Dresner MA *et al.* Scalp-recorded EEG localization in MRI volume data. *Brain Topography* 1998; **10**:245–253.

51. Lagerlund TD, Sharbrough FW, Jack CR, Jr. *et al.* Determination of 10–20 system electrode locations using magnetic resonance image scanning with markers. *Electroencephalography and Clinical Neurophysiology* 1993;**86**:7–14.

52. Yoo SS, Guttmann CR, Ives JR *et al.* 3D localization of surface 10–20 EEG electrodes on high resolution anatomical MR images. *Electroencephalography and Clinical Neurophysiology* 1997;**102**:335–339.

53. Rodin E, Rodin M, Boyer R, Thompson J. Displaying electroencephalographic dipole sources on magnetic resonance images. *Journal of Neuroimaging* 1997;**7**:106–110.

54. Scherg M, Ille N, Bornfleth H, Berg P. Advanced tools for digital EEG review: virtual source montages, whole-head mapping, correlation, and phase analysis. *Journal of Clinical Neurophysiology* 2002;**19**: 91–112.

55. Fletcher EM, Kussmaul CL, Mangun GR. Estimation of interpolation errors in scalp topographic mapping. *Electroencephalography and Clinical Neurophysiology* 1996;**98**:422–434.

56. Junghofer M, Elbert T, Tucker DM, Rockstroh B. Statistical control of artifacts in dense array EEG/MEG studies. *Psychophysiology* 2000;**37**:523–532.

57. Lins OG, Picton TW, Berg P, Scherg M. Ocular artifacts in EEG and event-related potentials. I: Scalp topography. *Brain Topography* 1993;**6**:51–63.

58. Berg P, Scherg M. Dipole models of eye movements and blinks.

*Electroencephalography and Clinical Neurophysiology* 1991;**79**:36–44.

59. Hyvarinen A, Oja E. Independent component analysis: algorithms and applications. *Neural Networks* 2000;**13**: 411–430.

60. Jung TP, Makeig S, Humphries C *et al.* Removing electroencephalographic artifacts by blind source separation. *Psychophysiology* 2000;**37**:163–178.

61. Jung TP, Makeig S, Westerfield M *et al.* Removal of eye activity artifacts from visual event-related potentials in normal and clinical subjects. *Clinical Neurophysiology* 2000;**111**:1745–1758.

62. Delorme A, Sejnowski T, Makeig S. Enhanced detection of artifacts in EEG data using higher-order statistics and independent component analysis. *Neuroimage* 2007;**34**:1443–1449.

63. Mantini D, Perrucci MG, Cugini S *et al.* Complete artifact removal for EEG recorded during continuous fMRI using independent component analysis. *Neuroimage* 2007;**34**:598–607.

64. Grouiller F, Vercueil L, Krainik A *et al.* A comparative study of different artefact removal algorithms for EEG signals acquired during functional MRI. *Neuroimage* 2007;**38**:124–137.

# Chapter 5

# Overview of analytical approaches

Thomas Koenig and Jiří Wackermann

## The general model

The aim of this chapter is to introduce a structured overview of the different possibilities available to display and analyze brain electric scalp potentials. First, a general formal model of time-varying distributed EEG potentials is introduced. Based on this model, the most common analysis strategies used in EEG research are introduced and discussed as specific cases of this general model. Both the general model and particular methods are also expressed in mathematical terms. It is however not necessary to understand these terms to understand the chapter.

The general model that we propose here is based on the statement made in Chapter 3, stating that the electric field produced by active neurons in the brain propagates in brain tissue without delay in time. Contrary to other imaging methods that are based on hemo-dynamic or metabolic processes, the EEG scalp potentials are thus "real-time," not delayed and not a-priori frequency-filtered measurements. If only a single dipolar source in the brain were active, the temporal dynamics of the activity of that source would be exactly reproduced by the temporal dynamics observed in the scalp potentials produced by that source. This is illustrated in Figure 5.1, where the expected EEG signal of a single source with spindle-like dynamics in time has been computed. The dynamics of the scalp potentials exactly reproduce the dynamics of the source. The amplitude of the measured potentials depends on the relation between the location and orientation of the active source, its strength and the electrode position. To translate the temporal dynamics of a given source to scalp potentials, one therefore merely has to apply a constant factor. Given the source configuration and the electrode positions, this factor can be computed, which is called the forward problem of the EEG[1,2]. For a series of sources and electrodes, the factors that are obtained when solving the forward problem are called lead-field.

Mathematically, this can be expressed as follows:

$$U_{t \times e} = s_{t \times 1} v_{1 \times e} \tag{1}$$

where $U$ is the time by channel matrix of measurements, $s$ is a column vector describing the dynamics of the neuronal activity across time, $v$ is a row vector describing the spatial distribution of the signal across the scalp, $e$ is the number of electrodes and $t$ is the number of time points. The resulting $U$ is a time by channel matrix of potentials that we would measure across time and electrodes.

In the case of several sources, the scalp field produced by two or more different dipolar sources is the sum of the scalp fields produced by these sources. Therefore, the temporal

*Electrical Neuroimaging*, ed. Christoph M. Michel, Thomas Koenig, Daniel Brandeis, Lorena R.R. Gianotti and Jiří Wackermann. Published by Cambridge University Press. © Cambridge University Press 2009.

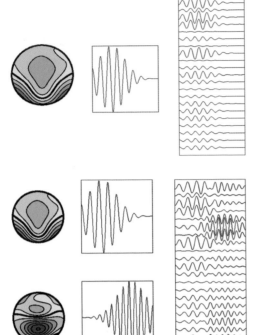

**Figure 5.1** The left graph shows the topography of a single process, the middle graph the temporal behavior of the process, and the right graph the EEG that would be recorded. All channels in the EEG show the same temporal behavior, but with different scaling.

**Figure 5.2** As in Figure 5.1, the left graph shows the maps of two processes, the middle graphs show the temporal behavior of the two processes, and the right graph the resulting multichannel EEG. The EEG at each channel is now a weighted mixture of both processes.

dynamics of the scalp potentials produced by these different sources also sum up. In other terms, assume that there are two sources and that the scalp field each source produces is known: to know the scalp field that is produced when both sources are simultaneously active, a weighted sum of the temporal dynamics of the two sources has to be computed for each scalp site, whereas the weights are given by the lead-field of the two sources (Figure 5.2).

In general, the EEG scalp potentials are thus weighted sums of the dynamics of some unknown number of intracerebral processes. Taking up the mathematical formulation above (Eqn 1), we now have:

$$U_{t \times e} = S_{t \times m} V_{m \times e} \qquad (2)$$

Where $S$ is now a matrix describing the dynamics of each neuronal activity across time, $m$ is the number of processes and $V$ is the lead-field matrix corresponding to each source configuration. The resulting $U$ is again a time by channel matrix of potentials that we would measure across time and electrodes.

This formulation has two important implications. First, the general model does not guarantee a unique solution, which implies that additional objectives may have to be introduced. Second, the formulation implies that there is no interaction of the spatial distribution of the source fields and the temporal dynamics of the sources. It is thus possible to discuss the spatial distribution and the temporal evolution of EEG data independently.

For the analysis of EEG data, one would typically aim to disentangle this mixture of signals in order to separate the different processes. In most studies, the unmixing of the data should be such that the results yield a comprehensive interpretation that should be supported by statistical inference. This means on one hand that the processes to be identified are physiologically plausible, limited to those that are relevant and that tend to be reproducible across the experiment. On the other hand, the dynamics of these processes should be expressed such that they contain, in a limited set of features, a maximal amount of relevant information, and suppress irrelevant information.

For example, when comparing EEG epochs that have been randomly selected during different sleep states, a Fast Fourier Transformation of the data is useful, because the results will not contain any latencies (that were random due to the arbitrary selection of the epoch onsets), but are maximally sensitive to changes in frequency distribution, where changes are expected. Furthermore, not necessarily all events visible in the data need to be accounted for, and a noise term for the unaccounted part of the data is introduced.

In our general model, for the analysis of EEG data, a limited set of possible temporal dynamics, and a limited set of scalp distributions are introduced. Each scalp distribution can potentially show any combination of the set of temporal dynamics. In mathematical terms, the proposed general model for the decomposition of EEG is shown in Eqn 3:

$$U_{t\times e} = D_{t\times w}C_{w\times n}V_{n\times e} + \varepsilon_{t\times e} \tag{3}$$

where

- $U$ is a two-dimensional, time by electrode matrix.

- $D$ is a set of signal patterns, i.e. functions of time. According to the usage in the literature, we will call $D$ the *dictionary*, and a single curve of the dictionary will be called a *word* of the dictionary. The dictionary is a two-dimensional, number of time points by number of words ($w$) matrix. The different words of the dictionary are by convention scaled to unit variance.

- $V$ is a set of spatial distributions, i.e. a set of voltage difference patterns on the scalp. We will call $V$ the *topographies*. The topographies are contained in a two-dimensional matrix with number of topographies ($n$) by number of ($e$). They can be displayed as topographic maps. As with the dictionary, the different topographies are by convention scaled to unit variance.

- The matrix $C$ is a set of *coefficients* that establish the relation between the dictionary and the topographies. If the topographies are defined such that they represent the spatial distribution of the processes that we are interested in, and if the dictionary is such that it represents the temporal dynamics of our interest, the coefficient matrix links these two. It indicates how much of each combination of words and topographies there is in the data. The coefficient matrix is thus quantitative, and is what is mostly used as a dependent variable in statistics. The coefficients matrix is a two-dimensional, number of words by number of topographies matrix.

- A *noise* term $\varepsilon$ may be used to account for variance that is not accounted for by the rest of the equation. Often, this noise term is minimized by some optimization of the other terms.

In the model described above, there is no interaction of spatial distribution and temporal dynamics. It is thus possible to construct a scheme of different EEG analysis methods displayed in a two-dimensional array, or "matrix." One dimension enumerates models of the temporal dynamics of the recorded potentials. The other dimension contains models for the spatial distribution of the potentials. Each of the different analysis methods is located in one cell of the matrix, depending on the specific model of spatial distribution it uses, and on the specific approach to describe the temporal dynamics of the data. Each analysis method is thus considered as a combination of specific spatial and temporal models of the data. In parts, this matrix has been proposed earlier[3].

The scheme allows the reader to make an appropriate choice of analysis strategies that fit the specific research questions. On the other hand, it allows researchers to schematize and eventually also predict the trends in the methodological developments of the field.

To illustrate the idea, let us assume we are interested in activity in the motor cortex associated with some simple movement. We have a rather precise hypothesis on the location and orientation of the sources based on our knowledge about the motor cortex. Furthermore, the literature tells us that we can expect task-related, transient EEG oscillations around the time the movement is performed. We have thus a rather precise idea in what form we want our data to be represented, both in terms of temporal dynamics (we expect transient oscillations) and in terms of spatial distribution (we want to measure the motor cortex).

In the above model, this implies specific choices of a dictionary and a set of topographies. In our present case, we would obviously choose a dictionary that is well suited to represent transient oscillations, which would be wavelets. The topographies should be chosen such that they are as specific for the motor cortex as possible; they could thus be constructed using a forward solution of sources in the motor cortex. Our analysis would thus investigate wavelet-like temporal behavior of topographies that are compatible with activity in the motor cortex.

## Temporal elements (model waveforms)

The choice of the dictionary determines the features that are used to describe the time-course of the data. The dictionary should be constructed such that all events of interest can be suitably represented by a combination of words; in mathematical terms, the dictionary has to be "complete." The fact that some dictionary is able to represent some temporal dynamics does however not imply that the assumptions contained in the dictionary actually hold for the data, because another dictionary containing other assumptions may explain the same dynamics equally well. The choice of a dictionary can therefore not only be based on a good fit between data and dictionary, although a poor fit is a good argument to question the choice of the dictionary. The choice of dictionary should be driven by a correspondence between the – assumed – properties of the temporal dynamics of the data, and the – well known – properties of the dictionary. For example, when analyzing event-related potentials, the typical assumption is that events in the brain stereotypically occur at a specific time before or after an observable event. The appropriate dictionary should therefore give precise information in time.

The number of currently used dictionaries is quite small. The most common dictionaries are briefly discussed below.

## Delta elements

The Delta dictionary consists of the most simple time functions, in the following called delta elements. A delta element is zero everywhere except at one time point at a given latency, $t_i$,

$$\delta_i(t) = \begin{cases} 1 & \text{for } t = t_i, \\ 0 & \text{otherwise} \end{cases} \tag{4}$$

**Figure 5.3** Example of a single delta element with a latency of 340 ms.

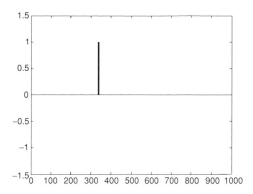

**Figure 5.4** A sinewave (right), obtained from a vector with length a (left) rotating constantly with 3 cycles (3 Hz) per second. The phase of the oscillation is determined by the phase-angle $\phi$. The left diagram is called a Nyquist diagram.

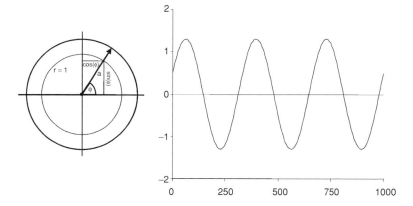

The complete dictionary consists of $n$ elements, $\delta_i (i = 0, \ldots, n − 1)$. Then, trivially, any observed time series can be expressed as a linear combination of delta elements,

$$u(t) = \sum_i u_i \delta_i(t) \tag{5}$$

An example of a delta element is shown in Figure 5.3. A delta element $\delta_i$ applied to a time series "picks up" exactly the value $u_i$ at the time coordinate $t_i$, and is "blind" to all other values. The representation of a signal in terms of delta elements thus preserves the time resolution (as determined by the sampling rate). On the other hand, the image of a delta element in the frequency domain (i.e. its Fourier spectrum – see below) is a constant function of frequency. Consequently, the representation of data via delta dictionary has no defined frequency resolution.

## Sinewave elements

A salient feature of EEG signals is their oscillatory character: the time series appear as "roughly" periodic functions of time. It is thus sensible to seek a representation of data in terms of strictly periodic time functions, in particular, trigonometric functions.

The outstanding role of trigonometric functions becomes evident from a geometric representation of the *harmonic motion*. Consider a vector of constant length $a$, rotating in a plane at a constant angular velocity (Figure 5.4), exerting one full rotation (angle $2\pi$) per time period $P$. The frequency of the motion is $f = 1/P$, which is sometimes convenient to express in angular units as so-called circular frequency, $\omega = 2\pi f$. The momentary angle $\phi$ at time instant $t$ is thus

$$\phi(t) = \omega t + \phi_0 \tag{6}$$

where $\phi_0 = \phi(0)$. A projection of the vector onto axis $x$ is then a periodic function of time,

$$x(t) = a \cos \phi(t) = a \cos (\omega t + \phi_0). \tag{7}$$

Similarly, a projection onto axis y is

$$y(t) = a \sin \phi(t) = a \sin (\omega t + \phi_0), \tag{8}$$

and, generally, parallel projections in any fixed direction can be expressed as a linear combination of the sine and cosine terms. A graphic representation of the harmonic motion is then a sinewave (Figure 5.4) with *amplitude a*, wave-number per time unit, or *frequency* $f = \omega/(2\pi)$, and *phase* $\phi_0$. Obviously, change of the phase results in a shift of the sinewave along the time axis and does not change the amplitude.

What makes the harmonic motion that important for mathematical representation of EEG signals? It is, firstly, the fact that harmonic motion is produced by (undamped) linear oscillators, that is, physical systems formally described by the differential equation

$$\frac{d^2 y}{dt^2} = -\omega^2 y \tag{9}$$

as, for instance, a swinging pendulum, a vibrating mass on a spring, or oscillations in electronic LC circuits. Secondly, there is an elaborated theory (going back to J.B.J. Fourier) concerning the representation of *any* periodic process as a linear combination of 'pure' harmonic components; symbolically,

$$u(t) = \sum_k a_k \cos(\omega_k t + \phi_k). \tag{10}$$

This is, essentially, the background idea of the representation of time series in terms of sinewave functions with discrete circular frequencies, $\phi_k = 2\pi k/N$, for $k = 0, 1, \ldots,$ $N - 1$, where $N$ is the number of data points in a given analysis epoch of duration $T = N/f_{\text{samp}}$. For each element, the amplitude $a_k$ and the phase $\phi_k$ corresponding to the circular frequency $\omega_k$ are uniquely determined (Fourier analysis). Conversely, given a complete set of amplitudes (Fourier coefficients) and phases, $\{(a_k, \phi_k)\}_{k=0, 1, \ldots, N-1}$, the corresponding time series $u(t0), \ldots, u(t_{N-1})$ can be reconstructed via Eqn 10 (Fourier synthesis).

In principle, the dictionary corresponds to the classical (discrete) Fourier transformation (FFT); it consists of oscillations at given discrete frequencies, $\omega_k$, extending over the entire analysis epoch $T$, and normalized to the sum of squares equal to unity. Trivially, a representation of a strictly periodic signal with frequency $f = \omega_k/(2\pi)$ has a single non-zero Fourier coefficient $a_k$, with all other coefficients equal to zero (single-line or "monochromatic" spectrum). Therefore the Fourier representation identifies uniquely signal components in terms of frequency, with no time resolution.

Where only contributions of singular frequency components are of interest, but the phase information is irrelevant, the Fourier representation can be reduced by computing power spectrum (squares of Fourier coefficients for single frequencies), or further by taking sums of squared amplitudes across a defined frequency band (band-specific power). Naturally, the sum of squared amplitudes over all frequencies is identical with the total power of the signal.

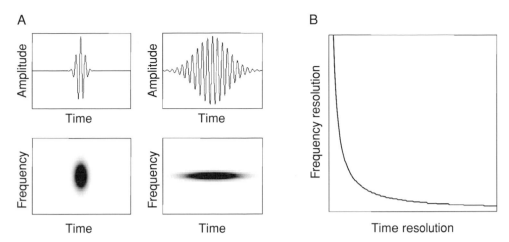

**Figure 5.5** Gabor functions and resolution in time and frequency. A. In the upper row, two Gabor functions constructed with the same frequency, but envelopes with different width. The lower rows shows at what frequencies and time points these Gabor functions would pick up signals. The left, shorter Gabor function has a better time resolution, while the right Gabor function has a better frequency resolution. The relation of time and frequency resolution is shown in (B).

These techniques are preferably employed where variations of frequency composition of the EEG over longer recordings are of interest, as for example in sleep research, studies of brain development, pharmaco-EEG and resting states.

## Wavelets and Gabor functions

The delta dictionary and Fourier dictionary are two extreme variants of possible signal representations in terms of time and frequency resolution: delta elements preserve the time resolution but provide no frequency domain information, while Fourier representation resolves data into frequency components but provides no localization in time. Consequently, their utility is restricted to special cases where either time or frequency information is of exclusive interest.

In studies of real brains operating in real-world conditions (in particular, cognitive functioning), both aspects of brain electrical activity are of importance. Variations of brain states in time are reflected by variations of spatio-temporal patterns of EEG oscillations, varying over time. For the sake of representation of time-varying, transient oscillatory activities, so-called wavelet dictionaries have been constructed, providing a compromise between time and frequency resolution. A wavelet is a pattern of temporal dynamics of limited temporal duration that can be shifted along the real-time axis (for temporal localization of transient events), and can be compressed or extended in time by a scaling factor. As a result, the amount of the signal represented by the wavelet can be visualized as a function of two variables, time offset and scaling factor, usually in the form of intensity-coded two-dimensional plots (See Figures 7.9 and 7.10)

Obviously, changing the time scale by factor $b$ corresponds to a change of frequency scale by factor $1/b$. A progressive scale change by factors $b = 2, 4, \ldots, 2n$, results in a rather rough frequency resolution. This is avoided by using dictionaries consisting of so-called Gabor functions, which provide an optimal compromise between uncertainty in time and frequency. Gabor functions are sinewave elements of freely defined frequency, modulated by a

Gaussian envelope; adjusting the envelope width properly, an optimal trade-off between time and frequency resolution can be obtained (Figure 5.5). The output of Gabor transformations can be further post-processed analogous to the Fourier transformation (see above), so that contributions of different frequencies or frequency bands can be traced as a function of time.

## Spatial elements (model topographies)

The choice of topographies determines how the spatial distribution of the data is described. Contrary to the choice of a dictionary, there are well-established, physics-based models of when and how intracerebral neuronal activity produces potential differences on the scalp and how these potential differences are distributed. These models are called *forward models*[1,2]. Forward models play a crucial role when it comes to arguing whether a chosen set of topographies is physically plausible or not. Topographies that are not compatible with brain electric activity in terms of physics can be identified and conclusions lacking a physical basis can be objectively rejected. Forward models, however, do not help to make a selection among different sets of topographies if all of these sets are in accordance with the forward model, and with the data.

As with dictionaries, the choice of a set of topographies cannot solely be based on a good fit between data and physically plausible topographies. The set of topographies has to meet some further – assumed – objectives. These objectives can either be of statistical nature[4–7], or such that they maximize the fit with some assumed properties of the intracerebral distribution of neural activity[8,9]. The usefulness of these objectives is then up to debate, and can eventually be validated based on external evidence.

## Single channels

In our formalism (Eqn 3), the channel by channel analysis corresponds to representation of EEG data by means of "singular distribution maps," that is, topographies which have the value 1 at the given electrode position, and zero everywhere else. These topographies are thus spatial analogs of delta elements in a time domain. Physically, such maps are not plausible; even a point source in the brain creates a spatially distributed field that extends over the entire scalp. In general, multiple sources may affect the same electrode so that potentials recorded at that electrode are superpositions of potentials generated by different processes at different intracerebral locations. The often-made assumption that voltage differences at a scalp site indicate differences in activity of the underlying brain tissue lacks a physiological rationale and implies a source model that is not validated and false in the general case. Single-channel analyses may serve to describe global phenomena, but are generally unsuited for conclusions in brain-space unless there is good evidence that the analysis isolates only the processes of interest (i.e. by measuring specific ERP components).

Technically, the signal recorded at one electrode is always the potential difference between the location of the electrode and the location of the reference electrode. The recorded signal thus depends not only on the location of the electrode, as intended, but also on the position of the reference electrode. This is usually undesired and often neglected.

## Spatial factor analysis (PCA, ICA, PLS)

The common idea of spatial factor analyses is to produce so-called *factors* that are constituted as a weighted sum of the recorded channels. The weighted sum of electrode potentials for some factor is called the *factor load* or *factor score*, and usually varies with time. In Eqn 3, the weights used to compute the factor scores correspond to the topographies.

The search for the factors aims at the best possible fit of a given data-set, that is, at a minimal residual that is not accounted by the model. Additional criteria such as maximal correlation with an external variable or higher-order independence of factor loads can be optionally applied.

The simplest and most commonly used variant of spatial factor analyses is the *principal component analysis* (PCA)[4,10,11]. The PCA solution has the special property that the first factor accounts for the maximum possible amount of data variance, and each next factor (the 2nd, 3rd, etc.) accounts for the maximum possible residual (i.e. not yet represented) variance. The factors identified by the PCA are always orthogonal, and the time series of factor scores are statistically uncorrelated. The number of factors identified by the PCA is lower than or equal to the number of EEG channels; factors contributing little to the explained variance may be neglected, which usually leads to a considerable dimension reduction. The PCA is useful to identify the main source of variance (the first principal component). Furthermore, the form of the variance distribution across the PCA factors provides information about spatial complexity of the data. (For details, see Chapter 9.)

The PCA can be seen as a special instance of signal de-correlation, that is, the cross-correlations between activities corresponding to separate factors are minimized (in the case of the PCA, in fact cancelled). Cross-correlation, however, is just a linear measure of interdependence between signals; there may still be higher-order relations, for example, quadratic relations. The method to remove these higher-order relations is called *independent component analysis* (ICA)[7]. The objective of the ICA is sometimes illustrated by the so-called "cocktail party problem," where the task is to decompose a sound recording from a party into contributions of individuals, talking independently of each other. As with the PCA, the ICA produces a weight coefficient for each factor and channel. The number of factors that the ICA extracts is lower than or equal to the number of channels in the data.

The ICA can be very useful if there are good reasons to assume that the biological nature of a factor is such that this factor is likely to be independent from the remaining part of the data. Good examples for such factors are artifacts such as eye-blinks[12], or interictal spikes[13,14]. The possibility of decomposing an EEG into a number of statistically independent factors does not, however, necessarily imply that there are indeed a similar number of independent processes in the brain.

Details for the computation of spatial EEG factors have been given elsewhere and software for these analyses is available[15]. One important issue to be considered when computing factor analyses is that one should avoid introducing dependencies into the data that contradict the objectives of the factor analysis. Such interdependencies are introduced, for example, by interpolating a channel by the surrounding channels, or by computing the average reference. This problem can be avoided by applying the factor analysis before additional interdependencies are introduced, or by reducing the number of factors to be identified.

Apart from analyses that optimize factors for minimal interdependence, there are methods that attempt to maximize the relation of a factor to be identified with some external variables. These variables often represent the experimental conditions[16]. This approach has been called partial least square (PLS) and is mentioned here for completeness; it will be discussed more thoroughly in Chapter 8, on statistics. As with PCA and ICA, the factor loads obtained by PLS are weighted sums of all channels. If more than one external variable is used, the resulting factors are uncorrelated in time and space.

## Spatial clusters

In the previous section, the analogy of the "cocktail party problem" was introduced, with all speakers talking independently. The problem solved by the ICA is the identification of each speaker. Let us now introduce a similar analogy pointing to another decomposition of multichannel scalp field data. Assume that all speakers of the party do not talk independently from each other, but interact in a very simple way, where only one speaker talks at the time and the others remain silent.

In Eqn (3), this implies that each word of the dictionary is assigned to a single topography, the coefficient matrix $C$ is such that in each row, all but one element are zero. In other words, we require the matrix $C$ to be sparse[17]. In the case of a delta-function dictionary, where each word of the dictionary corresponds to one moment in time, such a model allows only a single topography to occur at each moment in time.

Mathematically, one has to identify a set of topographies that explain a maximum amount of the variance of the data based on the given dictionary, under the constraint that each word of the dictionary is assigned to only one of these topographies. This problem is typically solved by cluster analysis, where each element of the data is assigned exclusively to one cluster. For the analysis of EEG and ERP data, existing clustering algorithms have been adapted[18]. A question that is of considerable importance when applying cluster analyses is how many clusters shall be identified. Spatial clusters in time and time-frequency-domain EEG and evoked potential data are covered by Chapters 6 and 7.

## Topographic component recognition (spatial filters)

Factor analysis and spatial clusters optimize the goodness of fit of the factors with the given data. One may also employ spatial factors obtained by other means, i.e. by an association to a stimulus condition or to another known event. The factor score obtained with such factors can then be taken as a measure for the presence of brain states resembling those associated with the condition or event of interest. This approach has been called topographic component recognition (TCR)[19] and can be considered as a spatial filter.

For example, in an experimental paradigm called N400, a violation of the subject's semantic expectancies produces a typical ERP effect around 400 ms after the stimulus called N400. A known N400 topography can thus be used as a topographic model of semantic violation in a new dataset: the more the spatial distribution of the data resembles the N400 topography, the more the brain-state associated with those data resembles a brain-state related to semantic violation. Within a given time window, one can thus construct a biological marker of semantic violation. This marker can then be quantified in various ways, e.g. by total amplitude or peak latency.

## Distributed inverse solutions

Information processing in the brain is spatially structured, and different brain functions are often localized in different regions. It is obviously interesting to search for topographies that preferably represent the activity from spatially delimited regions. This non-trivial problem is discussed in Chapter 3. Distributed inverse solutions are mentioned here because they typically contain a matrix of topographies that weight the data such that an estimate of activity at some voxel in the brain is obtained. In Eqn 3, the application of distributed inverse solutions corresponds to using a set of topographies that are constructed a priori based on a combination of physical and physiological models[20].

# Common properties of dictionaries and topographies

Dictionaries and sets of topographies can be formally studied and discussed in their general aspects, that is, their suitability to represent observed data. Therefore, we refer in the following to dictionaries and sets of topographies as "representation bases." It is desirable that data of interest can be mathematically expressed as linear combinations of the elements of the representation basis of our choice; i.e. signals can be constructed by superposition of time functions (words of a dictionary), and field distributions can be constructed by superposition of basis topographies. In this sense we speak of *completeness* of a given representation basis. A basis is complete if any dataset can be represented with respect to the basis with no residual error.

A complementary term to completeness is that of *uniqueness*. Theoretically, an "abundantly rich" representation basis may be suitable for representation of the same observed data by different combinations of different elements. To avoid ambiguity in data representation – and, consequently, in their interpretation – it is necessary that any dataset can be represented in only one way, thus yielding a unique set of coefficients with respect to the elements of a given basis.

Finally, we aim at a representation of data that is as efficient or "economical" as possible, that is, we wish the representation basis to consist of "no more elements than necessary." This rather fuzzy expression reflects an important aspect of data representation, namely, the trade-off between the size of the basis on the one hand, and the residual error on the other hand. Experience shows that a representation basis may not be capable of complete coverage of all observable datasets with zero residual, but does so with an acceptable error. To formalize this intuitive notion, we usually express the difference between the representable and the represented data by the residual variance relative to the total data variance. In this sense we may distinguish "incomplete" bases with non-zero but tolerable residual from "complete" bases sensu stricto. (Bases allowing for zero-residual, non-unique representations are sometimes referred to as "overcomplete." In such a case, additional objectives are needed to obtain a unique solution.)

An often discussed feature of representation bases is *orthogonality*. Orthogonality is a pair-wise relation: two elements, $e_1$ and $e_2$, of the basis are said to be orthogonal if representations of a dataset with respect to these elements are independent. In other words, eliminating the part of the data that is represented by $e_1$ does not affect the representation of the data by $e_2$, and vice versa. If all elements of a basis are mutually orthogonal, the basis itself is said to be orthogonal. (This intuitive definition should be sufficient for the purpose of the present chapter, as a rigorous definition of orthogonality would require a more advanced mathematical formalism.)

This property gives orthogonal bases their outstanding place among all other bases: since partial representations are independent, the total variance of an observed dataset can be uniquely represented (up to a minimal residual) as a sum of independent contributions of individual basis elements. If the dataset is reconstructed with zero error (complete basis), and the elements are normalized to unit variance, the variance of the representation is equal to the variance of the original data (Parseval's theorem). Typical examples of orthogonal representation bases are Fourier dictionaries in the time domain, and spatial principal

**Table 5.1** Scheme of the different EEG/ERP analysis methods, seen as combinations of specific spatial and temporal elements. Temporal elements are organized column-wise, spatial elements row-wise.

| | Delta elements | Sinewave elements | Wavelets and Gabor functions |
|---|---|---|---|
| Single channels | Single channel time-domain analysis: Peak amplitudes and latencies | Mapping of amplitude: power maps Analysis of phase: coherence | Single channel wavelet analysis, matching pursuit Event-related synchronization and desynchronization |
| Spatial factor analysis PCA, ICA, PLS | Spatial PCA, ICA Global descriptors | FFT approximation Global field synchronization | Wavelet synchronization |
| Spatial clusters | Microstate analysis | Identification of frequency bands based on topographies | Topographic time-frequency analysis |
| Topographic component recognition | ERP component recognition | | |
| Distributed inverse solutions | Time-domain distributed inverse solutions | Frequency-domain distributed inverse solutions | Time-frequency domain distributed inverse solutions |

components in the space domain. Orthogonal bases are thus always unique, but unique bases are not necessarily orthogonal.

The disadvantage of orthogonal bases is that the form of one element of the dictionary imposes constraints to the form of all subsequent elements of the dictionary. While these constraints are mathematically meaningful, they have no physiological significance. Consequently, many orthogonal bases applicable in mathematical physics find only limited or no use in representation of physiological data.

## Combinatorics of data-analytical approaches
Given the different possible spatial and temporal elements, we can now proceed to construct a scheme of all possible combinations (Table 5.1). The following is a brief review of the methods fitting the scheme, and discussion of their specific virtues and drawbacks.

## Single channel maps and delta-element dictionaries (waveshape analysis)
This combination is mentioned only for the sake of completeness. Obviously, this "representation" is identical to the original EEG data. Due to the limitations of the single channel representation discussed above, an unambiguous separation of processes occurring at different sites is often impossible. Furthermore, results obtained with single channels usually depend on the choice of the reference.

# Single channel maps and sinusoidal dictionaries (power maps and coherence)

Fourier analysis (FFT) carried out separately for each channel results in a set of amplitude coefficients and phases. These are usually summarized in the form of amplitude or power spectra. Extracting the power for a definite frequency (or frequency band) across channels, so-called power maps can be constructed.

FFT power mapping has become the standard analysis of continuous EEG without external events, where the analysis epochs are typically selected randomly in time. It has produced an abundant body of literature in research on development[21,22], neurology and psychiatry[23], sleep[24] and pharmacology[25,26]. To analyze data that have been randomly selected in time, the fact that a sinusoid dictionary has no resolution in time is convenient; the elements of the data are grouped by their frequency of oscillation, and not by the time they occur in the data. Since power maps are based on absolute values, they contain no polarity information, which limits the applicability of inverse solutions. Frequency domain inverse solutions typically take into account amplitude and phase of the data, and are not based on amplitude or power alone (see Chapter 3).

Whereas the traditional FFT spectral analysis focuses on amplitude or power, the phase component of the FFT result also contains useful and physiologically meaningful information. The stability of the phase relation between two time series is usually measured by coherence, which quantifies the relative common variance between the two channels separately for each frequency. High coherence between two signals at a given frequency may indicate a coupling between the activities at the two electrodes at that frequency. The fully carried-out frequency analysis yields coherence, on the one hand, and relative phase, on the other hand, as functions of frequency.

Coherence between two channels may be observed when there is functional coupling of two processes, or when a single process affects both channels simultaneously due to volume conduction or reference effects. This is a non-trivial, but insufficiently addressed issue in EEG research. As with single channel time-domain analysis, single channel frequency domain analysis is reference dependent.

# Single channel maps and wavelets

Wavelet analysis of EEG and ERP data has become increasingly popular, because it operationalizes the concept of transient oscillations that are assumingly associated with neurocognitive processes. By computing wavelet transformations in the single trials of evoked potential data and averaging the envelopes of the wavelets, it becomes possible to identify oscillatory events that occur before or after a stimulus, but that have a certain jitter in time, which leads to cancellation when the trials are averaged. The cancellation of signals by averaging becomes stronger the higher the frequency of the oscillations and the higher the jitter in time. Since the jitter in time probably increases with post-stimulus time, the frequency of events in typical ERPs decreases with post-stimulus latency. This can be avoided by using wavelet analysis and averaging of wavelet envelopes. The usage of the wavelet envelopes implies similar limitations as using the amplitude or power in frequency analysis: the polarity information of the data is lost, which limits the applicability of inverse solutions; and the results are reference dependent.

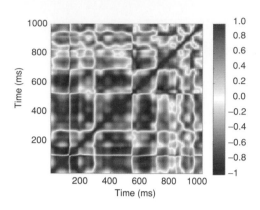

**Figure 5.6** Spatial correlation matrix of a multichannel single word evoked potential. There are prolonged periods during which all topographies are highly correlated, i.e. have assumingly similar active generators.

## Spatial factors and delta-function dictionaries

There is a line of research that has used spatial principal components[4,5,10] and independent components to isolate physiologically meaningful components from EEG and ERP data. This works well if there are good reasons to assume that the components of interest are uncorrelated or independent from the remaining part of the data, but this is often difficult to argue. Spatial principal components in time-domain EEG data have also been used to quantify the distribution of variance of EEG data, leading to a measure of spatial synchronization and complexity that is called Omega complexity (see Chapter 9).

## Spatial factors and sinusoidal dictionaries

As in time-domain EEG data, spatial principal components can also be used in frequency-domain EEG data to study spatial synchronization and complexity. Since in frequency-domain EEG data, the variance at each frequency is fully determined by the sine and cosine parts of the signals, there are only two spatial principal components per frequency bin. While the first principal component can be used to obtain the principal distribution of variance, the distribution of variance across the two factors is again an index of synchronization. It is called Global Field Synchronization (GFS) and is discussed in more detail in Chapter 7.

## Spatial factors and wavelets

If complex Gabor functions have been used to decompose an EEG, the result contains for each frequency and time window a sine and a cosine part. As in frequency-domain analysis it is then possible to compute GFS in time and frequency, yielding an index of global synchronization of brain processes as a function of time and frequency.

## Spatial clusters and delta functions (microstates)

When analyzing the change of topography with time in EEG and ERP data, it becomes apparent that these changes are not continuous across time, but that there are extended periods during which there is little change, often separated by brief periods of transition. This is well illustrated by the matrix of spatial correlation (Chapter 6) between all time points of a dataset that usually shows a sequence of delimited time periods during which all maps are highly correlated (Figure 5.6).

During periods where all maps are highly correlated, the brain field topography of the data has thus barely changed and there is little evidence for a change of generators in these time periods, which suggests that the functional state of the brain has remained stable. The data thus indicate that there is a sequence of states, each state lasting for some period, and not overlapping in time with the other states.

Such a dynamic is well captured by cluster analyses, where each element (in the present case each moment in time) is assigned exclusively to one cluster. Each cluster identified represents the ensemble of generators that have been simultaneously active during the time periods when the cluster has been observed.

The periods of stable topography identified by some criterion of map similarity have been called microstates. In ERP data, they have become useful to identify the latencies of spatially defined components associated with specific steps of information processing. A detailed account of microstate analysis is given in Chapter 6.

## Spatial clusters and sinusoidal dictionaries

Taking power maps as signatures for some set of generators oscillating at specific frequencies, one can begin to cluster power maps across frequency according to their similarity, yielding a data-driven identification of frequency bands. Although this argument is reasonable, it has rarely been employed[27].

## Spatial clusters and wavelets

When multichannel EEG and ERP data are decomposed using wavelets, each oscillation in the data is accounted for by one or more wavelets that overlap in time and frequency. If several wavelets account for the same events (i.e. for the same generators), they must have had the same spatial distribution across electrodes. Wavelets that account for the same processes can therefore again be identified using spatial clusters: wavelets that are assigned to the same cluster represent the same or a similar process in the brain. Although the methodology to apply spatial clustering to wavelet transformed data is available[28,29], it has rarely been applied systematically.

## Topographic component recognition and delta functions

Topographic component recognition (TCR) in time domain is often used in combination with time domain spatial cluster analysis. The topographies identified by the cluster algorithm are used as templates in the individual ERPs, such that individual microstate on- and offset latencies can be assessed and statistically compared. The TCR methodology will therefore be discussed further in combination with microstate analysis in Chapter 6.

## Distributed inverse solutions in time and frequency

For the issue of inverse solutions in time and frequency, we refer to Chapter 3.

## Conclusions

A specific choice of method determines what features of the data will be available, within which conceptual framework the results are represented, and which assumptions implied by the chosen method must be critically discussed. The two-dimensional scheme of analysis methods presented here allows the discussion of assumptions made about the temporal dynamics separately from those made about the spatial distribution of the data.

From a historical perspective, it becomes apparent that there is a trend from mathematically simple a-priori dictionaries and topographies towards more complicated dictionaries and topographies that are based on sometimes elaborate statistical or physical models.

# References

1. Fuchs M, Wagner M, Kastner J. Boundary element method volume conductor models for EEG source reconstruction. *Clinical Neurophysiology* 2001;**112**:1400–1407.

2. Mosher JC, Leahy RM, Lewis PS. EEG and MEG: forward solutions for inverse methods. *IEEE Transactions on Biomedical Engineering* 1999;**46**:245–259.

3. Koenig T, Hubl D, Mueller TJ. Decomposing the EEG in time, space and frequency: a formal model, existing methods, and new proposals. In Hirata K, ed. *International Congress Series 318 1232.* Amsterdam: Elsevier; 2002, pp. 317–321.

4. John ER, Easton P, Prichep LS, Friedman J. Standardized varimax descriptors of event related potentials: basic considerations. *Brain Topography* 1993;**6**:143–162.

5. John ER, Prichep LS, Easton P. Standardized varimax descriptors of event related potentials: evaluation of psychiatric patients. *Psychiatry Research* 1994;**55**:13–40.

6. Makeig S, Debener S, Onton J, Delorme A. Mining event-related brain dynamics. *Trends in Cognitive Science* 2004;**8**:204–210.

7. Makeig S, Jung TP, Bell AJ, Ghahremani D, Sejnowski TJ. Blind separation of auditory event-related brain responses into independent components. *Proceedings of the National Academy of Sciences USA* 1997;**94**: 10979–10984.

8. Ilmoniemi RJ. Models of source currents in the brain. *Brain Topography* 1993;**5**: 331–336.

9. Pascual-Marqui RD, Michel CM, Lehmann D. Low resolution electromagnetic tomography: a new method for localizing electrical activity in the brain. *International Journal of Psychophysiology* 1994;**18**:49–65.

10. Kayser J, Tenke CE. Trusting in or breaking with convention: towards a renaissance of principal components analysis in electrophysiology. *Clinical Neurophysiology* 2005;**116**:1747–1753.

11. Wackermann J. Beyond mapping: estimating complexity of multichannel EEG recordings. *Acta Neurobiologiae Experimentalis (Warszawa)*. 1996;**56**: 197–208.

12. Jung TP, Makeig S, Humphries C *et al.* Removing electroencephalographic artifacts by blind source separation. *Psychophysiology* 2000;**37**:163–178.

13. Kobayashi K, James CJ, Nakahori T, Akiyama T, Gotman J. Isolation of epileptiform discharges from unaveraged EEG by independent component analysis. *Clinical Neurophysiology* 1999;**110**: 1755–1763.

14. Urrestarazu E, Iriarte J, Artieda J *et al.* Independent component analysis separates spikes of different origin in the EEG. *Journal of Clinical Neurophysiology* 2006;**23**:72–78.

15. Delorme A, Makeig S. EEGLAB: an open source toolbox for analysis of single-trial EEG dynamics including independent component analysis. *Journal of Neuroscience Methods* 2004;**134**:9–21.

16. Lobaugh NJ, West R, McIntosh AR. Spatiotemporal analysis of experimental differences in event-related potential data with partial least squares. *Psychophysiology* 2001;**38**:517–530.

17. Koenig T, Studer D, Hubl D, Melie L, Strik WK. Brain connectivity at different time-scales measured with EEG. *Philosophical Transactions of the Royal Society London Series B Biological Sciences* 2005;**360**:1015–1023.

18. Pascual-Marqui RD, Michel CM, Lehmann D. Segmentation of brain electrical activity into microstates: model estimation and validation. *IEEE Transactions on Biomedical Engineering* 1995;**42**:658–665.

19. Brandeis D, Naylor H, Halliday R, Callaway E, Yano L. Scopolamine effects on visual information processing, attention, and event-related potential map latencies. *Psychophysiology* 1992;**29**:315–336.

20. Scherg M, Ille N, Bornfleth H, Berg P. Advanced tools for digital EEG review: virtual source montages, whole-head mapping, correlation, and phase analysis. *Journal of Clinical Neurophysiology* 2002;**19**: 91–112.

21. John ER, Ahn H, Prichep L *et al.* Developmental equations for the electroencephalogram. *Science* 1980;**210**:1255–1258.

22. John ER, Prichep LS, Fridman J, Easton P. Neurometrics: computer-assisted

differential diagnosis of brain dysfunctions. *Science* 1988;**239**:162–169.

23. Hughes JR, John ER. Conventional and quantitative electroencephalography in psychiatry. *Journal of Neuropsychiatry and Clinical Neuroscience* 1999;**11**:190–208.

24. Borbely AA, Achermann P. Sleep homeostasis and models of sleep regulation. *Journal of Biological Rhythms* 1999;**14**:557–568.

25. Herrmann WM. Development and critical evaluation of an objective for the electroencephalographic classification of psychotropic drugs. In Herrmann WM, ed. *Electroencephalography in Drug Research*. Stuttgart: Gustav Fisher; 1982, pp. 249–351.

26. Saletu B, Kufferle B, Grunberger J *et al.* Clinical, EEG mapping and psychometric studies in negative schizophrenia: comparative trials with amisulpride and fluphenazine. *Neuropsychobiology* 1994;**29**:125–135.

27. Finelli LA, Achermann P, Borbely AA. Individual 'fingerprints' in human sleep EEG topography. *Neuropsychopharmacology* 2001;**25**:S57–S62.

28. Koenig T, Marti-Lopez F, Valdes-Sosa P. Topographic time-frequency decomposition of the EEG. *Neuroimage* 2001;**14**:383–390.

29. Studer D, Hoffmann U, Koenig T. From EEG dependency multichannel matching pursuit to sparse topographic EEG decomposition. *Journal of Neuroscience Methods* 2006;**153**:261–275.

# Chapter 6

# Electrical neuroimaging in the time domain

Christoph M. Michel, Thomas Koenig and Daniel Brandeis

## Spatial analysis of the spontaneous EEG
### Resting state and neurocognitive networks

A publication entitled "A default mode of brain function"[1] initiated a new way of looking at functional imaging data. In this PET study the authors discussed the often-observed consistent *decrease* of brain activation in a variety of tasks as compared with the baseline. They suggested that this deactivation is due to a task-induced suspension of a default mode of brain function that is active during rest, i.e. that there exists intrinsic well-organized brain activity during rest in several distinct brain regions. This suggestion led to a large number of imaging studies on the resting state of the brain and to the conclusion that the study of this intrinsic activity is crucial for understanding how the brain works[2,3].

The fact that the brain is active during rest has been well known from a variety of EEG recordings for a very long time. Different states of the brain in the sleep–wake continuum are characterized by typical patterns of spontaneous oscillations in different frequency ranges and in different brain regions[4]. Best studied are the evolving states during the different sleep stages, but characteristic EEG oscillation patterns have also been well described during awake periods (see Chapter 1 for details). A highly recommended comprehensive review on the brain's default state defined by oscillatory electrical brain activities is provided in the recent book by György Buzsaki[5], showing how these states can be measured by electrophysiological procedures at the global brain level as well as at the local cellular level. Helmut Laufs and colleagues performed several excellent studies where these oscillations in the spontaneous EEG were correlated with the hemodynamic response function measured with fMRI[6–8]. This was made possible by systems that allow the recording of the EEG within the scanner and sophisticated algorithms that permit the elimination of the gradient and pulse artifact (see Chapter 10 for details). By using such a method Laufs and colleagues[7,8] showed that the intrinsic default mode networks described by Raichle and others were correlated with EEG power in different frequency bands. Thereby the different EEG frequencies correlated with distinct distributed patterns of fMRI activity that have characteristic response properties. In conclusion the EEG seems to be able to measure these resting states as well as the other imaging procedures, or even better because of the higher temporal resolution that allows the examination of the short-lasting fluctuations of these resting states.

It is clear that the brain is never at rest and that spontaneous mental activities continuously take place, even if they are not all consciously recalled. These spontaneous cognitive

*Electrical Neuroimaging*, ed. Christoph M. Michel, Thomas Koenig, Daniel Brandeis, Lorena R.R. Gianotti and Jiří Wackermann. Published by Cambridge University Press. © Cambridge University Press 2009.

activities or daydreams might at least partially represent the observed resting state activities in the functional imaging studies. It has been repeatedly demonstrated that complex mental activities are mediated by large-scale networks linking groups of neurons in separate cortical areas into functional entities[9-11]. It is reasonable to assume that these large-scale neuronal networks are not only active during effortful and attentive tasks, but also during spontaneous mental activities, i.e. stimulus-independent conscious thoughts. These large-scale neuronal networks might correspond to the neuronal workspace which is assumed to consist of a distributed set of cortical neurons, which physically integrate the multiple individual local processing neurons and form a discrete spatio-temporal pattern of activity[12-16]. These authors proposed that this neuronal workspace is the basic representation of conscious mental activities.

However, these large-scale neurocognitive networks have to flexibly and rapidly change depending on the momentary cognitive thought[9]. It is therefore required that they reorganize in different spatial patterns of coordination on a sub-second time scale[17]. Such sub-second changes of network functions cannot be studied with hemodynamic or metabolic functional imaging methods that work in the range of seconds or more, and are not captured by conventional EEG frequency power analysis that integrates the activity over seconds. Much better suited is the spatial analysis of the multichannel EEG because it measures the activity of large-scale neuronal networks at any moment in time with millisecond resolution.

The temporal coordination and the organization of these large-scale neuronal networks that have to grant both stability and plasticity have been widely discussed[18]. The main point of debate is whether cognitive processing occurs through a stream of discrete units or epochs or whether it is characterized as a continuous flow of neuronal activity[19]. There are many arguments that speak in favor of the proposal that neurocognitive networks rather evolve through a sequence of quasi-stable coordination states (for a discussion see Bressler & Tognali[17]). In the neuronal workspace model discussed above, it is proposed that episodes of coherent activity last a certain amount of time and are separated by sharp transitions. Only one such workspace representation is active at any given time[13,15]. This model adequately fits the observation of functional microstates of the brain that we will explain in the following section (discussed in Changeux & Michel[20]).

## Functional microstates of the brain

A striking observation when looking at a time series of scalp potential maps of the spontaneous EEG is that the topography of the map configuration does not randomly and continuously change as time elapses. The topography of the electric field and thus the configuration of the potential map remains stable for a certain length of time and then very abruptly changes into a new configuration in which it remains stable again (Figure 6.1). There is no continuous smooth transition from one landscape to the other but there are discrete segments of electrical stability separated by sharp transitions. Within a given period of stable configuration, the strength of the field increases and decreases, but the topography remains stable. This very fundamental observation was first described by Dietrich Lehmann and colleagues[21]. They proposed that these periods of stable electric field configurations reflect particular "steps" or "contents" of information processing, that is, they are the basic building blocks of the content of consciousness: "atoms of thoughts"[22,23] and gave them the name *functional microstates*. Thus, the functional microstates, expressed as periods of stable scalp electrical potential topographies, may be viewed as neural implementations of the elementary building blocks of consciousness content.

**Figure 6.1**
Demonstration of the stability of map topographies over time in the spontaneous EEG. Top: 42-channel spontaneous eyes-closed EEG of 12 s duration. Middle: Succession of maps over the 12 s. Only maps at GFP peaks are shown (i.e. about every 40–50 ms). The positions of the positive and negative maximum are connected. Bottom: Only the maxima positions are shown and connected, illustrating the periods of stability of these positions and thus stable map topographies. These periods are surrounded by boxes and marked in gray. Note the different durations and the fast transitions.

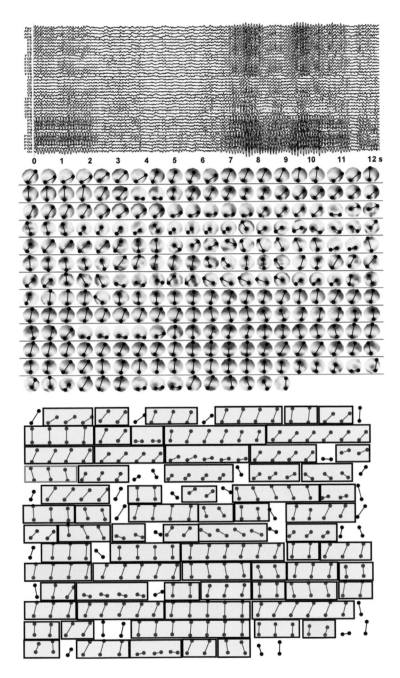

In other words, the functional microstates are viewed as the electrophysiological correlates of a process of global "conscious" integration at the brain-scale level discussed above (for detailed discussions see Baars[13], Fingelkurts[19], Changeux & Michel[20] and John[24]). A support for this hypothesis was given in a study where subjects were asked to recall spontaneous, conscious experiences after the presentation of a prompt signal[25]. The reports of the

113

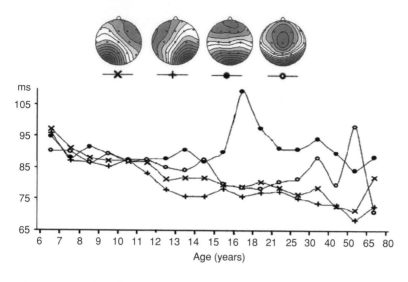

**Figure 6.2**
Microstate analysis of the spontaneous EEG of 496 subjects in different age range. The maps of the four dominant microstates are illustrated on top, and for each of them the duration across age is shown. The mean duration of the microstates is around 80–100 ms. One microstate dominates in duration during adolescence. From König et al.[26] with permission.

subjects were classified into imagery and abstract thoughts and it was shown that these two classes of thoughts differed significantly in the topography of the microstates just preceding the prompt, suggesting that the microstates reflect the momentary mental activity well.

The functional microstates of the spontaneous EEG last around 100 ms. A comprehensive analysis of close to 500 subjects between the age of 6 and 80 years revealed that the mean microstate duration is around 80–150 ms[26], confirming earlier studies with a smaller number of subjects[25,27]. The duration is somewhat longer in children but stabilizes in adulthood[26] (see Figure 6.2). This duration of around 100 ms again makes them good candidates for the electrophysiological manifestation of these global episodes of conscious experience. It agrees with the observation that sequentially presented stimuli are not perceived as separate when they follow each other within less than 80 ms[28], and that a stimulus can be successfully masked by another stimulus when presented with a latency of less than 100 ms[29,30].

The topographies of the functional microstates are strikingly simple and similar across different studies. Only 4–8 classes of distinct topographies are needed to explain most of the data[27,31].

Numerous studies examined the structure of functional microstates in the spontaneous EEG and their influence by age, drugs, pathologies or specific mental conditions. The parameters that were studied were the number of microstates, the duration of microstates and the syntax, i.e. the rules of succession of microstates over time. Patients with schizophrenia showed a reduced number and a shortening of some classes of microstates[32–34], that reversed with medication[35]. Depressed patients showed reduced duration and also increased repetition of microstates[36]. The EEG of Alzheimer patients was characterized by decreased duration and increased number of microstates with additional maps with frontal maxima[37,38]. In healthy subjects, sulpiride, an antipsychotic drug, increased microstate duration, while diazepam, a sedative and anxiolytic drug, changed the topography of the microstates[39]. Katayama et al.[40] demonstrated decreased duration of some microstate classes and increased duration of others during deep hypnosis.

Most interesting is a recent study by Lehmann et al.[41] showing disturbed syntax of the microstate succession in first-episode, medication-naïve schizophrenic patients. It is intriguing to propose that the syntax of microstates is crucial to come up with a meaningful and coherent "mental plot." If each microstate represents a certain information-processing step, the sequence, i.e. syntax, of these steps defines the appropriateness of the whole mental process, just as a correct sequence of words is needed to build a proper sentence and several correct sentences to build an understandable story. The study of the syntax of spontaneous functional microstates is in our opinion a most promising tool for understanding human thinking.

## Methods used to analyze microstates of the spontaneous EEG

Different methods have been used in the past to define the temporal sequence of microstates of the spontaneous EEG map series. Most of the studies in the 1990s used the map descriptors defined in Chapter 2 to describe the topography of each momentary map, i.e. the location of the negative and positive extreme or the location of the negative and positive centroid in the two- or three-dimensional electrode space. The trajectory of these map descriptors over time were then inspected. By defining certain spatial windows around the descriptors, moments where one of them significantly changed position could be detected and defined as a window border[27,31,42].

Pascual-Marqui and colleagues[43] proposed a statistical approach that is based on the calculation of the global map dissimilarity, i.e. the spatial correlation between maps (see Chapter 2). This parameter was used for performing a cluster-analysis that groups together maps with high spatial correlation and determines for each number of clusters the most representative topographies that best explain the variance in the data. A modified K-means cluster analysis was proposed that includes in a nested iterative way the following steps (see also[44] for detailed explanations).

First, it randomly selects a predefined number of maps from the data as initial prototype maps. Each of these prototype maps is then compared with all the original maps and each time point is labeled as belonging to that prototype map it best correlated with (see the paragraph on spatial correlation in Chapter 2). All maps that were labeled with the same prototype map are then averaged together and form a new (synthetic) prototype map. A global measure of quality of these prototype maps is determined by calculating the global explained variance (GEV). The GEV is the sum of the explained variances (squared spatial correlation) weighted by the global field power at each moment in time. The new synthetic prototype maps are then fitted again to the original data and the map series is relabeled. New average maps are then determined and the GEV is calculated again. The relabeling is repeated until the GEV converges to a limit. Once this is reached, the whole process is repeated with newly selected maps from the data. Out of several hundreds of repetitions, the prototype maps with maximal GEV are kept. Finally, the procedure is redone with increasing numbers of prototype maps. This iterative procedure is illustrated in Figure 6.3. The last question concerns the number of prototype maps that best explain the data. In Pascual-Marqui *et al.*[43] a cross-validation criteria was proposed that optimizes between GEV and the degrees of freedom. Other criteria for determining the optimal number of clusters can be used (for example the Krzanowski and Lai criterion introduced in Murray *et al.*[44]).

Several alternative cluster analysis methods are possible to determine the most dominant spatial components in map series, such as agglomerative hierarchical clustering[44], principal component analysis[45–47], independent component analysis[48,49], or a mixture of Gaussian algorithms that we will discuss below in the section on single trial analysis. The crucial aspect in the microstate approach is not so much the way the dominant maps are selected, but the assumption that only one spatial map configuration is present at one moment in time, and

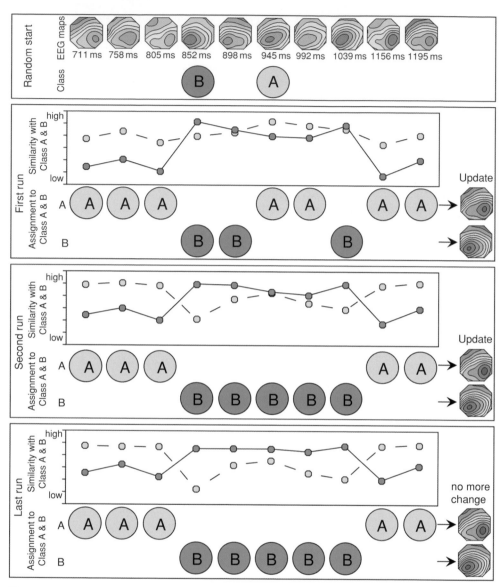

**Figure 6.3** Example of the identification of two microstate classes using a K-means cluster analysis. The top row shows the data to be analyzed, consisting of 10 EEG maps observed at moments of local maxima of the global field power. From this, two maps are randomly selected as initial microstate maps A and B. In the first run of the analysis, the similarity of all maps of the data to the initial microstate maps is computed using the squared correlation coefficient. Each map of the data is assigned to the best-fitting microstate map, as indicated by the labeled green and yellow circles. Each microstate map is then updated, by computing the first spatial principal component of all the maps that were assigned to this microstate map. The assignment and recomputation of the microstate maps is then repeated (second and third run). This is repeated until no further change in assignment is observed. Since the result might depend on the initial random selection, the entire procedure is repeated several times and the solution with the best overall fit is retained. Modified after Koenig et al.[33] with permission.

that the components do not overlap. This assumption is implemented in the labeling procedure, where each time frame is labeled with only one of the prototype maps, the one it best correlates with.

It is important to note that this one-or-no labeling procedure results in very structured time series, where each prototype map is present during a certain period of time, i.e. that the prototype maps are not randomly distributed in time. This result supports the idea of sequential functional microstates representing distinct functional processes. It is important to note that the functional microstate model by no means implies that only one area in the brain is active at one moment in time and that mental activity is a strictly sequential process. Many different areas can be active during a given microstate and many areas can be common to several states. But all the simultaneously active neuronal populations in the brain together generate one and only one global potential map on the scalp surface at one given moment in time. This global potential map is a manifestation of all simultaneously active brain processes. If two or more such processes are active at the same time and at the same frequency and phase, it is unlikely that they do this independently; it is, on the contrary, quite likely that some defined interaction of these processes will take place. The different interacting processes may therefore be considered as a single meta-process that is represented by a single scalp field topography. The objective that is deduced from this argument is thus that the processes to be isolated do not overlap. Figure 6.4 illustrates the stability of the map topography when two sources are simultaneously active, but not when they are temporally shifted.

There are some particularities when using the cluster analysis for spontaneous EEG as compared with the more common application to evoked potentials (see below). Most important is that polarity of the maps is ignored in the spontaneous EEG. Oscillations in the spontaneous EEG are at least partly due to reciprocal interaction of excitatory and inhibitory neurons in local circuit loops, leading to polarity-oscillating dipole generators that produce fields of both polarities. In fact, maps at successive times of maximal global field power frequently show similar landscape configurations but with reversed polarity[27,50]. Since we are interested in the change of topography of the field (indicating changes in the configuration of the generators) these polarity oscillations are considered as irrelevant. Formally, polarity is ignored by ignoring the sign of the spatial correlation coefficients (i.e. by squaring them). The map that best represents a cluster of maps is equal to the first principal component of all member maps. The result of microstate segmentation of spontaneous EEG is illustrated in Figure 6.5. It shows that a given microstate can encompass several polarity inverses of maps with otherwise similar topography.

The second particularity when segmenting the spontaneous EEG is the large number of maps as well as the low signal-to-noise ratio, particularly in unfiltered EEG. To overcome these two problems it has been suggested that the data be reduced to the time points of maximal global field power. There are two good reasons to do that: first, maps at maximal GFP have highest signal-to-noise ratio. They represent the maximum of amplitude of the oscillations. Second, the map topographies tend to be stable around maximal GFP and reverse polarity or change topography around the time of minimal GFP. This can also be seen in Figure 6.5. The GFP curve below the EEG traces show that the GFP follows the periodicity of the oscillation. The dissimilarity is inversely correlated with the GFP. It is low during high GFP and has peaks during low GFP. Consequently, the segmentation using the K-means cluster analysis shows segments that remain stable during high GFP and change during low GFP. For the purpose of microstate segmentation of a long period of spontaneous EEG it is therefore reasonable to reduce the data to the GFP peaks as it has been done in the 12 s epoch in Figure 6.1.

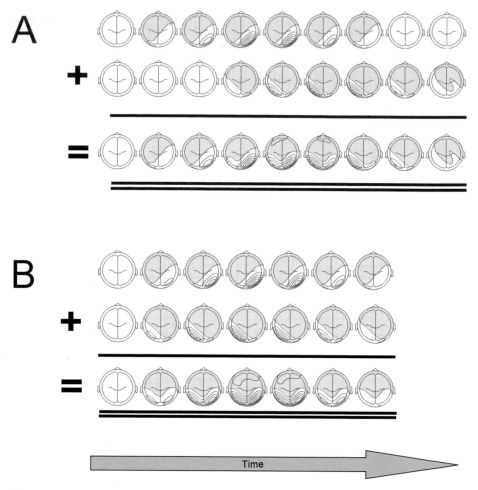

**Figure 6.4** Model examples illustrating the effects of nonsimultaneous (A) and simultaneous (B) activity in different brain regions on the temporal stability of scalp fields. In both examples, the maps in the upper row show the scalp fields associated with a source in the left occipital cortex over some time, and the maps in the middle row show the scalp fields associated with a source in the left occipital cortex over the same time. The lower row always shows the momentary scalp field maps resulting from both sources; it is always the sum of the scalp fields of the two sources. In the model shown in (A) the activity of the right source peaks before the activity of the left source. The maps resulting from both sources show continuous transitions from a scalp field that is predominated by the right source to a mixture of both sources to a scalp field predominated by the left source. In the model shown in (B), both sources peak at the same time. The maps resulting from both sources are thus always a mixture of both sources, but do not change their configuration over time. The temporal alignment of EEG sources is the assumed mechanism that leads to the observation of microstates in real data. The models have been constructed using the DipoleSimulator software.

## Spatial analysis of evoked potentials

Averaging of the EEG time-locked to specific external events results in characteristic potential fluctuations with relatively fixed latencies and polarities, called evoked (EP) or event-related (ERP) potentials. Evoked potentials are widely used in cognitive research as well as clinical applications. Many comprehensive textbooks describe the recording techniques, the analysis methods and the applications in clinics[51,52], as well as in cognitive research[53,54].

**Figure 6.5** K-means cluster analysis of spontaneous EEG. All single traces of a 4 s eyes-closed 42-channel EEG are shown on top. The two traces below show the global field power (GFP) and global map dissimilarity (GMD). Note that GMD is low during high GFP and shows peaks during low GFP. Below the overlapped map series the result of the K-means cluster analysis is shown. Four maps were found to best describe the period in terms of cross-validation. Each one is present during a certain period of time. Sometimes they only include one GFP peak, but often they span over several GFP peaks. This is shown in the enlarged epoch on the bottom with the maps at each GFP peak and their location of the positive and negative maximum. Note that the polarity inverses at each GFP peak but not the topography. No obvious relation between the dominant EEG frequency and the microstate segment borders can be seen.

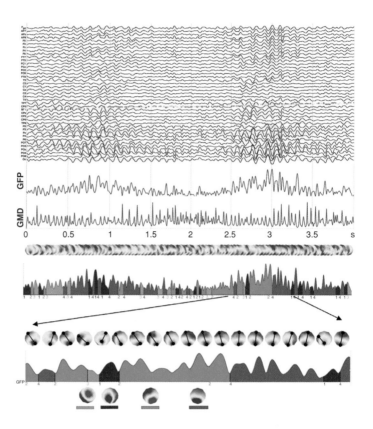

Traditionally, ERPs are described in terms of waveform features, i.e. as positive or negative deflections at certain latencies and certain electrode positions, called components. The functional significance of these components has been concluded from their sensitivity to experimental variables such as stimulus features or task demands. Thus, components are traditionally defined by their morphology, scalp distribution and sensitivity to experimental variables[55]. A large variety of components resulted from this definition with labels that referred either to their latency and polarity (e.g. P100), their localization on the scalp (e.g. early left anterior negativity) or their functional significance (e.g. mismatch negativity).

With the development and wider use of multichannel ERP recording systems some of these traditional definitions are challenged. This particularly concerns the morphology of the waveform, since it strongly depends on the position of the recording electrode as well as the position of the reference electrode (see Chapter 2; see also the discussions in Murray et al.[44] and Michel et al.[56]). Also, it is not easy to integrate the fact that other electrodes might show clear "components" at the same latency and that they can also and sometimes even independently be manipulated by the experimental variables. This has led to considerable confusion because components are sometimes defined with the same latency but peaking at different electrodes with opposite polarity. It is possible that these components are indeed generated in two different regions of the brain, but it could also be that they just reflect the opposite poles of the volume-conducted activity of one dipole generator.

In order to avoid these confusions, many experimenters decided to not take into account the full information that is available with the multichannel recordings, but to select only certain "important" electrodes and analyze the amplitudes at certain "expected" latencies that are known to best define the component of interest. While this pre-selection approach allows an easy comparison with existing literature it does not take full advantage of the additional information that multichannel recordings can provide.

The alternative to this rather narrow-minded definition of components as waveform peaks at certain electrodes is to characterize ERPs by a sequence of evoked electric field maps and to define a component as a specific distribution of the electric field at a given moment in time or during a certain time period. The basic support for this approach comes from the biophysical fact that different topographies of the scalp potential field are caused by different configurations of intracranial generators[57,58]. It is therefore reasonable to assume that different generator configurations reflect at least partly different functional states of the brain. Consequently, differences in map configuration over time or between conditions indicate that different functional processes were activated.

In the following, different methods used to analyze multichannel ERP data are demonstrated and their advantages and limitations are discussed. To this end, the analysis of a real dataset with these methods is illustrated. The data consist of 41-channel recordings in 12 subjects who performed an explicit semantic decision task where pairs of words were sequentially presented on a computer screen and subjects had to decide by button press whether the words were semantically related or not[59,60].

## Multichannel waveform analysis

Based on previous literature it is highly expected that the semantically unrelated words evoke a so-called N400 component in the ERP, a negative deflection on vertex electrodes at around 400 ms[61]. Conventional waveform analysis would check the appearance of the N400 in our data set by comparing the amplitudes between the ERPs of related vs. unrelated words in a time window around 400 ms at central electrode sites. This analysis indeed revealed significantly more negative potentials in this latency window for unrelated as compared with related words over central sites when measured against the average reference (Figure 6.6).

But instead of restricting the analysis to certain electrodes and a certain time window, the amplitude comparison can be extended to all electrodes and all time points[62-64]. Parametric (t-tests) or nonparametric (randomization test) statistics can thereby be applied. This comprehensive exploratory statistical analysis is illustrated in Figure 6.7A. It confirms the N400 effect by showing a long period of significant amplitude differences around 400 ms. By extending the analysis to all electrodes, it reveals that the effect is significant not only at central sites, but also at other electrodes that were not included in the previous restricted analysis. The extension of the analysis to all time points also reveals an earlier differential response between related and unrelated words at around 120–150 ms that is significant at many electrodes, particularly at electrodes over parietal and central regions. This effect is of course not seen when the analysis is restricted to later time periods. It is also not seen when restricting the analysis to the component peaks, because the difference is actually significant *between* two components (between the P100 and the N160). Finally, it would disappear when accepting only significant results that last for long time periods, such as the 40 ms proposed by Rossell *et al.*[65]. Indeed these authors also found this early ERP difference between related and unrelated words on the few electrodes that they analyzed, but because the effect did not fit into the time criteria, it was not further investigated.

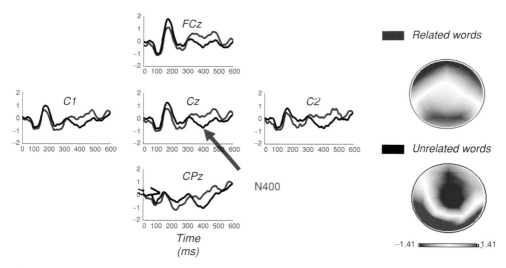

**Figure 6.6** Conventional waveform analysis of the ERP in the semantic priming paradigm. The ERPs are shown for four central electrodes. Traces are drawn for related (blue), and for unrelated (black) words. A clear negative voltage is seen for unrelated words around 400 ms, the N400 component. The mean map around this period is shown for both conditions, indicating that the N400 is not just increased amplitude of the same map, but completely different topographies.

While this amplitude analysis provides a concise summary of the entire data set, it bears several important limitations. First (as explained in Chapter 2) the analysis completely depends on the reference. Changing the reference will drastically change the results[44,56]. Second, the large number of statistical tests (41 electrodes × 300 time frames) poses the question of correction for multiple testing. Bonferroni corrections for number of electrodes and time points would be very drastic and would not consider the fact that the data are spatially and temporally highly correlated. A less severe way is to only accept effects that last for a given amount of time[65]. A third problem with the amplitude analysis of all channels is that the observed effects can be due to global amplitude modulations of the same generators, or due to changes in the spatial configuration of the generators, i.e. amplitude and topographic differences cannot be distinguished. One more problem with single channel amplitude tests is that a generator usually makes a positive and a negative pole, depending on the reference. Analysis of variance on the amplitudes, with the electrodes as one factor and the experimental conditions as the other factors, should therefore usually result in conditions by electrode interactions. Main effects are either because only a single pole of the generators making the effect has been looked at, or worse, are due to generators affecting the reference. A final but not less relevant problem concerns the possibility that a latency shift can provide statistical differences, i.e. that the same sequence of processes is activated by the two conditions, but that one is shifted in latency with respect to the other. This can lead to significant differences over time and space.

## Analysis of field strength and topography
Chapter 2 introduced two important global measures of the electric map that were first proposed by Lehmann and Skrandies[66]: global field power (GFP) and global map dissimilarity (GMD). These global measures can be used to test for differences of field strength and/or field topography of the ERPs between the two conditions at each moment in time. The test of

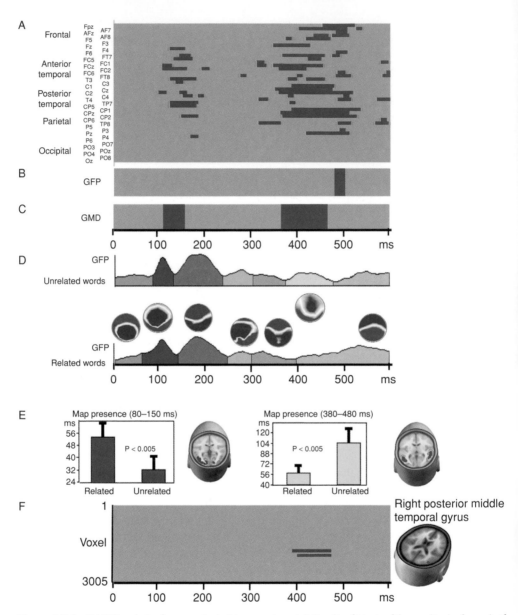

**Figure 6.7** Spatial ERP analysis of a semantic decision experiment. A. Results of t-tests of the amplitudes for each of the 42 electrodes and each time point between the ERPs to semantically related and unrelated words. B. A t-test of the global field power (GFP), indicating periods of significant map strength differences. C. Randomization test between the global map dissimilarities (GMD), revealing periods of significant map topography differences (for all tests: N = 12, P < 0.05 for at least 20 ms). D. Microstate segmentation using K-means clustering. Periods of stable topography are marked under the GFP curves of the two conditions. Same colors indicate same maps. E. Result of the fitting of the maps to the single subjects and testing the difference of map presence between the two conditions. The P100 map between 80–150 ms was present significantly longer in the ERP of related words, and the N400 map between 380–480 ms in the ERPs of unrelated words. The images beside the statistics show the areas of maximum activity estimated by a distributed linear inverse solution (LAURA). F. Statistical parametric mapping in the inverse space for each voxel and each time point. Significantly stronger activation for unrelated words was found at 400–500 ms in the right posterior middle temporal cortex.

GFP differences is straightforward and can be based on parametric (t-test) or nonparametric randomization tests just as for the single channel traces. However, testing topographic differences using the GMD is a little more complicated because the GMD is a single measure of difference between two maps (distance between two vectors representing each map), rather than a separate measure for each condition. Therefore mean and standard error of topography for each condition cannot be calculated. The way to overcome this problem is to perform a nonparametric randomization test based on the GMD values. This is done in the following way (see also Murray *et al.*[44]): (1) assigning the maps of the single subject in a randomized fashion to different experimental conditions (i.e. permutations of the data), (2) recalculating the group-average ERPs, and (3) recalculating the resulting GMD value for these "new" group-average ERPs. The number of permutations that can be made with a group-average ERP based on $n$ participants is $2^n$. The GMD value from the actual group-average ERPs is then compared with the values from the empirical distribution to determine the likelihood that the empirical distribution has a value higher than the GMD from the actual group-average ERPs. This procedure is then repeated for each time point. In a within-subject design, the permutation of the maps is done within the subjects, while in a group comparison the permutation is done across subjects. The statistical analyses described here are valid for comparison of two conditions or two groups. Analysis of variance with multiple factors can also be performed on topography comparisons. More detailed explanations on topographic statistical analysis methods are given in Chapter 8.

The results of the GFP and GMD tests for our data example are shown in Figure 6.7B and C. They show that the early effect is due to topographic differences without differences in field strength, while the late effect is due to both differences in topography as well as field strength. This analysis has several advantages as compared with the above waveform tests. First, it is reference-independent, because it is based on the spatial variation of the potential field. Second, GFP and GMD are one-number measures that are based on all electrodes and therefore are less prone to type 1 errors due to multiple testing or type 2 errors due to overcorrection. And third, they can distinguish between differences in topography and thus of the underlying generators, and differences in strength of fields with similar topography.

However, each time point is still tested independently, and thus corrections for multiple testing in time might be needed. Most used is the definition of a time window during which the effect has to remain significant. Also, the last problem described above for the waveform analysis still applies: latency shifts between the two conditions can lead to significant differences in both GFP and GMD. Thus even if this analysis leads to significant GMD effects in both time windows in our example, it does not allow us to conclude whether different neuronal processes were activated by related as compared with unrelated words in these two time periods, or whether latency shifts of the same processes led to these effects.

## Microstate analysis

We have seen above that EEG map series are typically characterized by sequential periods of stable map topographies separated by short transitions, the so-called functional microstates, and we have proposed that each of these microstates in the ongoing EEG represents a basic building block of information processing. These periods of stable map topographies are even more obvious in the averaged evoked potentials, as demonstrated in numerous studies over the last 15 years[56,44,68]. When looking at time series of evoked potential maps it is very obvious that they are characterized by sequential periods of low global dissimilarity and stable map topographies. During a period of stable topography, map strength (GFP) typically increases and decreases. As for the spontaneous EEG described above, topography changes usually occur during low GFP (this is however not always the case in the ERP). Typically, maps tend to be stable around the prototypical components of the ERPs, but some of the later ERP components are often divided into two or more topographies (see for example Brandeis *et al.*[69] for a demonstration of an early and late N400 map).

In light of the above discussion on the meaning of the microstates in the spontaneous EEG, it is proposed that each microstate of the evoked potential represents a certain information processing step that leads from perception to action. While several parallel activations are possible and most likely, there seems to be a certain sequence of information processing, probably related to the integration of the information at different complexity levels. Each integration step lasts a certain period of time, and consequently leads to a period of stable map topography.

Based on this very stable observation of microstates in evoked potential map series, the spatial K-means cluster analysis described above for the spontaneous EEG is also very efficiently applicable to the evoked potentials. The microstate segmentation of the ERPs thereby proposes to define ERP components in terms of the sequentially appearing map topographies instead of the sequentially appearing peaks at certain electrodes. Thus waveform morphology is not a defining attribute of a component any more, only the scalp distribution, i.e. the spatial configuration of the scalp potential field. Since different configurations are caused by different intracranial generator distributions[58], the characterization of ERPs as a sequence of spatially distinct maps aims to define the different large-scale neuronal networks that are activated by the incoming information. As for the spontaneous EEG, the microstate analysis of the ERP proposes that each global network is activated during a certain period of time and is then replaced by a new network that remains stable. These different networks can of course have many active areas in common, but the contribution of each of the active areas has changed or some areas are replaced or are not active any more, leading to new map topographies.

The spatial cluster analysis allows us to define the most dominant topographies in a given ERP map series, and the fitting by means of spatial correlation allows us to define when each of these topographies is present in the data[43,44]. Consequently, the influence of experimental variables on the appearance or disappearances of these topographies, on their temporal sequence, their strength or their duration, can be tested[70].

This is illustrated with the data of the semantic priming experiment analyzed above. The K-means cluster analysis was applied simultaneously to the grand mean maps of both conditions. The Krzanowski–Lai criterion[44] identified seven clusters as being the optimal number of clusters to explain the data, resulting in seven prototype maps. Fitting these maps to the data by means of spatial correlation indicated that all but one of them appeared in both conditions during the same time segments. However, one map only appeared in the ERPs of unrelated words, covering a time period between 380–480 ms. Figure 6.7D shows this segmentation of the ERPs as colored areas under the GFP curve of each condition. Same colors indicate the same prototype maps. The maps of each of these segments are also illustrated. The analysis suggests that the N400 is not due to increased amplitude of the same component, but that it actually represents a unique microstate with a unique topography. It suggests that unrelated words evoke an *additional* functional microstate, an additional processing step. It is reasonable to assume that this additional processing step leads to the significantly longer reaction time to unrelated as compared with related words.

The initial statistical analysis of all electrodes and time points (Figure 6.7A) as well as the topographic randomization test (Figure 6.7C) revealed a second period of difference between the conditions at around 120–150 ms. The microstate analysis did not indicate that different maps represented this period in the two conditions. However, the display in Figure 6.7D suggests that this early difference is due to a different type of effect, namely that the same microstate with the same map topography is active for a longer period in the ERP to related as compared with unrelated words. The microstate covers the period between the P100 and the N160 component.

Both observed effects of this microstate analysis on the grand mean data need statistical confirmation. One way to do this is to fit the cluster maps determined in the grand mean data to the single ERPs of each subject and each condition and to test whether some of the maps indeed significantly better represent one or the other condition in a given time period[70,71]. This approach has been introduced as topographic component recognition (TCR) by Brandeis et al.[72], and was initially used to determine the latency of a given component map. Different parameters can be determined by this fitting procedure and can then be statistically tested between the conditions. For example, it can be determined whether a given map explains more of the variance in the ERPs of one condition, whether it is more often present in one condition or whether it covers a different time segment or peaks at different latencies in one rather than the other condition. In designs with multiple conditions, these parameters can be tested using conventional analysis of variance statistics.

In our example, this statistical analysis indeed revealed two significant effects, namely that map number 2 was present significantly longer in the ERPs of related than of unrelated words, and that map number 6 was present longer in the ERPs of unrelated than of related words. This confirms the finding proposed from the grand mean analysis and leads to two distinctly different conclusions: in an early time period between 120 and 150 ms, the related words prolong the activation of the neuronal network that is implicated in visual access to word content, and in a later period, the unrelated words evoke an additional process, probably related to memory retrieval and additional cognitive analysis.

As shown above, the early effect is not seen in an analysis restricted to the peak of the components at given electrodes. In the waveforms (Figure 6.4) this effect is seen by a "wider" component and thus a later beginning of the next component.

## Source analysis

The last step of the spatial ERP analysis consists of the estimation of the putative sources of each of the different map topographies. In previous studies this source analysis has been performed at different levels. The first and most direct one is to apply a source localization algorithm to each of the prototype maps that characterize the different functional microstates (see Michel et al.[68] for examples). It has to be noted that the prototype maps are "synthetic" maps that represent the mean of the maps over a certain period. The map does not exist in exactly this topography in the real data and the sources estimated from this map are not necessarily those that were active in the real data. A somewhat more prudent way is to calculate the distributed inverse solution of each subject for the time period where the microstate appeared and then to average the inverse solutions over subjects. The result of this analysis is shown in Figure 6.7E for the two microstates for which the preceding analyses indicated significant differences, i.e. the P100 and the N400 microstates. For the first map this analysis revealed activation in the inferior occipital gyrus (Brodmann area 19), stronger in the right than the left hemisphere. This region has been described as the visual word form area[73]. The

N400 map shows strong bilateral activation in the middle temporal gyrus (Brodmann area 22). These areas have repeatedly been described as prominent sources of the N400 component[65,74].

An alternative strategy is to directly perform statistical analysis in the inverse space, i.e. to calculate the distributed inverse solution for each subject, each condition and each time point and statistically compare the source waveforms of each solution point between conditions. This can be done in exactly the same way as for the real recordings of the scalp potentials. However, the solution space usually consists of thousands of "virtual electrodes" and thus the number of tests and the question of correction for multiple testing becomes even more important. One way to circumvent this problem is to only look at certain areas of interest or average the activity in certain regions of interest[75,76]. In Figure 6.7F such reduction is not done. It shows the result of the statistical comparison of the activity in each voxel at each time point between the two conditions. Only the period around the N400 component revealed voxels with significantly different activity between the two conditions. They were localized in the right middle temporal gyrus. Thus while the N400 component per se shows bilateral activation in this paradigm, a significantly stronger activity for unrelated as compared with related words during this late time period is suggested to be located in the right hemisphere. This is in agreement with a number of studies that have shown activation of right posterior temporal regions during semantic tasks[65,77–80]. However, this result does not imply that the N400 component is generated in the right posterior temporal lobe. It is the difference between related and nonrelated words in our experimental paradigm that evokes this activation difference. Other paradigms can evoke differences in other areas during the same time period, such as left frontal areas in a sentence-reading paradigm[81].

## Applications of spatial ERP analysis methods

The spatial analysis strategies described here have been applied to many different ERP studies and have provided new insights into the spatio-temporal dynamics of information processing. Most of the basic topographical analysis methods (such as GFP, GMD, microstate segmentation) have been used for many years[82–85]. The more statistical approaches and fitting procedures, as well as the source analysis strategies, have been introduced more recently[44,47,56,68,71]. Most recent applications concerned sensory perceptions and integration[86–96], motor functions[97–99], attention[100,101], memory[102–104], language[59,105–110], emotion[111,112], face recognition[113,114], and mental imaging[70,115–118].

An important aspect of the analysis strategy (besides the fact that it is based on the whole electrode array) is that it is free from a-priori definition of components (and thus time periods) of interest. Because of this temporal openness, many of the above listed studies revealed very early different activation patterns (even earlier than 100 ms) for relatively complex stimulus features. Such early differential responses were found between novel and repeated faces[60,119] between semantically related vs. unrelated word pairs[60] (see also Figure 6.7), between nouns and verbs[120], between emotional vs. neutral words[110], for visual stimuli paired with an auditory cue[104], for visual stimuli located on the same side as a preceding angry face[111], for degraded faces[90], for repeated images that were previously accompanied by sounds[104], and efficient vs. inefficient visual searches[88]. Similar early differential neuronal responses (as described by different map topographies) were described in the auditory domain[93,121]. All these studies led to the conclusion that early ERP components can no longer be considered as purely "exogenous" and independent of cognitive demands.

On the contrary, they are already very profoundly modulated by higher cognitive brain functions, supporting the idea of fast top-down mechanisms influencing the visual cortex activity[122-124]; for a review see Michel et al.[60]).

## State-dependent information processing and pre-stimulus baseline

Event-related potential analysis traditionally assumes that all observed activity is evoked by the stimulus and is constant and similar across repetitions. The activity before the stimulus is considered to be random and irrelevant for stimulus processing. Therefore, most often a pre-stimulus baseline correction is applied, i.e. the EEG after the stimulus is subtracted from the EEG before the stimulus. Thus ERPs are usually averaged difference-waves or difference maps between post- and pre-stimulus activity (see also Chapter 2).

However as discussed above with respect to the spontaneous EEG, the neuronal activity varies in time in the millisecond range and reflects the momentary functional state of the resting brain. There is ample evidence that these fluctuations of the momentary brain states influence the ability to perform any given task and to perceive, process or react to internal or external signals, i.e. that sensory and cognitive processing is highly state-dependent. For example, animal studies have revealed a link between specific patterns of early visual cortex activity at baseline before visual stimulus onset, and the size or latency of the neuronal response to the forthcoming stimulus[125-127], as well as whether the stimulus reaches awareness[128-130]. In humans, spontaneous fluctuations at pre-stimulus baseline, that occur within areas of the visual network and account for differential behavioral or neuronal responses to identical visual stimuli, have been documented using EEG/MEG[131-136] or fMRI techniques[137,138]. Note that these state-dependent effects are unlikely to be explained by changes in the general alertness level over trials, since the predictive brain activity patterns vary across studies in topography and with the behavioral paradigms, which indicates that activation of different neuronal networks underlies these results. Therefore, the temporal variability of neuronal activity cannot be considered noise, without any functional significance, and cannot be ignored in the exploration of brain function.

As discussed above, the functional microstates of the spontaneous EEG are proposed to represent the momentary mental state of the brain and are thus ideal to determine state-dependent information processing. This has been done in the studies by Lehmann et al.[139] and Kondakor et al.[140,141]. They demonstrated that the morphology and topography of several ERP components to physically identical stimuli are different when averaged separately to different classes of microstates at the moment of stimulus presentation. Microstate analysis was also used by Müller et al.[142] to study illusory multistable motion perception. They found a specific microstate class that was more significantly present before the presentation of the stimulus that was marked as changed motion direction. In addition, the global complexity increased during this pre-stimulus period, indicating an increased number of uncorrelated processes in the brain (see Chapter 9). Together with previous results on spectral changes of the EEG before perceptual changes[143] the authors interpret their findings as indication for micro-fluctuations in vigilance and attention that influence perception.

While these first studies indicated that stimulus processing varies in dependency on the momentary microstate of the brain at stimulus presentation, they did not show that this leads to differences in performance. Two recent studies directly demonstrated such behavioral consequences. In the first study[144] 22 healthy subjects (11 women) performed a bilateral lexical

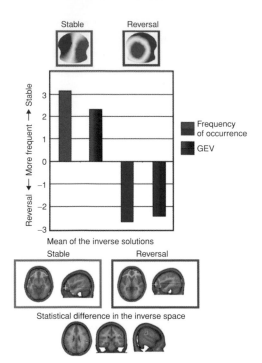

**Figure 6.8** Microstate analysis of the 256-channel EEG just before subjects indicated reversal of the perception of a Necker cube, compared with the period before stable perception. Two maps were found that significantly double dissociated the two conditions, both in terms of frequency of occurrence and in global explained variance (GEV). The maps are shown on top. On the bottom the mean of the inverse solutions over subjects for the two conditions are shown (minimum norm). The last row shows the results of statistical parametric mapping. One area in the right inferior posterior cortex was significantly more strongly activated when subjects subsequently indicated perceptual reversal.

decision task with very short presentation of emotional and neutral words and nonwords. Previous studies showed a clear recognition advantage for emotional words, an advantage that was particularly important when the words were presented to the left visual field[110,145]. A 128-channel EEG was continuously recorded while subjects performed this task. The maps at the last GFP peak just before stimulus arrival were determined for each trial and these different maps were classified using the K-means cluster analysis and cross-validation statistics. Twelve different map configurations were identified. These maps were further reduced into two classes based on the location of their maximum and minimum potentials. When comparing the emotional word advantage between trials that were preceded by one against the other map class, it became clear that this advantage was most significant after one class of maps, and this only in men, not in women.

The second study[146] used this methodological approach to test whether the momentary microstate immediately before stimulus presentation indicates how a physically unique but perceptually ambiguous stimulus will be perceived. The use of such stimuli was inspired by the studies of Müller et al.[142,143] described above; intermittent presentation of a Necker cube was used. An EEG was recorded from 256 channels in 12 subjects. Subjects indicated by button press whether the perception of the cube changed with respect to the previous presentation. K-means cluster analysis of all pre-state maps, and fitting the cluster maps to the individual trials revealed two maps that double dissociated perceptual reversals from perceptual stability. Distributed inverse solutions were calculated for all trials that were labeled with one or the other of these two maps and statistically compared across subjects. This yielded activity confined to a region in the right inferior parietal cortex that was significantly more active before a perceptual reversal. The results of this study are summarized in Figure 6.8.

In conclusion, the studies described above clearly indicate that the momentary state of the brain just before stimulus presentation defines the fate of the stimulus, both in terms of brain structures that are processing it and in terms of the way the subject responds to it. These results strongly cast doubt on the validity of averaging the EEG over trials and even more on the pre-stimulus baseline correction. They provide strong arguments for the development of methods that allow the analysis of single-trial evoked potentials, discussed in the next section.

## Spatial single-trial ERP analysis

Instead of averaging the evoked potentials and thereby assuming stationarity of the stimulus response, several approaches have focused on the development of analysis methods for single-trial data[101,147–149]. Analysis of ERP at single-trial level allows the addressing of a number of important issues. First of all, as discussed above, it allows the investigation of the possibility that different processing strategies are used by the brain, depending on its momentary state. It also allows the study of the effects of learning, vigilance and attention modulation[150–152]. Second, identifying the evoked components in the single-trial epochs allows the study of possible synchronization mechanisms underlying communication among brain areas for perception, working memory and sensorimotor integration[9,153–155]. The fundamental advantages offered by a single-trial analysis have driven several propositions about how to uncover the stimulus-related activity embedded in the ongoing complex EEG.

The most popular (and debated) approach is probably the one based on independent component analysis (ICA)[156,157]. This technique relies on the hypothesis that brain activity is the result of a superimposition of a number of independent activities weighted by a certain set of spatial coefficients. An ICA can provide an estimation of components in a number less than or equal to the number of electrodes and is in principle able to uncover any independent activities provided that no more than one source has Gaussian distribution. The main success of this technique is in the area of detection and elimination of artifacts in the EEG or MEG, including eye-blink artifacts, cardiac artifacts and muscle activity[158–161]. An important use of the ICA is in elimination of the cardiac pulse artifact in the EEG recorded in an MRI scanner[162–164]; see also Chapter 10. Clearly in all these cases the hypothesis of independence between these components from the rest of the brain activity holds very well, and several studies suggest that ICA is the most powerful approach for artifact detection.

However, the use of the ICA to disentangle the various components of brain activity in general is more problematic because the hypothesis of independence is difficult to accept. Indeed, cross-talk between unifocal brain activities and within distributed neural networks is certainly one of the main principles of brain organization, and a fundamental mechanism for generating coherent and functionally integrated mental states[165]. Nevertheless, ICA has been applied to the concatenated single-trial ERP data with the aim of separating multichannel data into a sum of independent activities[48,49]. Each of these components is represented by a potential map representing the strength of the volume-conducted component activity at each scalp electrode and the time course of its activity in every single trial. The physiological meaningfulness of these isolated component maps is argued by the resemblance between the scalp map and the projections of a single dipole[49,166,167]. However, the main limitation of ICA is that it cannot uncover components that are dynamically coupled, a situation that occurs in any parallel process and distributed activity in the brain, and therefore it is likely to be useful only in specific experimental circumstances.

An important argument for the application of ICA has been made with respect to the debate about the evoked and induced activity reflected in the ERP. It has been proposed that the incoming stimulus induces "phase resetting" of ongoing EEG rhythms in each trial and that averaging these phase-coherent rhythms produces the ERP[168,169], and that the ICA can identify those components that are responsible for the phase resetting mechanism. Doubts on this phase resetting theory are provided by direct studies of single-trial, intracortical activity in awake, behaving monkeys and calculation of current source density profiles across the different cortical layers. These studies show that an incoming stimulus evokes an additive, neural-population response in each trial and that these stimulus-evoked activities contribute predominantly to the evoked potential[170].

Numerous other approaches have been developed for single trial analysis. Methods that were used are blind source separation algorithms[171,172], differentially variable component analysis[149], Kalman filter methods[173], wavelet decomposition and time-frequency based methods[148,174]. These techniques are typically developed in the context of a brain–computer interface where the goal is classifying online single electrical responses[175,176]. In all these methods, the single response analysis is mainly based on features of the brain activity in their temporal or frequency domain. Often overlooked is the information conveyed by the spatial characteristic of the overall electric field measured at the scalp.

De Lucia *et al.*[177,178] recently proposed a single-trial approach for EEG analysis purely based on the topographic features of the multichannel data. It is founded on the above-discussed fact that the spontaneous EEG and the evoked potentials have a well-defined structure of temporally stable topographies (the microstates) and that these topographic stabilities can be easily identified in the ongoing EEG. This method is based on a similar principle to the microstate analysis, namely that the evoked response activity in the single trials can be modeled as a set of clusters of topographies without explicit assumption on their temporal behavior. However, because of the low signal-to-noise ratio in the single trials, a simple K-means cluster analysis as described above for the averaged evoked potentials will not allow differentiation of the evoked from the spontaneous microstates. De Lucia *et al.*[177] proposed to model the overall electrical response, including event-related and ongoing activity, as a mixture of Gaussians, i.e. as a set of clusters having Gaussian distribution in an $N$-dimensional space, where $N$ is the number of the electrodes in the montage. The computation needs to be initialized by a K-means algorithm which iteratively improves the estimation of means, covariances and priors of the $Q$ Gaussians until the likelihood reaches a plateau. For each time point and trial it then provides $Q$ conditional probabilities that relate the topographies to the clusters. Finally each time point and trial are labeled with the cluster with which they have highest conditional probability. The result of this analysis is illustrated in Figure 6.9.

The analysis showed that without making any assumption about the temporal behavior of the EEG signal, a significant modulation of single responses in comparison to the baseline activity can be uncovered as consistent topographic patterns of activity in time and across trials. The method makes minimal use of a-priori constraints and allows the identification of significant map presence and periods of difference across conditions.

## Spatio-temporal analysis of interictal epileptic activity

A particular application of the spatio-temporal analysis procedures described above concerns the analysis of epileptiform activity, where the main aim is to localize the primary epileptogenic focus and differentiate it from secondary foci due to propagation. It is well

**Figure 6.9** Spatial-single-trial analysis of auditory event-related potentials. Top: checkerboard-like representation in which each time point and trial are labeled with the cluster having the highest conditional probability. Note the periods of stable labeling with one and the same map across single trials. Bottom: Average conditional probability of each of the five clusters for which the topographies are illustrated below the probability plot. Modified from De Lucia *et al.*[177] with permission from the author.

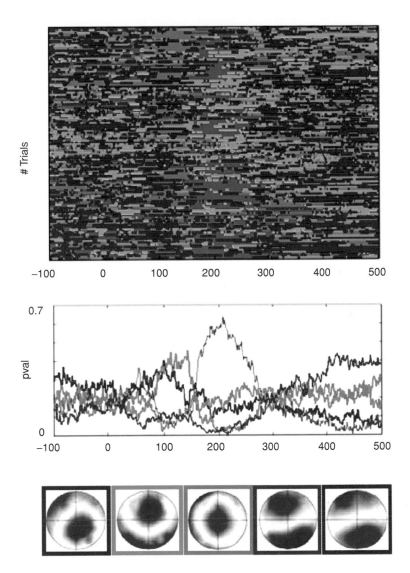

known that not only seizure activity propagates, but also interictal spike activity[179]. Intracranial recordings have shown that secondary spike foci occur in areas that are well connected by fiber tracts to the primary epileptogenic region[180,181] and can for example include propagations from the mesial to lateral and anterior to posterior temporal lobe[182] as well as from the temporal lobe to orbitofrontal regions[183]. Dipole modeling of scalp EEG spike data has also repeatedly described propagation of interictal activity within and between temporal lobes[184–186]. These very fast propagations within the *c.* 100–200 ms that a spike-wave complex lasts are one of the main reasons why EEG-linked fMRI for localization of the epileptic focus often reveals several areas of BOLD responses[187,188]. Only in combination with other information can the primary focus be identified based on the fMRI. One of these other methods is electrical neuroimaging with its inherent high temporal resolution[185,189–199]; for a review

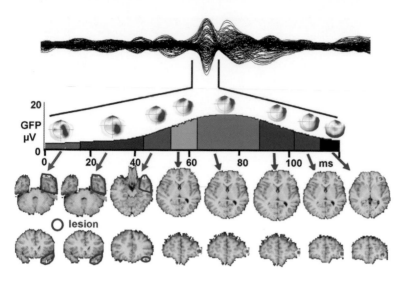

**Figure 6.10** Spatial K-means cluster analysis of an averaged spike recorded from 128 electrodes. Seven clusters were identified with distinct map topographies. Source localization of these maps reveal maximal activity within the epileptogenic and later resected lesion during the rising phase of the spike, but not at the peak of the spike. Modified after Lantz et al.[191] with permission.

see Michel et al.[67]. However, methods are needed that allow identification of the beginning of epileptic activity.

Lantz et al.[191] proposed to use the spatial K-means cluster analysis approach described above for microstate segmentation to identify initiation and propagation of interictal activity. In this study, 128-channel interictal activity was recorded in 16 patients suffering from pharmaco-resistant partial epilepsy. All patients had clear MRI lesions and were seizure-free after epilepsy surgery, thus allowing an unambiguous location of the epileptic focus. Several spikes were visually identified in each patient and averaged. Then the spatial K-means cluster analysis described above was applied to periods of ±60 ms around the spike peak. The cluster analysis defined the different dominant maps in this period and the time segment during which they appeared. A linear inverse solution method called EPIFOCUS[190,200] was then applied to each segment map. The inverse solutions were calculated in a solution space defined by each patient's own MRI, using an anatomically constrained spherical head model (SMAC[201]). The maximum of the source localization was determined for each segment map and the distance of the maximum to the resected lesion was determined (Figure 6.10). The analysis of all 16 patients revealed that only in eight of the 16 patients was the source within the lesion during the entire rising phase of the spike, including the spike peak. In the remaining cases, source locations were outside the lesion either in the very beginning, or at the later phases of the spike. It is important to note that in five cases the source at the peak of the spike was outside the lesion. Only at around 50% rising time of the spike were the sources of all patients within the lesion. This confirms earlier reports that the spike peak might include propagated activity[184] and does not make it the best candidate for epileptic source localization, despite the good signal-to-noise ratio.

Another strategy to define the onset area of interictal activity has been proposed[194,197]. It is based on statistical nonparametric (randomization) or parametric (t-test) mapping in the source space. LORETA analysis has been used in Zumsteg et al.[197] and the LAURA algorithm in Sperli et al.[194]. The method is illustrated with one example in Figure 6.11. First, inverse solutions are calculated for each single spike and each time point around the spike, including a sufficiently long pre-spike period. The activity during this pre-spike period is considered as

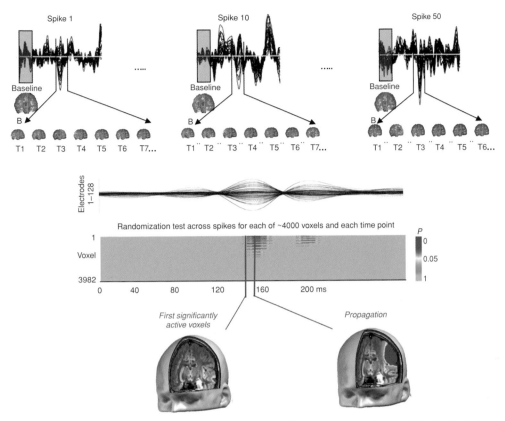

**Figure 6.11** Illustration of the statistical parametric mapping analysis of interictal epileptic activity. Distributed inverse solutions are calculated for each time point in a period around the spike peak for each individual spike, and for a baseline period before the spike. For each time point, each voxel and each spike the difference to the baseline is calculated and paired t-tests are computed. The time point of first significant active voxels is considered as representing the initial activity in the primary focus (here the left lateral temporal lobe). The additional significant active voxels are considered as propagated activity (here in the parietal lobe).

baseline. Differences between the activity during the spike and during the baseline are then calculated for each solution point and each time point. This allows the determination of the time point when the first significant activation appears and the location of the solution points that are significant during this first time point. It also allows the study of propagation patterns by looking at subsequent time points and identifying other solution points that become activated during the spike. Confirming the findings discussed above, both studies[194,197] showed that the first significant activity is found during the rising phase of the spike and that these first significantly active solution points identify the epileptic focus very well.

## Conclusion

This chapter has illustrated the advantages that spatio-temporal analysis of multichannel EEG and ERP provide to study spontaneous, evoked and pathological brain functions. The fact that the temporal progression of brain electric activity can be described as a sequence of microstates with stable map topographies makes it reasonable to consider these microstates as the neurophysiological manifestation of the basic building blocks of spontaneous or evoked mental functions. The spatial segmentation procedures adapted from pattern recognition algorithms permits researchers to mathematically describe and efficiently differentiate these microstates in time and between experimental conditions. Together with powerful distributed source analysis methods the microstate analysis allows the description of the active large-scale neuronal networks of the brain in the sub-second range.

Concerning the spontaneous EEG, it is challenging to propose that these functional microstates describe the subsequent blocks of conscious global neuronal workspace activity. In the analysis of event-related potentials (averaged or single trials), these microstates are an alternative way to describe the different components that are evoked by the stimuli. In the analysis of clinical electrical activity, such as interictal discharges, microstate analysis allows us to reliably define the location of initial pathological activity and differentiate it from propagated activity.

We also illustrated the possibility of directly performing the temporal analysis in the source space. While it is still more prudent to stay as close as possible to the real recorded data, the potential that source localization procedures offer cannot be neglected. Distributed source localization algorithms are becoming more and more reliable, due to improved and physiologically more plausible source models, better realistic head models and of course much higher numbers of electrodes. It would be most interesting to see applications of the microstate segmentation algorithms in the inverse space and to directly look for temporally stable patterns of distributed large-scale neuronal networks.

# References

1. Raichle ME, MacLeod AM, Snyder AZ et al. A default mode of brain function. *Proceedings of the National Academy of Sciences USA*. 2001;**98**:676–682.

2. Raichle ME, Snyder AZ. A default mode of brain function: a brief history of an evolving idea. *Neuroimage* 2007;**37**: 1083–1090; discussion 1097–1089.

3. Fox MD, Raichle ME. Spontaneous fluctuations in brain activity observed with functional magnetic resonance imaging. *Nature Reviews Neuroscience* 2007;**8**:700–711.

4. Lopes da Silva F. Neural mechanisms underlying brain waves: from neural membranes to networks. *Electroencephalography and Clinical Neurophysiology* 1991;**79**:81–93.

5. Buzsaki G. *Rhythms of the Brain*. Oxford: Oxford University Press; 2006.

6. Laufs H, Krakow K, Sterzer P et al. Electroencephalographic signatures of attentional and cognitive default modes in spontaneous brain activity fluctuations at rest. *Proceedings of the National Academy of Sciences USA* 2003;**100**:11053–11058.

7. Laufs H, Kleinschmidt A, Beyerle A et al. EEG-correlated fMRI of human alpha activity. *Neuroimage* 2003;**19**:1463–1476.

8. Laufs H, Holt JL, Elfont R et al. Where the BOLD signal goes when alpha EEG leaves. *Neuroimage* 2006;**31**:1408–1418.

9. Bressler SL. Large-scale cortical networks and cognition. *Brain Research. Brain Research Reviews* 1995;**20**:288–304.

10. Mesulam MM. From sensation to cognition. *Brain* 1998;**121**:1013–1052.

11. Fuster JM. The cognit: a network model of cortical representation. *International Journal of Psychophysiology* 2006;**60**:125–132.

12. Baars BJ. *In the Theater of Consciousness: The Workspace of the Mind*. Oxford: Oxford University Press; 1997.

13. Baars BJ. The conscious access hypothesis: origins and recent evidence. *Trends in Cognitive Science* 2002;**6**:47–52.

14. Dehaene S, Kerszberg M, Changeux JP. A neuronal model of a global workspace in effortful cognitive tasks. *Proceedings of the National Academy of Sciences USA*. 1998; **95**:14529–14534.

15. Dehaene S, Sergent C, Changeux JP. A neuronal network model linking subjective

reports and objective physiological data during conscious perception. *Proceedings of the National Academy of Sciences USA* 2003;**100**:8520–8525.

16. Dehaene S, Naccache L. Towards a cognitive neuroscience of consciousness: basic evidence and a workspace framework. *Cognition* 2001;**79**:1–37.

17. Bressler SL, Tognoli E. Operational principles of neurocognitive networks. *International Journal of Psychophysiology* 2006;**60**:139–148.

18. Grossberg S. The complementary brain: unifying brain dynamics and modularity. *Trends in Cognitive Science* 2000;**4**:233–246.

19. Fingelkurts AA. Timing in cognition and EEG brain dynamics: discreteness versus continuity. *Cognitive Processes* 2006;**7**:135–162.

20. Changeux J-P, Michel CM. Mechanism of neural integration at the brain-scale level. In Grillner S, Graybiel AM, eds. *Microcircuits*. Cambridge: MIT Press; 2004, pp. 347–370.

21. Lehmann D, Ozaki H, Pal I. EEG alpha map series: brain micro-states by space-oriented adaptive segmentation. *Electroencephalography and Clinical Neurophysiology* 1987;**67**:271–288.

22. Koukkou M, Lehmann D. An information-processing perspective of psychophysiological measurements. *Journal of Psychophysiology* 1987;**1**:109–112.

23. Lehmann D. Brain electric fields and brain functional states. In Friedrich R, Wunderlin A, eds. *Evolution of Dynamical Structures in Complex Systems*. Berlin: Springer; 1992, pp. 235–248.

24. John ER. A field theory of consciousness. *Conscious Cognition* 2001;**10**:184–213.

25. Lehmann D, Strik WK, Henggeler B, Koenig T, Koukkou M. Brain electric microstates and momentary conscious mind states as building blocks of spontaneous thinking: I. Visual imagery and abstract thoughts. *International Journal of Psychophysiology* 1998;**29**:1–11.

26. Koenig T, Prichep L, Lehmann D *et al.* Millisecond by millisecond, year by year: normative EEG microstates and

developmental stages. *Neuroimage* 2002; **16**:41–48.

27. Wackerman J, Lehmann D, Michel CM, Strik WK. Adaptive segmentation of spontaneous EEG map series into spatially defined microstates. *International Journal of Psychophysiology* 1993;**14**:269–283.

28. Efron R. The minimum duration of a perception. *Neuropsychologia* 1970;**8**:57–63.

29. Libet B. The experimental evidence of subjective referral of a sensory experience backward in time. *Philosophy and Science* 1981;**48**:182–197.

30. Sergent C, Dehaene S. Neural processes underlying conscious perception: experimental findings and a global neuronal workspace framework. *Journal of Physiology, Paris* 2004;**98**:374–384.

31. Strik WK, Lehmann D. Data determined window size and space-oriented segmentation of spontaneous EEG map series. *Electroencephalography and Clinical Neurophysiology* 1993;**87**:169–174.

32. Kinoshita T, Strik WK, Michel CM *et al.* Microstate segmentation of spontaneous multichannel EEG map series under diazepam and sulpiride. *Pharmacopsychiatry* 1995;**28**:51–55.

33. Koenig T, Lehmann D, Merlo MC *et al.* A deviant EEG brain microstate in acute, neuroleptic-naive schizophrenics at rest. *European Archives in Psychiatry and Clinical Neuroscience* 1999;**249**:205–211.

34. Strelets V, Faber PL, Golikova J *et al.* Chronic schizophrenics with positive symptomatology have shortened EEG microstate durations. *Clinical Neurophysiology* 2003;**114**:2043–2051.

35. Kikuchi M, Koenig T, Wada Y *et al.* Native EEG and treatment effects in neuroleptic-naive schizophrenic patients: time and frequency domain approaches. *Schizophrenia Research* 2007;**97**:163–172.

36. Strik WK, Dierks T, Becker T, Lehmann D. Larger topographical variance and decreased duration of brain electric microstates in depression. *Journal of Neural Transmission General Section* 1995; **99**:213–222.

37. Dierks T, Jelic V, Julin P *et al.* EEG-microstates in mild memory

impairment and Alzheimer's disease: possible association with disturbed information processing. *Journal of Neural Transmission* 1997;**104**:483–495.

38. Strik WK, Chiaramonti R, Muscas GC *et al.* Decreased EEG microstate duration and anteriorisation of the brain electrical fields in mild and moderate dementia of the Alzheimer type. *Psychiatry Research* 1997;**75**:183–191.

39. Kinoshita T, Michel CM, Yagyu T, Lehmann D, Saito M. Diazepam and sulpiride effects on frequency domain EEG source localisations. *Neuropsychobiology* 1994;**30**:126–131.

40. Katayama H, Gianotti LR, Isotani T *et al.* Classes of multichannel EEG microstates in light and deep hypnotic conditions. *Brain Topography* 2007;**20**:7–14.

41. Lehmann D, Faber PL, Galderisi S *et al.* EEG microstate duration and syntax in acute, medication-naive, first-episode schizophrenia: a multi-center study. *Psychiatry Research* 2005;**138**:141–156.

42. Lehmann D, Wackermann J, Michel CM, Koenig T. Space-oriented EEG segmentation reveals changes in brain electric field maps under the influence of a nootropic drug. *Psychiatry Research* 1993; **50**:275–282.

43. Pascual-Marqui RD, Michel CM, Lehmann D. Segmentation of brain electrical activity into microstates: model estimation and validation. *IEEE Transactions on Biomedical Engineering* 1995;**42**:658–665.

44. Murray MM, Brunet D, Michel CM. Topographic ERP analyses: a step-by-step tutorial review. *Brain Topography* 2008; **20**:249–264.

45. Skrandies W. Data reduction of multichannel fields: global field power and principal component analysis. *Brain Topography* 1989;**2**:73–80.

46. Spencer KM, Dien J, Donchin E. Spatiotemporal analysis of the late ERP responses to deviant stimuli. *Psychophysiology* 2001;**38**:343–358.

47. Pourtois G, Deplanque S, Michel C.M. *et al.* Beyond the conventional event-related brain potential (ERP): exploring the time-course of visual

emotion processing using topographic and principal component analyses. *Brain Topography* 2008;**20**:265–277.

48. Makeig S, Westerfield M, Jung TP *et al.* Functionally independent components of the late positive event-related potential during visual spatial attention. *Journal of Neuroscience* 1999;**19**:2665–2680.

49. Makeig S, Debener S, Onton J, Delorme A. Mining event-related brain dynamics. *Trends in Cognitive Science* 2004;**8**:204–210.

50. Lehmann D. Multichannel topography of human alpha EEG fields. *Electroencephalography and Clinical Neurophysiology* 1971;**31**:439–449.

51. Regan D. *Human Brain Electrophysiology: Evoked Potentials and Evoked Magnetic Fields in Science and Medicine.* Amsterdam: Elsevier; 1989.

52. Chiappa KH, ed. *Evoked Potentials in Clinical Medicine.* 3rd edn. Philadelphia: Lippincott-Raven; 1997.

53. Luck SJ. *An Introduction to the Event-Related Potential Technique.* Cambridge, MA: MIT Press; 2005.

54. Handy TC. *Event-Related Potentials: A Methods Handbook.* Cambridge, MA: MIT Press; 2004.

55. Donchin E, Isreal JB. Event-related potentials and psychological theory. *Progress in Brain Research* 1980;**54**:697–715.

56. Michel CM, Murray MM, Lantz G *et al.* EEG source imaging. *Clinical Neurophysiology* 2004;**115**:2195–2222.

57. McCarthy G, Wood CC. Scalp distributions of event-related potentials: an ambiguity associated with analysis of variance models. *Electroencephalography and Clinical Neurophysiology* 1985;**62**:203–208.

58. Vaughan HGJ. The neural origins of human event-related potentials. *Annals of the New York Academy of Sciences* 1982; **388**:125–138.

59. Khateb A, Annoni JM, Landis T *et al.* Spatio-temporal analysis of electric brain activity during semantic and phonological word processing. *International Journal of Psychophysiology* 1999;**32**:215–231.

60. Michel CM, Seeck M, Murray MM. The speed of visual cognition. *Supplement in Clinical Neurophysiology* 2004;**57**:617–627.

61. Kutas M, Hillyard SA. Reading senseless sentences: brain potentials reflect semantic incongruity. *Science* 1980;**207**:203–205.

62. Guthrie D, Buchwald JS. Significance testing of difference potentials. *Psychophysiology* 1991;**28**:240–244.

63. Seeck M, Mainwaring N, Cosgrove R et al. Neurophysiologic correlates of implicit face memory in intracranial visual evoked potentials. *Neurology* 1997;**49**:1312–1316.

64. Molholm S, Ritter W, Murray MM et al. Multisensory auditory-visual interactions during early sensory processing in humans: a high-density electrical mapping study. *Brain Research Cognitive Brain Research* 2002;**14**:115–128.

65. Rossell SL, Price CJ, Nobre AC. The anatomy and time course of semantic priming investigated by fMRI and ERPs. *Neuropsychologia* 2003;**41**:550–564.

66. Lehmann D, Skrandies W. Reference-free identification of components of checkerboard-evoked multichannel potential fields. *Electroencephalography and Clinical Neurophysiology* 1980;**48**:609–621.

67. Michel CM, Grave de Peralta R, Lantz G et al. Spatio-temporal EEG analysis and distributed source estimation in presurgical epilepsy evaluation. *Journal of Clinical Neurophysiology* 1999;**16**:225–238.

68. Michel CM, Thut G, Morand S et al. Electric source imaging of human brain functions. *Brain Research. Brain Research Reviews* 2001;**36**:108–118.

69. Brandeis D, Lehmann D, Michel CM, Mingrone W. Mapping event-related brain potential microstates to sentence endings. *Brain Topography* 1995;**8**:145–159.

70. Pegna AJ, Khateb A, Spinelli L et al. Unravelling the cerebral dynamics of mental imagery. *Human Brain Mapping* 1997;**5**:410–421.

71. Michel CM, Seeck M, Landis T. Spatiotemporal dynamics of human cognition. *News in Physiological Science* 1999;**14**:206–214.

72. Brandeis D, Naylor H, Halliday R, Callaway E, Yano L. Scopolamine effects on visual information processing, attention, and event-related potential map latencies. *Psychophysiology* 1992;**29**:315–336.

73. Cohen L, Lehericy S, Chochon F et al. Language-specific tuning of visual cortex? Functional properties of the Visual Word Form Area. *Brain* 2002;**125**:1054–1069.

74. Salmelin R. Clinical neurophysiology of language: the MEG approach. *Clinical Neurophysiology* 2007;**118**:237–254.

75. Ortigue S, Thut G, Landis T, Michel CM. Time-resolved sex differences in language lateralization. *Brain* 2005;**128**:E28; author reply E29.

76. James CE, Britz J, Vuilleumier P, Hauert CA, Michel CM. Early neuronal responses in right limbic structures mediate harmony incongruity processing in musical experts. *Neuroimage* 2008;**42**:1597–1608.

77. Bottini G, Corcoran R, Sterzi R et al. The role of the right hemisphere in the interpretation of figurative aspects of language. A positron emission tomography activation study. *Brain* 1994;**117**:1241–1253.

78. Kuperberg GR, McGuire PK, Bullmore ET et al. Common and distinct neural substrates for pragmatic, semantic, and syntactic processing of spoken sentences: an fMRI study. *Journal of Cognitive Neuroscience* 2000;**12**:321–341.

79. St George M, Kutas M, Martinez A, Sereno MI. Semantic integration in reading: engagement of the right hemisphere during discourse processing. *Brain* 1999;**122**:1317–1325.

80. Rossell SL, Bullmore ET, Williams SC, David AS. Brain activation during automatic and controlled processing of semantic relations: a priming experiment using lexical-decision. *Neuropsychologia* 2001;**39**:1167–1176.

81. Schulz E, Maurer U, van der Mark S et al. Impaired semantic processing during sentence reading in children with dyslexia: combined fMRI and ERP evidence. *Neuroimage* 2008;**41**:153–168.

82. Lehmann D, Skrandies W. Spatial analysis of evoked potentials in man – a review. *Progress in Neurobiology* 1984;**23**:227–250.

83. Skrandies W. Global field power and topographic similarity. *Brain Topography* 1990;**3**:137–141.

84. Skrandies W. EEG/EP: new techniques. *Brain Topography* 1993;**5**:347–350.

85. Brandeis D, Lehmann D. Event-related potentials of the brain and cognitive processes: approaches and applications. *Neuropsychologia* 1986;**24**:151–168.

86. Morand S, Thut G, Grave de Peralta R *et al.* Electrophysiological evidence for fast visual processing through the human koniocellular pathway when stimuli move. *Cerebral Cortex* 2000;**10**:817–825.

87. Ducommun CY, Murray MM, Thut G *et al.* Segregated processing of auditory motion and auditory location: an ERP mapping study. *Neuroimage* 2002;**16**:76–88.

88. Leonards U, Palix J, Michel C, Ibanez V. Comparison of early cortical networks in efficient and inefficient visual search: an event-related potential study. *Journal of Cognitive Neuroscience* 2003;**15**:1039–1051.

89. Pegna AJ, Khateb A, Murray MM, Landis T, Michel CM. Neural processing of illusory and real contours revealed by high-density ERP mapping. *Neuroreport* 2002;**13**:965–968.

90. Pegna AJ, Khateb A, Michel CM, Landis T. Visual recognition of faces, objects, and words using degraded stimuli: where and when it occurs. *Human Brain Mapping* 2004;**22**:300–311.

91. Murray MM, Foxe JJ, Higgins BA, Javitt DC, Schroeder CE. Visuo-spatial neural response interactions in early cortical processing during a simple reaction time task: a high-density electrical mapping study. *Neuropsychologia* 2001;**39**:828–844.

92. Murray MM, Molholm S, Michel CM *et al.* Grabbing your ear: rapid auditory-somatosensory multisensory interactions in low-level sensory cortices are not constrained by stimulus alignment. *Cerebral Cortex* 2005;**15**:963–974.

93. Murray MM, Camen C, Gonzalez Andino SL, Bovet P, Clarke S. Rapid brain discrimination of sounds of objects. *Journal of Neuroscience* 2006;**26**:1293–1302.

94. Murray MM, Imber ML, Javitt DC, Foxe JJ. Boundary completion is automatic and dissociable from shape discrimination. *Journal of Neuroscience* 2006;**26**:12043–12054.

95. De Santis L, Clarke S, Murray MM. Automatic and intrinsic auditory "what" and "where" processing in humans revealed by electrical neuroimaging. *Cerebral Cortex* 2007;**17**:9–17.

96. De Santis L, Spierer L, Clarke S, Murray MM. Getting in touch: segregated somatosensory what and where pathways in humans revealed by electrical neuroimaging. *Neuroimage* 2007;**37**:890–903.

97. Thut G, Hauert CA, Morand S, Seeck M, Landis T, Michel C. Evidence for interhemispheric motor-level transfer in a simple reaction time task: an EEG study. *Experimental Brain Research* 1999;**128**:256–261.

98. Thut G, Hauert CA, Viviani P *et al.* Internally driven versus externally cued movement selection: a study on the timing of brain activity. *Cognitive Brain Research* 2000;**9**:261–269.

99. Caldara R, Deiber MP, Andrey C *et al.* Actual and mental motor preparation and execution: a spatiotemporal ERP study. *Experimental Brain Research* 2004;**159**:389–399.

100. Khateb A, Michel CM, Pegna AJ, Landis T, Annoni JM. New insights into the Stroop effect: a spatio-temporal analysis of electric brain activity. *Neuroreport* 2000;**11**:1849–1855.

101. Gonzalez Andino SL, Michel CM, Thut G, Landis T, Grave de Peralta R. Prediction of response speed by anticipatory high-frequency (gamma band) oscillations in the human brain. *Human Brain Mapping* 2005;**24**:50–58.

102. Schnider A, Valenza N, Morand S, Michel CM. Early cortical distinction between memories that pertain to ongoing reality and memories that don't. *Cerebral Cortex* 2002;**12**:54–61.

103. Schnider A, Mohr C, Morand S, Michel CM. Early cortical response to

behaviorally relevant absence of anticipated outcomes: a human event-related potential study. *Neuroimage* 2007;**35**:1348–1355.

104. Murray MM, Michel CM, Grave de Peralta R *et al.* Rapid discrimination of visual and multisensory memories revealed by electrical neuroimaging. *Neuroimage* 2004;**21**:125–135.

105. Khateb A, Michel CM, Pegna AJ *et al.* The time course of semantic category processing in the cerebral hemispheres: an electrophysiological study. *Cognitive Brain Research* 2001;**10**:251–264.

106. Khateb A, Michel CM, Pegna AJ *et al.* Processing of semantic categorical and associative relations: an ERP mapping study. *International Journal of Psychophysiology* 2003;**49**:41–55.

107. Khateb A, Pegna AJ, Landis T *et al.* Rhyme processing in the brain: an ERP mapping study. *International Journal of Psychophysiology* 2007;**63**:240–250.

108. Khateb A, Abutalebi J, Michel CM *et al.* Language selection in bilinguals: a spatio-temporal analysis of electric brain activity. *International Journal of Psychophysiology* 2007;**65**:201–213.

109. Wirth M, Horn H, Koenig T *et al.* Sex differences in semantic processing: event-related brain potentials distinguish between lower and higher order semantic analysis during word reading. *Cerebral Cortex* 2007;**17**:1987–1997.

110. Ortigue S, Michel CM, Murray MM *et al.* Electrical neuroimaging reveals early generator modulation to emotional words. *Neuroimage* 2004;**21**:1242–1251.

111. Pourtois G, Thut G, Grave de Peralta R, Michel C, Vuilleumier P. Two electrophysiological stages of spatial orienting towards fearful faces: early temporo-parietal activation preceding gain control in extrastriate visual cortex. *Neuroimage* 2005;**26**:149–163.

112. Gianotti LR, Faber PL, Schuler M *et al.* First valence, then arousal: the temporal dynamics of brain electric activity evoked by emotional stimuli. *Brain Topography* 2008;**20**:143–156.

113. Caldara R, Thut G, Servoir P *et al.* Face versus non-face object perception and the 'other-race' effect: a spatio-temporal event-related potential study. *Clinical Neurophysiology* 2003;**114**:515–528.

114. Thierry G, Martin CD, Downing P, Pegna AJ. Controlling for interstimulus perceptual variance abolishes N170 face selectivity. *Nature Neuroscience* 2007;**10**: 505–511.

115. Petit LS, Pegna AJ, Harris IM, Michel CM. Automatic motor cortex activation for natural as compared to awkward grips of a manipulable object. *Experimental Brain Research* 2006;**168**:120–130.

116. Overney LS, Michel CM, Harris IM, Pegna AJ. Cerebral processes in mental transformations of body parts: recognition prior to rotation. *Brain Research. Cognitive Brain Research* 2005;**25**:722–734.

117. Blanke O, Mohr C, Michel CM *et al.* Linking out-of-body experience and self processing to mental own-body imagery at the temporoparietal junction. *Journal of Neuroscience* 2005;**25**:550–557.

118. Arzy S, Thut G, Mohr C, Michel CM, Blanke O. Neural basis of embodiment: distinct contributions of temporoparietal junction and extrastriate body area. *Journal of Neuroscience* 2006;**26**:8074–8081.

119. Seeck M, Michel CM, Mainwaring N *et al.* Evidence for rapid face recognition from human scalp and intracranial electrodes. *Neuroreport* 1997;**8**:2749–2754.

120. Koenig T, Lehmann D. Microstates in language-related brain potential maps show noun-verb differences. *Brain and Language* 1996;**53**:169–182.

121. Tardif E, Murray MM, Meylan R, Spierer L, Clarke S. The spatio-temporal brain dynamics of processing and integrating sound localization cues in humans. *Brain Research* 2006;**1092**:161–176.

122. Thorpe S, Fize D, Marlot C. Speed of processing in the human visual system. *Nature* 1996;**381**:520–522.

123. Schroeder CE, Mehta AD, Givre SJ. A spatiotemporal profile of visual system activation revealed by current source density analysis in the awake macaque. *Cerebral Cortex* 1998;**8**:575–592.

124. Bullier J. Integrated model of visual processing. *Brain Research. Brain Research Review* 2001;**36**:96–107.

125. Arieli A, Sterkin A, Grinvald A, Aertsen A. Dynamics of ongoing activity: explanation of the large variability in evoked cortical responses. *Science* 1996;**273**:1868–1871.

126. Fries P, Neuenschwander S, Engel AK, Goebel R, Singer W. Rapid feature selective neuronal synchronization through correlated latency shifting. *Nature Neuroscience* 2001;**4**:194–200.

127. van der Togt C, Spekreijse H, Super H. Neural responses in cat visual cortex reflect state changes in correlated activity. *European Journal of Neuroscience* 2005;**22**:465–475.

128. Super H, van der Togt C, Spekreijse H, Lamme VA. Internal state of monkey primary visual cortex (V1) predicts figure-ground perception. *Journal of Neuroscience* 2003;**23**:3407–3414.

129. van der Togt C, Kalitzin S, Spekreijse H, Lamme VA, Super H. Synchrony dynamics in monkey V1 predict success in visual detection. *Cerebral Cortex* 2006;**16**:136–148.

130. Womelsdorf T, Fries P, Mitra PP, Desimone R. Gamma-band synchronization in visual cortex predicts speed of change detection. *Nature* 2006;**439**:733–736.

131. Ergenoglu T, Demiralp T, Bayraktaroglu Z et al. Alpha rhythm of the EEG modulates visual detection performance in humans. *Brain Research. Cognitive Brain Research* 2004;**20**:376–383.

132. Hanslmayr S, Sauseng P, Doppelmayr M, Schabus M, Klimesch W. Increasing individual upper alpha power by neurofeedback improves cognitive performance in human subjects. *Applied Psychophysiology and Biofeedback* 2005;**30**:1–10.

133. Babiloni C, Vecchio F, Bultrini A, Luca Romani G, Rossini PM. Pre- and poststimulus alpha rhythms are related to conscious visual perception: a high-resolution EEG study. *Cerebral Cortex* 2006;**16**:1690–1700.

134. Thut G, Nietzel A, Brandt SA, Pascual-Leone A. Alpha-band electroencephalographic activity over occipital cortex indexes visuospatial attention bias and predicts visual target detection. *Journal of Neuroscience* 2006;**26**:9494–9502.

135. Rihs TA, Michel CM, Thut G. Mechanisms of selective inhibition in visual spatial attention are indexed by alpha-band EEG synchronization. *European Journal of Neuroscience* 2007;**25**:603–610.

136. Romei V, Brodbeck V, Michel C et al. Spontaneous fluctuations in posterior {alpha}-band EEG activity reflect variability in excitability of human visual areas. *Cerebral Cortex* 2008;**18**:2010–2018.

137. Ress D, Backus BT, Heeger DJ. Activity in primary visual cortex predicts performance in a visual detection task. *Nature Neuroscience* 2000;**3**:940–945.

138. Fox MD, Snyder AZ, Zacks JM, Raichle ME. Coherent spontaneous activity accounts for trial-to-trial variability in human evoked brain responses. *Nature Neuroscience* 2006;**9**:23–25.

139. Lehmann D, Michel CM, Pal I, Pascual-Marqui RD. Event-related potential maps depend on prestimulus brain electric microstate map. *International Journal of Neuroscience* 1994;**74**:239–248.

140. Kondakor I, Pascual-Marqui RD, Michel CM, Lehmann D. Event-related potential map differences depend on the prestimulus microstates. *Journal of Medical Engineering and Technology* 1995;**19**:66–69.

141. Kondakor I, Lehmann D, Michel CM et al. Prestimulus EEG microstates influence visual event-related potential microstates in field maps with 47 channels. *Journal of Neural Transmission* 1997;**104**:161–173.

142. Müller TJ, Koenig T, Wackermann J et al. Subsecond changes of global brain state in illusory multistable motion perception. *Journal of Neural Transmission* 2005;**112**:565–576.

143. Müller TJ, Federspiel A, Fallgatter AJ, Strik WK. EEG signs of vigilance fluctuations preceding perceptual flips in multistable illusionary motion. *Neuroreport* 1999;**10**:3423–3427.

144. Mohr C, Michel CM, Lantz G et al. Brain state-dependent functional hemispheric

specialization in men but not in women. *Cerebral Cortex* 2005;**15**:1451–1458.

145. Graves R, Landis T, Goodglass H. Laterality and sex differences for visual recognition of emotional and non-emotional words. *Neuropsychologia* 1981;**19**:95–102.

146. Britz J, Landis T, Michel CM. Right parietal brain activity precedes perceptual alternation of bistable stimuli. *Cerebral Cortex* 2009;**19**:55–65.

147. Makeig S, Westerfield M, Jung TP *et al.* Dynamic brain sources of visual evoked responses. *Science* 2002;**295**:690–694.

148. Quian Quiroga R, Garcia H. Single-trial event-related potentials with wavelet denoising. *Clinical Neurophysiology* 2003; **114**:376–390.

149. Knuth KH, Shah AS, Truccolo WA *et al.* Differentially variable component analysis: identifying multiple evoked components using trial-to-trial variability. *Journal of Neurophysiology* 2006;**95**:3257–3276.

150. Jongsma ML, Eichele T, Van Rijn CM *et al.* Tracking pattern learning with single-trial event-related potentials. *Clinical Neurophysiology* 2006;**117**:1957–1973.

151. Quian Quiroga R, van Luijtelaar EL. Habituation and sensitization in rat auditory evoked potentials: a single-trial analysis with wavelet denoising. *International Journal of Psychophysiology* 2002;**43**:141–153.

152. Quian Quiroga R, Snyder LH, Batista AP, Cui H, Andersen RA. Movement intention is better predicted than attention in the posterior parietal cortex. *Journal of Neuroscience* 2006;**26**:3615–3620.

153. Singer W. Synchronization of cortical activity and its putative role in information processing and learning. *Annual Review of Physiology* 1993;**55**:349–374.

154. Engel AK, Fries P, Singer W. Dynamic predictions: oscillations and synchrony in top-down processing. *Nature Review Neuroscience* 2001;**2**:704–716.

155. Lee KH, Williams LM, Breakspear M, Gordon E. Synchronous gamma activity: a review and contribution to an integrative neuroscience model of schizophrenia. *Brain Research. Brain Research Review* 2003;**41**:57–78.

156. Bell AJ, Sejnowski TJ. An information-maximization approach to blind separation and blind deconvolution. *Neural Comput* 1995;**7**:1129–1159.

157. Hyvarinen A, Oja E. A fast fixed-point algorithm for independent component analysis. *Neural Computation* 1997;**9**: 1483–1492.

158. Vigario RN. Extraction of ocular artefacts from EEG using independent component analysis. *Electroencephalography and Clinical Neurophysiology* 1997;**103**:395–404.

159. Barbati G, Porcaro C, Zappasodi F, Rossini PM, Tecchio F. Optimization of an independent component analysis approach for artifact identification and removal in magnetoencephalographic signals. *Clinical Neurophysiology* 2004;**115**:1220–1232.

160. Delorme A, Makeig S. EEGLAB: an open source toolbox for analysis of single-trial EEG dynamics including independent component analysis. *Journal of Neuroscience Methods* 2004;**134**:9–21.

161. Mantini D, Franciotti R, Romani GL, Pizzella V. Improving MEG source localizations: an automated method for complete artifact removal based on independent component analysis. *Neuroimage* 2008;**40**:160–173.

162. Nakamura W, Anami K, Mori T *et al.* Removal of ballistocardiogram artifacts from simultaneously recorded EEG and fMRI data using independent component analysis. *IEEE Transactions on Biomedical Engineering* 2006;**53**:1294–1308.

163. Mantini D, Perrucci MG, Cugini S *et al.* Complete artifact removal for EEG recorded during continuous fMRI using independent component analysis. *Neuroimage* 2007;**34**:598–607.

164. Grouiller F, Vercueil L, Krainik A *et al.* A comparative study of different artefact removal algorithms for EEG signals acquired during functional MRI. *Neuroimage* 2007;**38**:124–137.

165. Womelsdorf T, Schoffelen JM, Oostenveld R *et al.* Modulation of neuronal interactions through neuronal synchronization. *Science* 2007;**316**:1609–1612.

166. Onton J, Delorme A, Makeig S. Frontal midline EEG dynamics during working memory. *Neuroimage* 2005;**27**:341–356.

167. Onton J, Westerfield M, Townsend J, Makeig S. Imaging human EEG dynamics using independent component analysis. *Neuroscience and Biobehavioral Reviews* 2006;**30**:808–822.

168. Makeig S. Response: event-related brain dynamics – unifying brain electrophysiology. *Trends in Neuroscience* 2002;**25**:390.

169. Jansen BH, Agarwal G, Hegde A, Boutros NN. Phase synchronization of the ongoing EEG and auditory EP generation. *Clinical Neurophysiology* 2003;**114**:79–85.

170. Shah AS, Bressler SL, Knuth KH et al. Neural dynamics and the fundamental mechanisms of event-related brain potentials. *Cerebral Cortex* 2004;**14**: 476–483.

171. Belouchrani A, Abed-Merain K, Cardoso J-F, Moulines E. A blind source separation technique using second-order statistics. *IEEE Transactions on Signaling Processes* 1997;**5**:434–444.

172. Barbati G, Sigismondi R, Zappasodi F et al. Functional source separation from magnetoencephalographic signals. *Human Brain Mapping* 2006;**27**:925–934.

173. Georgiadis SD, Ranta-aho PO, Tarvainen MP, Karjalainen PA. Single-trial dynamical estimation of event-related potentials: a Kalman filter-based approach. *IEEE Transactions on Biomedical Engineering* 2005;**52**:1397–1406.

174. Wang Z, Maier A, Leopold DA, Logothetis NK, Liang H. Single-trial evoked potential estimation using wavelets. *Computers in Biology and Medicine* 2007;**37**:463–473.

175. Bai O, Lin P, Vorbach S et al. Exploration of computational methods for classification of movement intention during human voluntary movement from single trial EEG. *Clinical Neurophysiology* 2007;**118**:2637–2655.

176. Muller KR, Tangermann M, Dornhege G et al. Machine learning for real-time single-trial EEG-analysis: from brain-computer interfacing to mental state monitoring. *Journal of Neuroscientific Methods* 2008;**167**:82–90.

177. De Lucia M, Michel CM, Clarke S, Murray MM. Single-trial topographic analysis of human EEG: a new 'image' of event-related potentials. *Proceedings of the IEEE/EMBS Region 8 International Conference on Information Technology Applications in Biomedicine*, ITAB 2007; article 4407353, pp 95–98.

178. De Lucia M, Michel CM, Clarke S, Murray MM. Single subject EEG analysis based on topographic information. *International Journal of Bioelectromagnetism* 2007;**9**: 168–171.

179. Alarcon G, Guy CN, Binnie CD et al. Intracerebral propagation of interictal activity in partial epilepsy: implications for source localisation. *Journal of Neurology, Neurosurgery and Psychiatry* 1994;**57**:435–449.

180. Engel J, Jr. Intracerebral recordings: organization of the human epileptogenic region. *Journal of Clinical Neurophysiology* 1993;**10**:90–98.

181. Alarcon G, Seoane JJG, Binnie CD et al. Origin and propagation of interictal discharges in the acute electrocorticogram. Implications for pathophysiology and surgical treatment of temporal lobe epilepsy. *Brain* 1997;**120**:259–282.

182. Ebersole JS. Non-invasive pre-surgical evaluation with EEG/MEG source analysis. *Electroencephalography and Clinical Neurophysiology Supplement* 1999;**50**:167–174.

183. Merlet I, Gotman J. Reliability of dipole models of epileptic spikes. *Clinical Neurophysiology* 1999;**110**:1013–1028.

184. Scherg M, Bast T, Berg P. Multiple source analysis of interictal spikes: goals, requirements, and clinical value. *Journal of Clinical Neurophysiology* 1999;**16**:214–224.

185. Huppertz HJ, Hoegg S, Sick C et al. Cortical current density reconstruction of interictal epileptiform activity in temporal lobe epilepsy. *Clinical Neurophysiology* 2001;**112**:1761–1772.

186. Merlet I, Garcia-Larrea L, Gregoire MC, Lavenne F, Mauguière F. Source propagation of interictal spikes in temporal lobe epilepsy. Correlations between spike dipole modelling and

[18F]fluorodeoxyglucose PET data. *Brain* 1996;**119**:377–392.

187. Seeck M, Lazeyras F, Michel CM *et al.* Non invasive epileptic focus localization using EEG-triggered functional MRI and electromagnetic tomography. *Electroencephalography and Clinical Neurophysiology* 1998;**106**:508–512.

188. Lantz G, Spinelli L, Menendez RG, Seeck M, Michel CM. Localization of distributed sources and comparison with functional MRI. *Epileptic Disorders* 2001;**Special Issue**:45–58.

189. Lantz G, Michel CM, Pascual-Marqui RD *et al.* Extracranial localization of intracranial interictal epileptiform activity using LORETA (low resolution electromagnetic tomography). *Electroencephalography and Clinical Neurophysiology* 1997;**102**:414–422.

190. Lantz G, Grave de Peralta R, Gonzalez S, Michel CM. Noninvasive localization of electromagnetic epileptic activity. II. Demonstration of sublobar accuracy in patients with simultaneous surface and depth recordings. *Brain Topography* 2001;**14**:139–147.

191. Lantz G, Spinelli L, Seeck M *et al.* Propagation of interictal epileptiform activity can lead to erroneous source localizations: a 128 channel EEG mapping study. *Journal of Clinical Neurophysiology* 2003;**20**:311–319.

192. Lantz G, Grave de Peralta R, Spinelli L, Seeck M, Michel CM. Epileptic source localization with high density EEG: how many electrodes are needed? *Clinical Neurophysiology* 2003;**114**:63–69.

193. Michel CM, Lantz G, Spinelli L *et al.* 128-channel EEG source imaging in epilepsy: clinical yield and localization precision. *Journal of Clinical Neurophysiology* 2004;**21**:71–83.

194. Sperli F, Spinelli L, Seeck M *et al.* EEG source imaging in paediatric epilepsy surgery: a new perspective in presurgical workup. *Epilepsia* 2006;**47**:981–990.

195. Zumsteg D, Friedman A, Wennberg RA, Wieser HG. Source localization of mesial temporal interictal epileptiform discharges: correlation with intracranial foramen ovale electrode recordings. *Clinical Neurophysiology* 2005;**116**:2810–2818.

196. Zumsteg D, Andrade DM, Wennberg RA. Source localization of small sharp spikes: low resolution electromagnetic tomography (LORETA) reveals two distinct cortical sources. *Clinical Neurophysiology* 2006;**117**:1380–1387.

197. Zumsteg D, Friedman A, Wieser HG, Wennberg RA. Source localization of interictal epileptiform discharges: comparison of three different techniques to improve signal to noise ratio. *Clinical Neurophysiology* 2006;**117**:562–571.

198. Holmes MD, Brown M, Tucker DM. Are "generalized" seizures truly generalized? Evidence of localized mesial frontal and frontopolar discharges in absence. *Epilepsia* 2004;**45**:1568–1579.

199. Worrell GA, Lagerlund TD, Sharbrough FW *et al.* Localization of the epileptic focus by low-resolution electromagnetic tomography in patients with a lesion demonstrated by MRI. *Brain Topography* 2000;**12**:273–282.

200. Grave de Peralta Menendez R, Gonzalez Andino S, Lantz G, Michel CM, Landis T. Noninvasive localization of electromagnetic epileptic activity. I. Method descriptions and simulations. *Brain Topography* 2001;**14**:131–137.

201. Spinelli L, Andino SG, Lantz G, Seeck M, Michel CM. Electromagnetic inverse solutions in anatomically constrained spherical head models. *Brain Topography* 2000;**13**:115–125.

# Multichannel frequency and time-frequency analysis

Thomas Koenig and Roberto D. Pascual-Marqui

## Introduction and overview

Time series of EEG scalp potential differences typically appear to be composed of oscillations at various frequencies. Although the amplitude and spatial distributions of these oscillations may fluctuate in time, the quantification of these oscillations as a function of frequency and location (i.e. the multichannel spectral analysis of the EEG) is very reproducible within and across subjects and systematically varies depending on a series of physiologically interesting factors. To mention a few examples, EEG spectral analysis has been successfully employed to characterize a subject's age[1], state of arousal[2], the presence of neurological or psychiatric disorders[3], drugs[4,5] or task demand[6,7] as systematic deviations of spectral power from a norm.

In the present chapter, we will outline the possibilities of quantifying EEG oscillations with a special emphasis on those aspects that are specific for multichannel EEG. First, a methodological primer delineates the interdependencies among spectral amplitude, phase and recording montage. In addition, it also delineates what scalp signals we expect from one or several known oscillating sources in the brain. Next, we describe the currently employed analysis strategies: starting from the classic EEG spectral power mapping of measured EEG, we proceed to methods that take into account the relations of amplitude and phase between the different electrodes, which is an essential prerequisite for discussing the results in terms of sources and interactions of brain regions. Finally, we delineate possible methods for custom-tailored quantitative analyses of multichannel EEG oscillations and source localization in the frequency domain.

Electroencephalogram oscillations often are not continuous, but transient. The occurrence, amplitude and spatial distribution of such transient oscillations may vary spontaneously or in a systematic relation to some event. Many of these transient oscillations occur in the sub-second range and are not well accounted for by typical FFT-based analyses. The method of choice to characterize such transient EEG oscillations is the wavelet analysis that decomposes signals into oscillatory components with a limited duration in time[8]. As previously discussed in Chapter 5, we aim at wavelets that have an optimal resolution in time and frequency, whereas frequency is typically defined by sinusoidal oscillations. This objective is optimally met by so-called Gabor functions that are defined as real or complex exponentials (sine and cosine waves) that are modulated by a Gaussian envelope with a defined extent and peak time. This chapter will thus introduce systematically how to obtain meaningful descriptions and quantifiers of multichannel EEG data that have been submitted to a Gabor transformation.

*Electrical Neuroimaging*, ed. Christoph M. Michel, Thomas Koenig, Daniel Brandeis, Lorena R.R. Gianotti and Jiří Wackermann. Published by Cambridge University Press. © Cambridge University Press 2009.

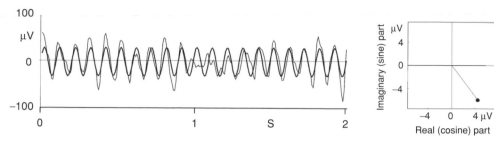

**Figure 7.1** A single channel of alpha EEG (gray line) and the 10 Hz complex exponential employed by the FFT to explain the variance at 10 Hz. The polar representation is at the right.

The FFT-based EEG analysis and the EEG analysis using Gabor functions are related: from a computational point of view, the results of a Gabor transformation with a defined Gaussian envelope are equivalent to those of an FFT applied to EEG data that has been amplitude modulated using the same envelope. Although computationally clumsy, this allows us to extend many of the arguments that will be made for FFT-transformed EEG data into Gabor-transformed EEG data. We will thus first introduce a series of arguments and methods that apply to the FFT-transformed data, and then transfer and extend them to Gabor-transformed EEG data.

## Frequency-domain EEG analysis
### Frequency, amplitude, power and phase of a single channel

Fourier transformation-based spectral analysis decomposes a signal into a weighted sum of sine and cosine functions with different frequencies and amplitudes. These continuous functions form the "atomic" elements or words of the dictionary of FFT-based spectral analysis.

In Chapter 5, we saw that for a given frequency, the resulting weights of the cosine and sine parts of the signal are the real and imaginary part of a complex exponential and can be represented as a point in a sine–cosine diagram (Figure 7.1).

By converting the Cartesian (XY) coordinates of such a point into polar coordinates, the point becomes represented by a radius and an angle. In polar coordinates, the radius of the point from the coordinate system's origin indicates the amplitude of the signal, and the angle between the vector connecting the point with the origin and the x-axis indicates the phase angle. This phase angle is directly proportional to the latency of the first maximum of the oscillation at the frequency of interest.

How does a change of the reference affect the spectral amplitude and phase at the different electrodes? The reference has by definition no amplitude; it is therefore by definition at the origin of the coordinate system. If several electrodes have been recorded against a common reference, the relation of amplitude and phase between the different electrodes can be visualized by entering the sine and cosine values of several electrodes into the polar plot.

Since the reference coincides by definition with the origin of the coordinate system, changing the reference is equivalent to changing the origin of the coordinate system. In Figure 7.2, the sine and cosine values of three electrodes at 10 Hz have been entered into a common plot. Each of the three electrodes has been used once as reference and is thus at the origin of the coordinate system and the other two channels have been recomputed against that reference. The spectral amplitude and the phase angles of the three signals against the reference are shown below the polar plot (Figure 7.2).

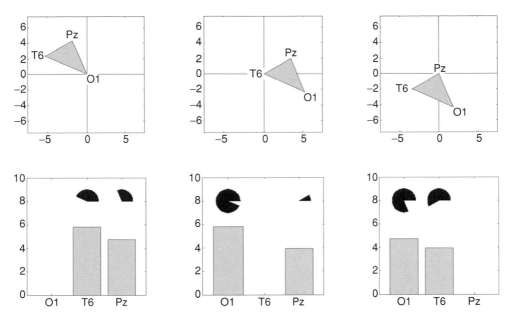

**Figure 7.2** The upper row shows the sine–cosine diagram of an EEG with three channels. Each channel has been used once as the recording reference (Left, O1; middle, T6; right, Pz). The triangle indicates the phase and amplitude relations among the channels. The lower row shows the amplitudes and phases corresponding to the sine–cosine diagrams against the reference.

An inspection of Figure 7.2 shows that a change of reference does not affect the phase and amplitude relationships between the electrodes. The gray triangle in the upper graph of Figure 7.2 represents these relationships. By changing the reference, the triangle changes neither in size nor geometry, but only in its position in the coordinate system. The absolute amplitude and phase at the different electrodes (as shown in the lower graph), however, change drastically when another reference is used. The observation that a change of reference changes the absolute phase and amplitude values in frequency-domain EEG, but does not affect the phase and amplitude relationship between the different EEG channels is analogous to the observation that in time-domain EEG data, a change of reference changes the potential values at the electrodes, but does not affect the potential differences between the electrodes. Mathematically, re-referencing in time- and frequency-domain EEG data must be analogous because both the transformation of data between the time domain and the frequency domain and the change of reference are linear operations.

The arguments and conclusions made about the reference in Chapter 2 thus apply equally to frequency-transformed EEG data. This means that:

(1) Spectral amplitudes strongly depend on the choice of reference, as illustrated in Figure 7.2.

(2) It is not possible to prove in general that some point on the scalp or elsewhere is electrically inactive and can therefore be used as the "correct" reference for EEG spectral analysis.

A desirable property of EEG data would be that across the entire head surface, the integral of all real (cosine) values and the integral of all complex (sine) values are always zero[9].

This is, however, not measurable. If a large part of the head has been covered by a sufficiently large number of approximately equally spaced electrodes, it can be approximated by setting the sums of all real and imaginary values to zero. This is equivalent to the computation of the common average reference or to centering the complex plane at the mean of all points. Analyses in frequency-domain EEG data that are based on the relationship of phase and amplitude between channels and not on absolute phase and amplitude are in general reference independent if properly done. This holds also for the computation of frequency-domain inverse solutions.

## Amplitude, power and phase of a single intracerebral oscillating source

In Chapter 3, it was shown that the activity of a point source instantaneously produces an electrical potential field that extends across the entire scalp. For a point source with a given position and a given orientation, one can compute a factor by which the activity at the source is multiplied to obtain the potential at a defined scalp position. The distribution of these factors across the scalp is called the lead field of the point source (see Chapter 3). The lead field is always dipolar (i.e. it has an area that has negative potentials and an area that has positive potentials, although these areas may not always be covered by the electrode array), while the amplitude of the potential varies depending on the scalp position and the strength, orientation and position of the point source. The computation of the lead field at the electrode array is called the forward solution (see Chapter 3).

The fact that the signal of a single source at a single electrode is always exactly proportional to the activity of the source itself implies that if only a single source is active, changes in the activity of the source result in exactly simultaneous and proportional changes of the signal at all electrodes.

Assume that we have a single point source that oscillates with some constant frequency and amplitude in the brain. What would the amplitudes and phase angles of the different electrodes look like in the complex plane? The fact that changes in the activity of a source occur simultaneously with the changes in the scalp potential field implies that the oscillations observed on the scalp are locked in time. Two different channels may pick up either the same or the opposite pole of the scalp electric field. Therefore, their oscillations may either be in phase (reach the maximum and minimum at the same moment in time) or in counterphase (while one channel reaches a maximum, the other one reaches a minimum). More precisely, among any pair of electrodes, we may only observe differences of phase angles that are either 0 or 180°. Finally, because for a given source, the amplitude of the scalp potential depends on the scalp position, different electrodes will show oscillations with different amplitudes. On the complex plane, this implies that all electrodes have either the same or the opposite phase angle and must therefore lie on a straight line that crosses the origin (reference) of the plane. The position of an electrode on that line in reference to any other electrode depends on the amplitude differences between the two electrodes and whether they are in phase or in counterphase. The orientation of the line on the complex plane depends only on the phase of the oscillation of the source and is random if the epoch has been selected at a random time interval (Figure 7.3).

## Amplitude, power and phase of several intracerebral oscillating sources

As we learned in Chapter 3, EEG scalp fields are additive: when several sources in the brain are simultaneously active, the resulting scalp field is equal to the sum of the scalp fields that each of the sources produces. For a given electrode, this means that the measured signal is the

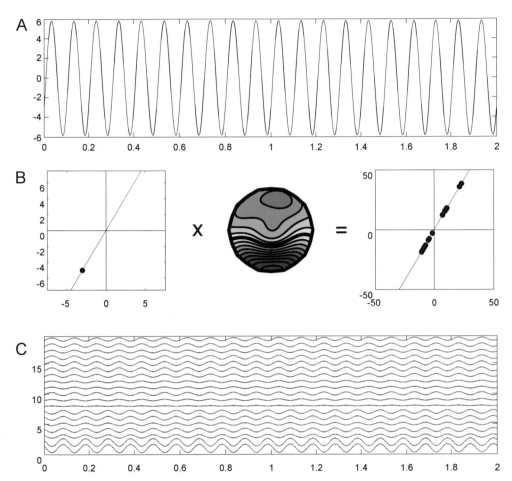

**Figure 7.3** Simulation of an EEG produced by a single, constantly oscillating intracerebral source. A. Oscillation of the source across time. B. Left graph shows the sine–cosine diagram of the oscillation shown in A. The central map in B shows the distribution of the scalp field produced by the assumed source. The resulting EEG potentials are shown in a sine–cosine diagram in B to the right, and as EEG traces in C.

sum of the signals of all active sources weighted by the forward solutions of these sources at the given electrode position. This also holds for frequency-transformed EEG data. If several sources in the brain oscillate at the same frequency, the sine and cosine values obtained by FFT transforming the resulting EEG are the sum of the sine and cosine values resulting from each of the oscillating sources (Figure 7.4).

## Amplitude and power of real EEG data

In the case of resting-state EEG, the amplitude of the signals is typically assumed to be of interest, while the phase information is mostly ignored. This is so because the phase of the signals at the electrodes is randomly distributed due to the fact that EEG epochs in resting EEG are selected at random time intervals. (Note that the phase-relationships between electrodes are not random, because they are determined by the configuration and interaction of intracerebral sources.) The method chosen to deal with such data has thus often been the

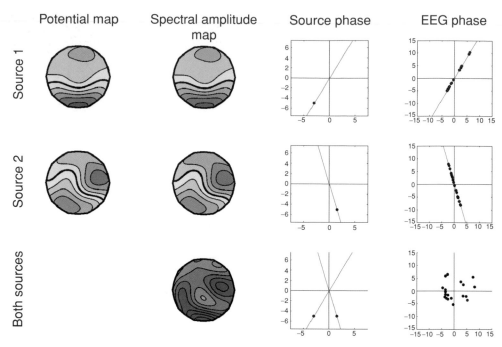

Potential map | Spectral amplitude map | Source phase | EEG phase

Source 1 | Source 2 | Both sources

**Figure 7.4** Simulation with two hypothetical sources oscillating at the same frequency, but with different phase. The left-most column shows the scalp fields produced by the sources and the next column shows the spectral amplitudes expected by the two sources and by the simultaneous activity of both sources. The graphs of the third and fourth columns show the sine–cosine diagrams of the sources and the EEG. Note that the spectral amplitude map obtained by combining both sources (second column, third row) is not the sum of the spectral amplitude maps obtained for each of the two sources.

mapping and comparison of averaged spectral amplitude or power maps. This has been very successful and sensitive for describing i.e. age-related EEG changes, changes related to fluctuating vigilance and sleep, drug-effects, or clinically relevant conditions such as neurological and psychiatric disorders[5,10–15]. An example comparing the spectral amplitudes of a patient with Alzheimer's dementia and a healthy control is shown in Figure 7.5.

Because the phase relationships between electrodes are lost, the spectral amplitudes and power are reference-dependent and inverse solutions to localize the sources cannot be applied. This is a major disadvantage of this method. For a recent discussion of reference effects on spectral power, see Yuvat-Greenberg et al.[16].

## Phase of real EEG data and measures of phase synchronization

In an ongoing EEG, the phase information at a given frequency and channel may eventually depend on some events, but is random in the classic case where the analysis epochs have been selected at random time intervals. There may nevertheless be strong phase interdependencies between channels and between frequencies. The interdependencies among channels may result from volume conduction and from the spontaneous coupling of brain regions with oscillating electric activity. Since the effects of volume conduction can be assumed to be relatively constant, the coupling among brain regions as a function of the subject's condition may systematically change the observed phase interdependencies. Quantifying and

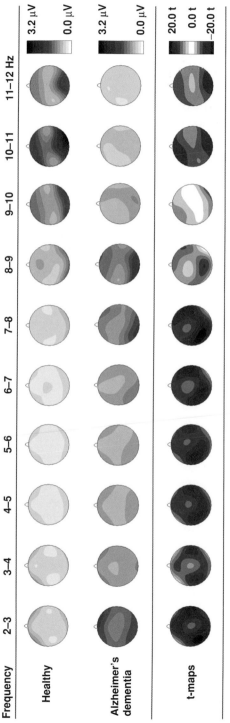

**Figure 7.5** shows average spectral amplitude maps of a healthy control (upper row) and a patient with Alzheimer's type dementia (lower row). The patient has higher spectral amplitude across large scalp areas in the delta and theta band, and lower spectral amplitude in the alpha band. This is illustrated by t-maps computed based on the averages and standard deviations over the single epochs of the two subjects.

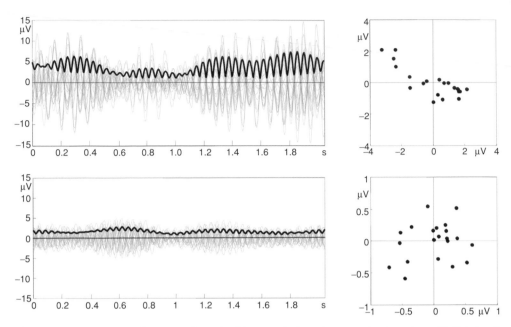

**Figure 7.6** Alpha-bandpass-filtered EEG from a healthy control subject (upper row) and a patient with Alzheimer's dementia. The graphs on the left show an overlay of the EEG traces and the global field power of the EEG, while the graphs on the right show the corresponding sine–cosine diagrams. The global field power curve is much more modulated in the control subject, indicating that the moments of maximal signal strength tend to coincide across electrodes. This is not the case in the patient's EEG. Furthermore, the sine–cosine diagrams show a preferential phase across electrodes for the control subject, but not for the patient.

comparing phase interdependencies between electrodes is thus a convenient way to measure the strength of coupling of activity between brain regions.

Figure 7.6 shows two examples of an alpha-bandpass-filtered EEG and its GFP on one side, and the sine–cosine diagram of all electrodes at the alpha frequency on the other side. One EEG is from a healthy control and the other is from a patient with dementia. In the control subject, the cloud of electrode entries in the sine–cosine diagram has an elongated shape, and electrodes showing large amplitudes (distances from the origin) appear to lie more or less on a line crossing the origin. The orientation of the cloud in the sine–cosine diagram is meaningless, because it depends on the randomly chosen onset of the epoch. The relationship among the phase angles of the different electrodes, however, depends on the temporal and spatial relationship between the oscillating generators in the brain. The fact that there is a phase that is predominating across electrodes can theoretically have two interpretations:

(1) There is a single source in the brain that accounts for a large proportion of the measured EEG. The phase of the EEG at the different electrodes is thus determined by the phase of this source (as is exemplified in Figure 7.3 above). The remaining part of the signal is random noise, i.e. noise with random amplitude and random phase that adds a spread to the electrode entries in the sine–cosine diagram in all directions, and thus transforms the initial line of entries into an elongated cloud. The amount of elongation of the cloud would thus depend on the signal-to-noise ratio of the EEG produced by that single source. A large signal-to-noise ratio would produce a more elongated cloud, and a low signal-to-noise ratio would produce a more circular cloud. Such a model is plausible

when there is good reason to assume one predominant source. Examples for such cases are, for example, pathological conditions such as epilepsy or tumors, or when a specific well-circumscribed brain region is stimulated at a fixed and rather fast frequency such that driving phenomena occur. The model is however unlikely in general cases, where presumably many generators are active simultaneously.

(2) There are several sources active that operate in an approximately phase-locked, zero-delay mode, such that they appear as a single meta-generator that hence produces a common phase across electrodes.

The observation that there is a predominant phase across electrodes is incompatible with the existence of several, similarly visible EEG generators that operate at independent phases. Given that there is a predominant phase across electrodes, and given that it is unlikely that this can be accounted for by a single source, this implies that at the given frequency, the brain electric oscillations visible to EEG synchronize across a major proportion of the active sources[17–19,20].

The patient with dementia shown in Figure 7.6 has considerably lower amplitudes of the signals, but the signals also appear to have less zero-phase synchronization in time. This becomes clearly apparent in the sine–cosine diagram, where there is little evidence for a common phase across electrodes. One may thus speculate that the changes we observe in EEG are at least partly due to a disorganization of oscillatory neural activity in time, and the reduction of signal amplitude may at least partly be caused by an increased cancellation of signals on the level of the EEG.

The differences observed in the sine–cosine diagram can be quantified on a global level by computing a principal component analysis (PCA) based on the two-dimensional positions of the electrode-entries in the sine–cosine diagram: the sum of the resulting two eigenvalues can be used as a simple indicator of cloud size, or global spectral amplitude. The shape of the cloud can be quantified using the normalized difference between the two eigenvalues. The more the eigenvalue of the first PC exceeds the eigenvalue of the second PC, the more the electrode entries are on a straight line, indicating a common phase across electrodes. If the first and the second eigenvalues are similar, a common phase across electrodes and thus across generators is absent. In order to avoid confounding the comparison of eigenvalues by the global amplitude of the signal, the difference between eigenvalues is normalized (divided) by global amplitude. The normalized difference between the two eigenvalues has been termed Global Field Synchronization (GFS,[18,19]) and is thus defined as follows:

$$GFS = (|V1 - V2|/(V1 + V2))$$

Global field synchronization ranges from 0 to 1, where high GFS values indicate the presence of a single, predominant phase over all electrodes, whereas low GFS indicates the absence of such a common phase. Global field synchronization is independent of the total power of the data and of the recording reference. As for the computation of GFP, the distribution of the scalp signals is not taken into account. Global field synchronization is a useful measure of synchronization of brain functions when no clear hypothesis about the distribution of sources of interest exists and yields a single, non-local measure of synchronization of brain functions. An example of results obtained with GFS is shown in Figure 7.7.

The measures of frequency-domain global amplitude and GFS are conceptually and mathematically closely related to the global descriptors introduced in Chapter 9, where global spectral amplitude corresponds to the Sigma descriptor and GFS corresponds to the Omega

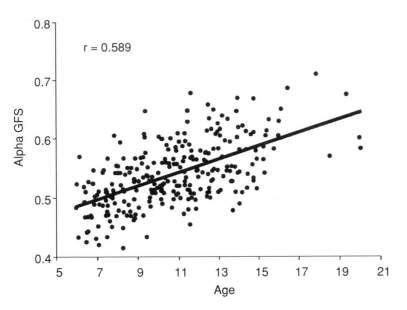

**Figure 7.7**
Alpha-band global field synchronization as function of age in healthy children. There is a strong positive correlation between alpha-band synchronization and age, indicating a progressively increasing degree of synchronization among brain regions.

descriptor. Since global spectral amplitude and GFS assess the shape of the cloud of electrode entries in the sine–cosine diagram, and since the shape of that cloud is independent of the reference, both measures are reference independent.

Apart from asking to what degree brain processes occur simultaneously, one may also ask whether two oscillations occur with a consistent delay in time, such that one may conclude that there is a flow of information among the two processes. This leads to the measure of coherence and is addressed below.

## Averaging of complex frequency-domain EEG data

In the simulations of EEG resulting from one or more oscillating point sources, we have learned that the phase and amplitude relationships among electrodes are entirely determined by the amplitude, location, orientation and phase relationship of the sources that produce the EEG. For many analysis purposes, and especially for the estimation of sources and the analysis of phase relationships of sources, it is therefore vital to preserve this information. On the other hand, we usually assume that the phase of the processes that we analyze is random in relation to the beginning of our analysis period. This is namely the case for the analysis of spontaneous EEG, where we select our analysis periods randomly, and it is also the typical assumption when analyzing event-related oscillations. If we had assumed that some event-related oscillations are phase locked, we would have the standard situation for evoked potentials and could proceed using the standard average ERP analysis strategies of Chapter 6. Our data therefore contain phase differences among electrodes that are relevant for our analysis, and phase information that is constant across all electrodes and presumably random. Due to this random factor, averaging of complex frequency-domain EEG data selected at random intervals would result in the same, usually massive cancellation of signals as in time-domain.

What we therefore need is a representation of frequency-transformed EEG data that contains all the phase and amplitude relationships among electrodes, but is invariant to changes of phase applied simultaneously to all electrodes. Such a representation is given by the so-called cross-spectral matrix. The cross-spectral matrix is a three-dimensional electrode-by-electrode-by-frequency matrix and corresponds to the variance-covariance matrix in time-domain data. For each pair of electrodes, the matrix contains the cross spectrum of one pair of electrodes. Mathematically, the cross spectrum between a pair of channels at one frequency is defined as the product of the frequency-transformed signal of one channel with the complex conjugate of the frequency-transformed signal of the other channel. This product is again a complex number. When considering the two frequency-transformed signals and their cross spectrum as a two-dimensional vector on the complex plane, the following properties emerge:

(1) The length of vector of the cross spectrum in the complex plane is the product of the length of the vectors representing the two signals.

(2) The orientation of this vector is equal to the difference of orientations (phases) of the two signals' vectors. It therefore represents the phase difference between the two signals.

(3) The cross spectrum of an electrode with itself is equal to the power of the electrode and has no imaginary part.

The above properties imply that adding the same random phase shift to both signals does not change their cross spectrum; the amplitude of both signals is not affected by the phase shift, and nor therefore by the length of the cross-spectral vector, and because the orientation of the cross-spectrum vector is the difference of the two signal vectors, rotating both vectors by a constant angle still yields the same difference of orientation and thus the same orientation of the cross-spectrum vector. Cross-spectral matrices therefore only contain the phase differences among electrodes, which is what we assume (a) to be related to physiology and (b) to consist of a relevant and constant signal, and some irrelevant and random noise. Averaging cross-spectral matrices across epochs will thus preserve the constant signal and gradually cancel the random noise.

Average cross-spectral matrices can serve several purposes. First, they can be used to compute frequency-domain inverse solutions, because they represent all the phase and amplitude relationships among all channels completely. Computing inverses based on averaged cross-spectral matrices is equivalent to computing inverse solutions at each time-point and in each epoch, frequency transforming the estimate at each voxel and then averaging across epochs. From a computational point of view, averaging cross-spectral matrices is much more efficient than averaging frequency-transformed inverses, because the estimation of inverse solutions usually results in a massive inflation of data to handle, and it is convenient to do this analysis step as late as possible.

Another application of average cross-spectral matrices is the assessment of the stability of phase differences. If it can be shown that at a given frequency, the phase difference between two processes is nonrandom across a series of repetitions, this suggests these processes are coupled by some mechanism and potentially interact functionally. In order to estimate whether the phase difference between two signals is nonrandom, one can thus compare the mean direction of the cross spectrum of the two signals across repetitions with its variance. This comparison leads to the measure of coherence[21-24]. Coherence has been applied to resting-state EEG[25,26] as well as to EEG recorded during tasks where changes of interaction of different brain regions were expected[24,27-30].

155

The major obstacle for the application of coherence to EEG data is the extraction of suited signals. In Chapter 3, it has been shown that there are strong intrinsic relationships among the signals recorded at different electrodes. These relationships result from the effects of volume conduction and the typically unknown effect of the choice of reference electrode[31], and depend on the configuration of active sources[32]. For an interpretation of coherence results in terms of changes of functional connectivity of brain regions, it is thus necessary to separate the presumably interacting processes in brain space, which is not a trivial problem[33]. The methods to resolve this problem have included the application of spatial filters[22,32], or estimation of local current density based on some inverse solution[34,35]. The available literature that has employed such techniques is still sparse.

## Frequency-domain source models (single phase and multiple phase)

Because the additivity of EEG data from different sources also holds in the frequency domain, the principles of source localization and inverse solution can also be applied to frequency-domain data. Distributed inverse solutions can thus be computed that fit a distribution of complex three-dimensional vectors such that their forward solution is compatible with the complex FFT values obtained at the scalp electrodes, and such that they meet some further specific objective of the chosen inverse solution such as sparseness for dipoles, spatial smoothness or some minimal norm for distributed inverse solutions[36-48]. Therefore, all the possibilities and restrictions of inverse solutions for time-domain data also apply to frequency-domain data, but frequency-domain inverse solutions are initially complex. An example of frequency-domain inverse solutions is given in Figure 7.8.

As pointed out above, the estimation of distributed inverse solutions of large numbers of frequency-domain EEG epochs is much more efficient when average cross-spectral matrices are computed first. For the technical details on the computation of inverse solutions based on cross-spectral matrices, see Frei *et al.*[36].

There is a special case in frequency-domain inverse solutions where the rules of inverse solutions in time domain do not fully hold: this is the fit of dipoles. As shown above, a single dipole cannot account for phase differences between electrodes. Before fitting single dipoles to frequency-domain EEG data, one has therefore to assure that the data that are fitted have a single common phase, or that dipoles are fitted such that they can account for phase differences. To obtain common phase data suited for a single dipole, a procedure called FFT approximation can be applied that projects all electrodes onto the first principal component of the cloud of electrode entries[49-52,74]. Alternatively, one may choose to fit two dipoles that are restricted to have the same position. One of these dipoles is fitted to account for the real part of the data, while the other is fitted to account for the complex part of the data. The position and the resulting three-dimensional complex vector then optimally explain the complex frequency-domain data on the scalp.

## Time-varying oscillations (wavelets)
### Relationship to frequency-domain analysis

Applying an FFT to EEG data assumes that the proportion of the data that we are interested in is stationary, i.e. that neither its amplitude nor its variance changes across time. In formal terms, stationarity means that the statistical properties of the data we are interested in are invariant to time shifts. This is typically not the case in EEG if transient oscillations occur

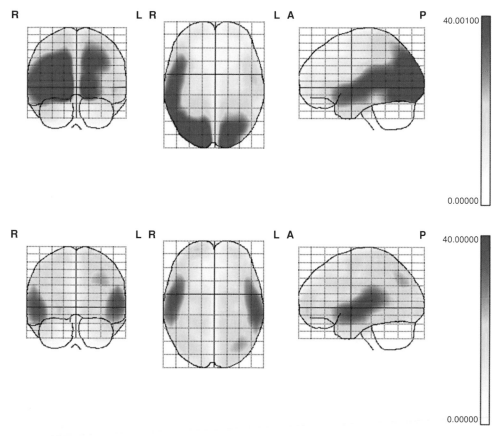

**Figure 7.8** This shows a sample frequency-domain inverse solution of EEG activity of the healthy control and of the patient with Alzheimer's dementia introduced in Figures 7.5 and 7.6 at 11 Hz. The patient shows the typical reduction of posterior alpha activity. Color coded is a glass-brain view of the spectral amplitude at each voxel on the cortex.

often, either spontaneously or induced by some event. By applying an FFT across the entire analysis period, one obtains an estimate of the average of these oscillations. Information on the variance of these oscillations across time is not available, and it remains open whether the obtained average really represents the typical event or just a mixture of different classes of events.

From this point of view, it may be useful to extend the methodological background provided above to the analysis of time-varying EEG oscillations. This can be achieved by modulating the EEG with some window function prior to applying an FFT. The resulting FFT decomposition is then representative only for that part of the data that has not been suppressed by the window. By systematically shifting the window across the analysis period and computing an FFT after each shift, a time-varying frequency decomposition of the EEG is obtained.

Theoretically, it is equivalent whether the window is applied to the EEG data or the complex exponentials are used to compute the FFT. Computationally, the modulation of the complex exponentials is more efficient. As already introduced in Chapter 5, a window function that is well suited for this type of analysis is the Gaussian function. Complex

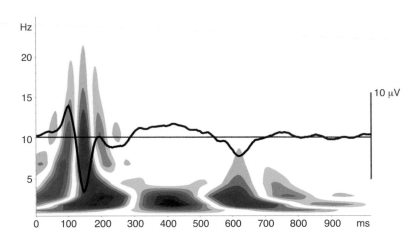

**Figure 7.9** Time frequency display of a single-channel averaged evoked potential. Blue indicates negative, red positive amplitudes. The overlay shows the trace of the channel, with its amplitude scale to the right.

exponentials that are modulated by a Gaussian envelope are called Gabor functions; the analysis of time series based on Gabor functions is called Gabor decomposition. When talking about multi-channel time-frequency decompositions of EEG data, we will thus essentially refer to a Gabor decomposition applied to all EEG channels and using initially complex Gabor functions. Using complex Gabor functions preserves the phase information, which is later important for source estimation and estimates of time-varying synchronization. Applying a Gabor transformation to an EEG channel will answer the question of how to weight each of the Gabor elements such that it represents the maximum possible amount of variance of the data. The obtained weights can be positive or negative and are equivalent to the covariance of the data with the wavelets.

## Display of single-channel time-frequency data

Applying a time-frequency decomposition to EEG or ERP data will thus tell us with what weight each of the employed wavelets is represented in the data. These weights alone are not very informative, because the information about time and frequency are still in the wavelets. What one would like to see is a representation of the signal's amplitude as a function of time and frequency.

To obtain the signal's time-varying amplitude at a given frequency, the weights obtained from the wavelet analysis can be back-transformed using only those wavelets that were constructed based on the frequency of interest. This is sometimes called wavelet layer extraction and is equivalent to applying a bandpass filter. For a complete representation of time-frequency data, this wavelet layer extraction is computed for each of the frequencies used to construct the wavelets.

The resulting two-dimensional time-frequency representations are typically shown using an intensity plot with a horizontal time axis and a vertical frequency axis (Figure 7.9). For the frequency axis, sometimes a logarithmic scale is used, because the frequency resolution decreases with increasing frequency.

Sometimes, one is merely interested in the strength of the signal and wants to disregard the phase of the oscillations[53]. In this case, it can be useful to back-transform the data using the previously obtained weights, but replacing the wavelets by the envelope of the wavelets. The resulting time-frequency decomposition is then always positive and much smoother in time, because it ignores the fast oscillations of the data (Figure 7.10).

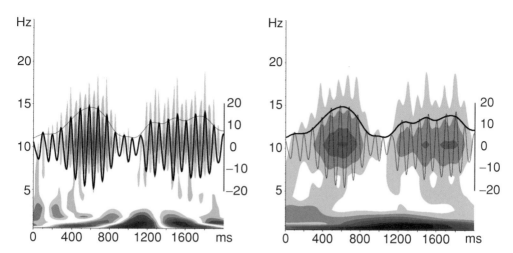

**Figure 7.10** Time-frequency display of a single-channel resting-state EEG with predominant alpha spindles. The left graph shows a display constructed with the wavelets, where the fast oscillations and polarity reversals are clearly visible. The right graph shows the same data, but the time-frequency display has been based on the envelope of the wavelets. The result is always positive, and the fast oscillations are not represented any more.

## Time-frequency analysis under different models of event-related brain activity

While the FFT analysis is time-sensitive only in regard to the phase of the oscillations and has no representation of transient fluctuations of the envelope of the signal, time-frequency analysis can represent both the phase of the oscillations and their envelope. Time-frequency decompositions have thus two intrinsic time scales, a fast one that is expressed as frequency and phase of oscillations, and a slow one that expresses the modulation of these oscillations. The different analysis strategies used when applying multichannel time-frequency decompositions to EEG and ERP data can be classified according to their assumptions of randomness of these two time scales. A scheme is shown in Figure 7.11. Note that the phase relationships between electrodes are never random, because they are determined by the forward solution of the active sources. We only tabulate randomness in relation to the external event.

In the remaining part of this section, we will now discuss the four possible combinations of dynamics on these two time scales and provide examples of typical applications (see also Friston et al.[54]).

### Envelope and phase are event-locked

This is the typical assumption made when evoked potentials are computed and analyzed using time-frequency decomposition: the relevant signals are assumed to have phase and envelope locked to the event of interest, and signals not meeting these criteria are considered as noise. Since both phase and envelope are assumed to be locked to the stimulus, no cancellation of the signals of interest should occur during averaging. It also makes no difference whether single trials are first transformed into the time-frequency domain and then averaged, or whether the averaged evoked potential is transformed into the time-frequency domain, because both averaging and the time-frequency transformation are linear operations. Assuming that the noise has a random phase while the signal has a constant phase also implies that the noise should have a zero mean, while the mean of the signal should

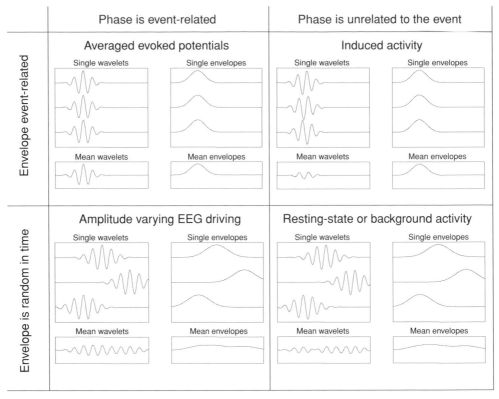

**Figure 7.11** Scheme of different applications of EEG time-frequency decompositions as function of the decomposition's sensitivity to fast and slow variations in the data.

be different from zero. In the evoked potential model, it is thus possible to compute signal-to-noise ratios and thus statistics across a series of trials without need of a further baseline condition[8,55,56]. Phase and amplitude relationship of the EEG to a stimulus has also received attention to clarify whether and how averaged event-related potentials are related to EEG phase resetting[57–61].

### Envelope is event-locked, but phase is random

This is the model that is typically referred to as induced activity or event-related synchronization (ERS)/event-related desynchronization (ERD)[53]. It is assumed that in a well-defined time window before or after an event, some EEG oscillations are enhanced or suppressed, but that the phase of these oscillations is not locked to the event, such that averaging of the signals would lead to a massive cancellation. In order to avoid such a cancellation of signals, one typically averages the envelope and not the signal. However, because the envelope is always positive, mean envelopes will always be larger than zero, whether there was some event-related activity or not. For statistics, it is thus necessary to record a baseline condition that contains no event or some type of control event, such that mean envelope differences between the condition of interest and the baseline condition can be computed. It is thus possible to see an event-related increase of activity, which is often called event-related synchronization (although it is strictly speaking not synchronization), or event-related decrease of activity (often called event-related desynchronization). Typical applications of this methodology are for example amplitude changes of the mu and beta rhythms over motor areas before and after a voluntary movement or spectral changes due to the perception of a stimulus[62–68], always compared with baseline activity.

### Envelope is random, but phase is event-locked

If there is a train of stimuli with short interstimulus intervals, one sometimes observes a phenomenon called driving, which means that in the EEG, oscillations appear that have the same frequency as the stimuli, that are locked to the stimulus, but that vary in amplitude. This would correspond to a model where the phase is event-related but the envelope is random. This view is rarely employed and reported here mainly for completeness, but might be worthwhile to be further explored. Given that such a model is correct and that the fluctuations of the envelope are of no interest, one may either compute event-related averages that would yield an approximately stationary mean signal, or equivalently, one may compute an FFT based on epochs that are locked to the stimuli and average the resulting complex numbers.

### Envelope and phase are random

Random envelope and phase are the typical assumptions in the case of spontaneous EEG, where oscillations at different frequency seem to be present with time-varying amplitudes. Since there is typically no external event that helps to isolate specific EEG events, there are two options to analyze such data: one may either choose to obtain an estimate of the average of the activity at a given frequency, disregarding the phase of the signal, or one may attempt to identify the spontaneously occurring events.

Estimating the average of activity is typically achieved by computing the mean of the absolute spectral amplitude or power after an FFT (EEG power mapping). It is methodologically simple, and has yielded an overwhelming body of very replicable and relevant literature (see above). It is however insensitive to the plausible assumption that there may be several types of oscillations with largely overlapping frequency spectra, but different sources and different functions.

In order to identify and separately quantify spontaneously occurring EEG events, it is necessary to employ methods that employ some pattern learning and recognition algorithms. An overview of these methods is given in the next section.

# Reduction of dimensions in frequency- and time-frequency-domain EEG data

## Reduction of dimensions in space based on map learning

Similarly to time- and frequency-domain data, multichannel time-frequency EEG data have an intrinsic redundancy across channels, both because of volume conduction that makes the same intracerebral process visible across a large proportion of all channels, and because several intracerebral sources might synchronize and show similar temporal dynamics. In order to lower the redundancy of the data and to obtain simple, complete and interpretable representations of the data, it is useful to decompose the data into a series of scalp-distributed EEG processes that are plausible candidates to represent functionally distinct intracerebral processes. This problem is very similar to the problem of decomposing time-domain EEG data, and many of the methods and arguments coincide.

How should such a meaningful EEG process be defined? A strong claim for defining criteria to separate different EEG processes can be made regarding delays between electrodes: since volume conduction is instantaneous, a scalp-distributed EEG process that corresponds to a single intracerebral source cannot have any delays between electrodes. Similarly, if several sources are simultaneously active, a scalp-distributed process corresponding to such an assembly of synchronized sources can by definition not produce delays between electrodes. If an EEG process to be identified is supposed to correspond either to a single source or to a synchronized network of sources, it must therefore not contain any delays between electrodes and can thus be accounted for by a real, noncomplex map of scalp potentials.

The argument that a decomposition of frequency- and time-frequency-domain EEG data should be based on noncomplex EEG scalp field distributions is useful, but not sufficient to obtain a unique decomposition, and further plausible objectives need to be introduced. One such objective can be constructed by considering the massive interdependence of intracerebral brain processes. If two or more such processes are active at the same time and at the same frequency and phase, it is unlikely that they do this independently; it is contrarily quite likely that some defined interaction of these processes will take place. The different interacting processes may therefore be considered as a single meta-process that is represented by a single scalp-field topography. The objective deduced from this argument is thus that the processes to be isolated do not overlap, i.e. that in frequency-domain data, they do not occur at the same frequency and phase, and in time-frequency-domain data, they do not occur at the same frequency, time and phase. On the other side, a single process may cover several frequency and time intervals, i.e. several wavelets.

The classic procedure to fit data to such a model is K-means clustering, where each observation is assigned to exactly one of a limited set of classes using a best-fit criterion[69]. In our case, a single observation is the spatial distribution of scalp voltages accounted for by a single, noncomplex wavelet or sinusoidal oscillation. The result is a set of prototypical scalp field configurations, and a weight matrix with the dimensions number of clusters by number of wavelets[70,71]. This weight matrix contains the contribution of each oscillation to each scalp field configuration. According to the clustering rule, for each oscillation, all but one weights are zero, and the non-zero weights indicate to which scalp-field configuration the oscillation has been assigned and how it needed to be scaled to fit the data.

To obtain a representation of the time-frequency patterns of activity assigned to a single class, the procedure is analogous to the one used to display single-channel activity, but instead of using the weights of a single channel to construct the display, one uses the weights obtained for the class of interest by the cluster analysis. As in the single-channel display, one may choose to base the reconstruction using the wavelets or the envelopes. An example is given in Figure 7.12.

## Reduction of dictionary size by dictionary learning

Dictionaries used for time-frequency analysis are typically over-complete, and a single event may be accounted for by a combination of more than one wavelet of the dictionary. If one aims at a one-to-one correspondence between oscillatory events in the data and words in the dictionary, adaptive dictionary learning algorithms have to be employed. These algorithms typically optimize the features of a single wavelet (i.e. the frequency and phase of the oscillation and the latency and extent of the envelope) for a maximal fit to the data[72,73]. All variance of the data that can be explained by the optimally fitting wavelet is then removed from the data and a next wavelet is fitted. The fitting and removal steps are repeated until a predefined

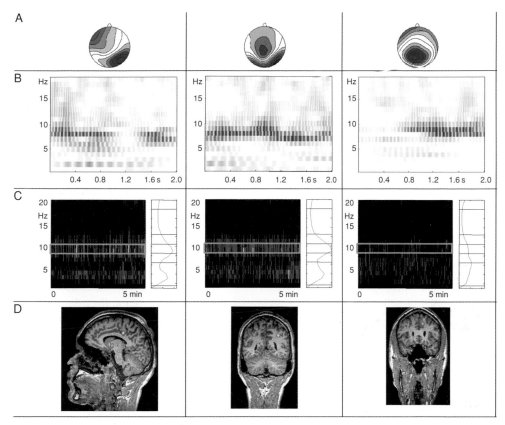

**Figure 7.12** Example of the application of K-means clustering to time-frequency decomposed EEG data for the identification of fMRI correlates of subcomponents of alpha activity. A. Prototypical maps obtained by clustering the wavelet weight topographies of resting-state EEG recorded in an fMRI scanner. B. Time-frequency plots of the loadings of the maps shown in A for a representative epoch of the data. There appear to be several, alternating types of alpha activity that appear in different clusters. C. Evolution of these different types of alpha activity across the entire analysis time. The graphs show an intensity plot obtained by averaging within each epoch the absolute amplitude of the signal across time. The blue box indicates the window used to construct the regressor for the fMRI data. D. BOLD correlates obtained for the regressors shown in C, after convolution with a hemodynamic response function.

stop criterion is met, for example until a certain amount of the total variance is explained. For EEG specific analyses, the goodness-of-fit criterion can be extended to include the well-known interdependencies of multichannel EEG into the optimization of the wavelets to be employed[71]. An example is given in Figure 7.13.

# Conclusions

This chapter has shown that many of the basic considerations that have to be made when analyzing time-domain data also hold when the data are transformed into frequency- and time-frequency-domain data. It is important to take into account that the instantaneity of the effects of intracerebral activity on the measured scalp potentials implies that in frequency-domain EEG data, potentials generated by the same source or by synchronized sources must have the same or opposite phase angle. By considering the phase relationships among all

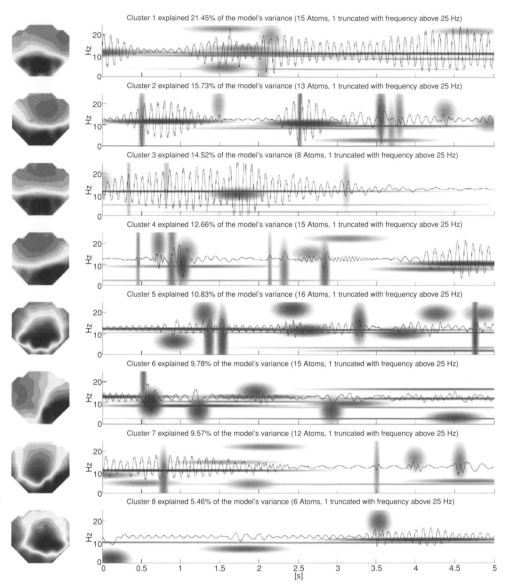

**Figure 7.13** Result of a multichannel matching pursuit decomposition of a resting-state EEG. The left panels show the intensity plots in the time-frequency plane of the Gabor functions obtained by optimizing their parameters for an optimal fit with the data. White areas indicate low, red values indicate high values of energy. The plots are overlaid by the corresponding representative waveforms. The left panels show the corresponding topographies obtained by clustering the spatial distributions of the weights of each of the fitted Gabor functions. (Reprinted from Studes *et al.*[71] with permission from Elsevier).

channels, it is then possible to construct frequency-domain inverse solutions and apply measures of phase-locking of neural generators. When multichannel time-frequency decompositions are applied, more than one type of oscillation can be accounted for, and methods similar to time-domain microstate analysis can be employed to identify a limited set of classes of EEG oscillations with a defined spatial distribution. Multichannel time-frequency analyses may thus be the methods of choice to link the well-known observations made in time-domain event-related potential analyses and the equally well known frequency-domain signatures of different modes of information processing in the brain.

# References

1. John ER, Ahn H, Prichep L et al. Developmental equations for the electroencephalogram. *Science* 1980;**210**:1255–1258.

2. Borbely AA, Achermann P. Sleep homeostasis and models of sleep regulation. *Journal of Biological Rhythms* 1999;**14**:557–568.

3. John ER, Prichep LS, Fridman J, Easton P. Neurometrics: computer-assisted differential diagnosis of brain dysfunctions. *Science* 1988;**239**:162–169.

4. Herrmann WM. Development and critical evaluation of an objective for the electroencephalographic classification of psychotropic drugs. In Herrmann WM, ed. *Electroencephalography in Drug Research.* Stuttgart: Gustav Fisher; 1982, pp. 249–351.

5. Saletu B, Anderer P, Saletu-Zyhlarz GM. EEG topography and tomography (LORETA) in the classification and evaluation of the pharmacodynamics of psychotropic drugs. *Clinical EEG and Neuroscience* 2006;**37**:66–80.

6. Fernandez T, Harmony T, Rodriguez M et al. EEG activation patterns during the performance of tasks involving different components of mental calculation. *Electroencephalography and Clinical Neurophysiology* 1995;**94**:175–182.

7. Gevins A, Smith ME, McEvoy L, Yu D. High-resolution EEG mapping of cortical activation related to working memory: effects of task difficulty, type of processing, and practice. *Cerebral Cortex* 1997;**7**:374–385.

8. Samar VJ, Swartz KP, Raghuveer MR. Multiresolution analysis of event-related potentials by wavelet decomposition. *Brain and Cognition* 1995;**27**:398–438.

9. Bertrand O, Perrin F, Pernier J. A theoretical justification of the average reference in topographic evoked potential studies. *Electroencephalography and Clinical Neurophysiology* 1985;**62**:462–464.

10. Adamis D, Sahu S, Treloar A. The utility of EEG in dementia: a clinical perspective. *International Journal of Geriatric Psychiatry* 2005;**20**:1038–1045.

11. Coburn KL, Lauterbach EC, Boutros NN et al. The value of quantitative electroencephalography in clinical psychiatry: a report by the Committee on Research of the American Neuropsychiatric Association. *Journal of Neuropsychiatry and Clinical Neuroscience* 2006;**18**:460–500.

12. John ER, Prichep LS. The relevance of QEEG to the evaluation of behavioral disorders and pharmacological interventions. *Clinical EEG and Neuroscience* 2006;**37**:135–143.

13. Mucci A, Volpe U, Merlotti E, Bucci P, Galderisi S. Pharmaco-EEG in psychiatry. *Clinical EEG and Neuroscience* 2006;**37**:81–98.

14. Prichep LS. Use of normative databases and statistical methods in demonstrating clinical utility of QEEG: importance and cautions. *Clinical EEG and Neuroscience* 2005;**36**:82–87.

15. Wolf H, Jelic V, Gertz HJ et al. A critical discussion of the role of neuroimaging in mild cognitive impairment. *Acta Neurologica Scandinavica Supplement* 2003;**179**:52–76.

16. Yuval-Greenberg S, Tomer O, Keren AS, Nelken I, Deouell LY. Transient induced gamma-band response in EEG as a manifestation of miniature saccades. *Neuron* 2008;**58**:429–441.

17. Gonzalez Andino SL, Grave de Peralta Menendez R, Lantz CM et al. Non-stationary distributed source approximation: an alternative to improve localization procedures. *Human Brain Mapping* 2001;**14**:81–95.

18. Koenig T, Lehmann D, Saito N et al. Decreased functional connectivity of EEG theta-frequency activity in first-episode, neuroleptic-naive patients with schizophrenia: preliminary results. *Schizophrenia Research* 2001;**50**:55–60.

19. Koenig T, Prichep L, Dierks T *et al.* Decreased EEG synchronization in Alzheimer's disease and mild cognitive impairment. *Neurobiology and Aging* 2005;**26**:165–171.

20. Jann K, Dierks T, Boesch C *et al.* BOLD correlates of EEG alpha phase-locking and the fMRI default mode network. *Neuroimage* 2009;**45**:903–916.

21. Nunez PL, Silberstein RB, Shi Z *et al.* EEG coherency II: experimental comparisons of multiple measures. *Clinical Neurophysiology* 1999;**110**:469–486.

22. Nunez PL, Srinivasan R, Westdorp AF *et al.* EEG coherency. I: Statistics, reference electrode, volume conduction, Laplacians, cortical imaging, and interpretation at multiple scales. *Electroencephalography and Clinical Neurophysiology* 1997;**103**:499–515.

23. Rappelsberger P, Petsche H. Probability mapping: power and coherence analyses of cognitive processes. *Brain Topography* 1988;**1**:46–54.

24. Rappelsberger P, Pfurtscheller G, Filz O. Calculation of event-related coherence – a new method to study short-lasting coupling between brain areas. *Brain Topography* 1994;**7**:121–127.

25. Leocani L, Comi G. EEG coherence in pathological conditions. *Journal of Clinical Neurophysiology* 1999;**16**:548–555.

26. Tauscher J, Fischer P, Neumeister A, Rappelsberger P, Kasper S. Low frontal electroencephalographic coherence in neuroleptic-free schizophrenic patients. *Biological Psychiatry* 1998;**44**:438–447.

27. Reiterer S, Hemmelmann C, Rappelsberger P, Berger ML. Characteristic functional networks in high versus low-proficiency second language speakers detected also during native language processing: an explorative EEG coherence study in 6 frequency bands. *Brain Research. Cognitive Brain Research* 2005;**25**:566–578.

28. Sarnthein J, von Stein A, Rappelsberger P *et al.* Persistent patterns of brain activity: an EEG coherence study of the positive effect of music on spatial-temporal reasoning. *Neurology Research* 1997;**19**:107–116.

29. Nolte G, Bai O, Wheaton L *et al.* Identifying true brain interaction from EEG data using the imaginary part of coherency. *Clinical Neurophysiology* 2004;**115**:2292.

30. Stam CJ, Nolte G, Daffertshofer A. Phase lag index: assessment of functional connectivity from multi channel EEG and MEG with diminished bias from common sources. *Human Brain Mapping* 2007;**28**:1178–1193.

31. Essl M, Rappelsberger P. EEG coherence and reference signals: experimental results and mathematical explanations. *Medical and Biological Engineering and Computing* 1998;**36**:399–406.

32. Srinivasan R, Nunez PL, Silberstein RB. Spatial filtering and neocortical dynamics: estimates of EEG coherence. *IEEE Transactions in Biomedical Engineering* 1998;**45**:814–826.

33. Winter WR, Nunez PL, Ding J, Srinivasan R. Comparison of the effect of volume conduction on EEG coherence with the effect of field spread on MEG coherence. *Statistics in Medicine* 2007;**26**:3946–3957.

34. Hoechstetter K, Bornfleth H, Weckesser D *et al.* BESA source coherence: a new method to study cortical oscillatory coupling. *Brain Topography* 2004;**16**:233–238.

35. Lehmann D, Faber PL, Gianotti LR, Kochi K, Pascual-Marqui RD. Coherence and phase locking in the scalp EEG and between LORETA model sources, and microstates as putative mechanisms of brain temporo-spatial functional organization. *Journal of Physiology Paris* 2006;**99**:29–36.

36. Frei E, Gamma A, Pascual-Marqui R *et al.* Localization of MDMA-induced brain activity in healthy volunteers using low resolution brain electromagnetic tomography (LORETA). *Human Brain Mapping* 2001;**14**:152–165.

37. Bosch-Bayard J, Valdes-Sosa P, Virues-Alba T *et al.* 3D statistical parametric mapping of EEG source spectra by means of variable resolution electromagnetic tomography (VARETA). *Clinical Electroencephalography* 2001;**32**:47–61.

38. di Michele F, Prichep L, John ER, Chabot RJ. The neurophysiology of attention-deficit/hyperactivity disorder. *International Journal of Psychophysiology* 2005;**58**:81–93.

39. Fernandez-Bouzas A, Harmony T, Fernandez T *et al.* Sources of abnormal

EEG activity in spontaneous intracerebral hemorrhage. *Clinical Electroencephalography* 2002;**33**:70–76.

40. Gianotti LR, Kunig G, Faber PL *et al.* Rivastigmine effects on EEG spectra and three-dimensional LORETA functional imaging in Alzheimer's disease. *Psychopharmacology* 2008;**198**:323–332.

41. Gianotti LR, Kunig G, Lehmann D *et al.* Correlation between disease severity and brain electric LORETA tomography in Alzheimer's disease. *Clinical Neurophysiology* 2007;**118**:186–196.

42. Gomez CM, Marco-Pallares J, Grau C. Location of brain rhythms and their modulation by preparatory attention estimated by current density. *Brain Research* 2006;**1107**:151–160.

43. John ER, Prichep LS, Kox W *et al.* Invariant reversible QEEG effects of anesthetics. *Conscious Cognition* 2001;**10**:165–183.

44. Koles ZJ, Flor-Henry P, Lind JC. Low-resolution electrical tomography of the brain during psychometrically matched verbal and spatial cognitive tasks. *Human Brain Mapping* 2001;**12**:144–156.

45. Lehmann D, Faber PL, Achermann P *et al.* Brain sources of EEG gamma frequency during volitionally meditation-induced, altered states of consciousness, and experience of the self. *Psychiatry Research* 2001;**108**:111–121.

46. Pascual-Marqui RD, Esslen M, Kochi K, Lehmann D. Functional imaging with low-resolution brain electromagnetic tomography (LORETA): a review. *Methods and Findings in Experimental and Clinical Pharmacology* 2002;**24 Suppl** C:91–95.

47. Pascual-Marqui RD, Lehmann D, Koenig T *et al.* Low resolution brain electromagnetic tomography (LORETA) functional imaging in acute, neuroleptic-naive, first-episode, productive schizophrenia. *Psychiatry Research* 1999;**90**:169–179.

48. Thatcher RW, North D, Biver C. Evaluation and validity of a LORETA normative EEG database. *Clinical EEG and Neuroscience* 2005;**36**:116–122.

49. Kinoshita T, Michel CM, Yagyu T, Lehmann D, Saito M. Diazepam and sulpiride effects on frequency domain EEG source locations. *Neuropsychobiology* 1994; **30**:126–131.

50. Lehmann D, Henggeler B, Koukkou M, Michel CM. Source localization of brain electric field frequency bands during conscious, spontaneous, visual imagery and abstract thought. *Brain Research Cognitive Brain Research* 1993;**1**:203–210.

51. Lehmann D, Michel CM. Intracerebral dipole source localization for FFT power maps. *Electroencephalography and Clinical Neurophysiology* 1990;**76**:271–276.

52. Michel CM, Lehmann D, Henggeler B, Brandeis D. Localization of the sources of EEG delta, theta, alpha and beta frequency bands using the FFT dipole approximation. *Electroencephalography and Clinical Neurophysiology* 1992;**82**:38–44.

53. Pfurtscheller G, Lopes da Silva FH. Event-related EEG/MEG synchronization and desynchronization: basic principles. *Clinical Neurophysiology* 1999;**110**:1842–1857.

54. Friston K, Henson R, Phillips C, Mattout J. Bayesian estimation of evoked and induced responses. *Human Brain Mapping* 2006;**27**: 722–735.

55. Demiralp T, Ademoglu A. Decomposition of event-related brain potentials into multiple functional components using wavelet transform. *Clinical Electroencephalography* 2001;**32**:122–138.

56. Heinrich H, Moll GH, Dickhaus H *et al.* Time-on-task analysis using wavelet networks in an event-related potential study on attention-deficit hyperactivity disorder. *Clinical Neurophysiology* 2001;**112**:1280–1287.

57. David O, Harrison L, Friston KJ. Modelling event-related responses in the brain. *Neuroimage* 2005;**25**:756–770.

58. Fell J, Dietl T, Grunwald T *et al.* Neural bases of cognitive ERPs: more than phase reset. *Journal of Cognitive Neuroscience* 2004;**16**:1595–1604.

59. Makeig S, Westerfield M, Jung TP *et al.* Dynamic brain sources of visual evoked responses. *Science* 2002;**295**:690–694.

60. Mazaheri A, Jensen O. Posterior alpha activity is not phase-reset by visual stimuli. *Proceedings of the National Academy of Sciences of the USA* 2006;**103**:2948–2952.

61. Sauseng P, Klimesch W, Gruber WR *et al.* Are event-related potential components generated by phase resetting of brain oscillations? A critical discussion. *Neuroscience* 2007;**146**:1435–1444.

62. Bai O, Lin P, Vorbach S *et al.* Exploration of computational methods for classification of movement intention during human voluntary movement from single trial EEG. *Clinical Neurophysiology* 2007;**118**:2637–2655.

63. Hald LA, Bastiaansen MC, Hagoort P. EEG theta and gamma responses to semantic violations in online sentence processing. *Brain Language* 2006;**96**:90–105.

64. Hsiao FJ, Lin YY, Hsieh JC *et al.* Oscillatory characteristics of face-evoked neuromagnetic responses. *International Journal of Psychophysiology* 2006;**61**:113–120.

65. Isoglu-Alkac U, Basar-Eroglu C, Ademoglu A *et al.* Alpha activity decreases during the perception of Necker cube reversals: an application of wavelet transform. *Biological Cybernetics* 2000;**82**:313–320.

66. Neuper C, Pfurtscheller G. Evidence for distinct beta resonance frequencies in human EEG related to specific sensorimotor cortical areas. *Clinical Neurophysiology* 2001;**112**:2084–2097.

67. Tzur G, Berger A. When things look wrong: theta activity in rule violation. *Neuropsychologia* 2007;**45**:3122–3126.

68. Yordanova J, Kolev V, Heinrich H *et al.* Developmental event-related gamma oscillations: effects of auditory attention. *European Journal of Neuroscience* 2002;**16**:2214–2224.

69. Pascual-Marqui RD, Michel CM, Lehmann D. Segmentation of brain electrical activity into microstates: model estimation and validation. *IEEE Transactions on Biomedical Engineering* 1995;**42**:658–665.

70. Koenig T, Marti-Lopez F, Valdes-Sosa P. Topographic time-frequency decomposition of the EEG. *Neuroimage* 2001;**14**:383–390.

71. Studer D, Hoffmann U, Koenig T. From EEG dependency multichannel matching pursuit to sparse topographic EEG decomposition. *Journal of Neuroscience Methods* 2006;**153**:261–275.

72. Durka PJ, Blinowska KJ. Analysis of EEG transients by means of matching pursuit. *Annals of Biomedical Engineering* 1995;**23**:608–611.

73. Mallat SG, Zhang Z. Matching pursuits with time-frequency dictionaries. *IEEE Transactions on Signal Processing* 1993;**41**:3397–3415.

74. Lehmann D, Ozaki H, Pal I. Averaging of spectral power and phase via vector diagram best fits without reference electrode or reference channel. *Electroencephalography and Clinical Neurophysiology* 1986;**64**:350–363.

# Statistical analysis of multichannel scalp field data

Thomas Koenig and Lester Melie-García

## Introduction

High density spatial and temporal sampling of EEG data enhances the quality of results of electrophysiological experiments[1-3]. Because EEG sources typically produce widespread electric fields (see Chapter 3) and operate at frequencies well below the sampling rate, increasing the number of electrodes and time samples will not necessarily increase the number of observed processes, but mainly increase the accuracy of the representation of these processes. This is namely the case when inverse solutions are computed.

As a consequence, increasing the sampling in space and time increases the redundancy of the data (in space, because electrodes are correlated due to volume conduction, and time, because neighboring time points are correlated), while the degrees of freedom of the data change only little. This has to be taken into account when statistical inferences are to be made from the data. However, in many ERP studies, the intrinsic correlation structure of the data has been disregarded. Often, some electrodes or groups of electrodes are a priori selected as the analysis entity and considered as repeated (within subject) measures that are analyzed using standard univariate statistics. The increased spatial resolution obtained with more electrodes is thus poorly represented by the resulting statistics. In addition, the assumptions made (e.g. in terms of what constitutes a repeated measure) are not supported by what we know about the properties of EEG data.

From the point of view of physics (see Chapter 3), the natural "atomic" analysis entity of EEG and ERP data is the scalp electric field. It represents the potential differences that a single generator or a set of simultaneously active generators produce on the scalp. (One can maintain this point of view even for statistics based on inverse solution, where the "atomic" entity is the activity of a voxel: because each voxel has a well-defined forward solution that is a scalp electric field, thinking in terms of voxels is initially equivalent to thinking in terms of scalp fields.)

Since on the scalp, the effects of intracerebral generators simply add up, one can also use additive models for statistical inference. For example, differences in active sources in two experimental conditions are directly reflected as the difference field between the scalp fields evoked by those two conditions[4,5]. The sources of the difference maps are thus identical to the differences of sources, although this might be difficult to show in praxis because the differences may be small and below the resolution of the currently available inverse solutions. Nevertheless, it is legitimate to use differences of scalp fields between conditions as representatives of sources differences between conditions.

*Electrical Neuroimaging*, ed. Christoph M. Michel, Thomas Koenig, Daniel Brandeis, Lorena R.R. Gianotti and Jiří Wackermann. Published by Cambridge University Press. © Cambridge University Press 2009.

In order to establish the statistical significance of experimental effects observed in scalp electric fields, standard multivariate statistical approaches such as MANOVAs[6] may be applied. To compute a MANOVA, it is however necessary to have more observations than variables (electrodes), which is not a realistic option in experiments with large numbers of electrodes. Another approach to these problems that has become increasingly popular in the field of multichannel EEG analyses is the usage of multivariate randomization statistics[7-13].

Randomization statistics are computationally expensive, but require very few assumptions, have a high statistical power and allow the construction of custom-tailored tests for specific questions of interest. In this chapter, we will first give a general introduction and a "toy" example of randomization statistics. Then, while we analyze an ERP dataset, we will gradually introduce a series of randomization tests that are conceptually derived from specific properties of ERP data. This analysis will include tests for the existence of a consistent topography across subjects, tests for scalp field differences in a multifactorial design, partial least squares, tests for correlations of the ERP data with a continuous behavioral variable, tests for the significance of the duration of effects across time and tests for the significance of differences of microstate assignment. The aim is to outline the possible strategies that are available to address the typical questions that arise during the analysis of ERP data, and to stimulate the reader's creativity when a novel problem arises. The analysis of the data will not be exhaustive, because that is not the intention of this chapter.

# Basic principles of randomization statistics and a "toy" example

As with most statistics, randomization statistics are tests of plausibility of the so-called null hypothesis. The null hypothesis postulates that the variance in the data is unrelated to some assumed structure in the data. The aim of a statistical test is to estimate the probability of the null hypothesis. If this probability is sufficiently low, the null hypothesis is rejected, and the alternative hypothesis is adopted, i.e. one assumes that the variance of the data is probably related to the assumed structure and says that the assumed structure has a significant effect in the data.

This general procedure thus requires two steps. First, test-statistics have to be introduced that measure to what extent the variance of the data is related to the assumed structure. In other words, the test-statistics yield some magnitude of the effect (the so-called effect size) of the assumed structure in the data. In a second step, it is estimated how likely it is that the observed effect size has been observed by chance. Classical statistics base the second step upon the theoretical distribution of the effect size under the null hypothesis, which implies that such a theoretical distribution exists and can be estimated.

Randomization statistics construct the distribution of the effect size under the null hypothesis by systematically destroying (randomizing) the assumed structure in the data and recomputing the effect size[14,15]. The randomized data are thus one instance of a set of observations that one could have made under the null hypothesis, and the effect size obtained from randomized data is by definition one instance of an effect size obtained under the null hypothesis. By repeating the randomization of the data and the computation of the effect size in the randomized data many times, one obtains an empirical distribution of the effect size that is by definition compatible with the null hypothesis. The observed effect size obtained in the actually observed data is then compared to the empirical distribution of the effect size under the null hypothesis. This gives us the likelihood that the observed effect size has been obtained while the null hypothesis was true[15]. If this likelihood is sufficiently low, we adopt the alternative hypothesis and say that the assumed structure has a significant effect on the data.

For those who are not so familiar with such explanations, here is a "toy" example to illustrate the two approaches. There is a saying that "Fortune favors fools," which has a rather pictorial correspondence in German, in which people say that "The most stupid farmer harvests the biggest potatoes." In order to put this hypothesis to a test, we can ask the most stupid farmer we can find to bring a bag of his potatoes, and ask a farmer with average IQ to do the same. As outlined above, we have to choose test statistics that quantify to what degree the potatoes of the fool are larger than those of the farmer with normal intelligence. We could, for example, choose the test statistics to be the mean volume of all potatoes in the bag. Let us assume that the mean volume of the potatoes of the fool is actually larger than that of his colleague. In classical statistics, we would proceed to find the theoretical distribution of potato volume, based on the sample of potatoes we have in the two bags. We could for example claim that potato volume has a normal Gaussian distribution and estimate the width of this normal distribution based on the variance of potato volume in the two bags. Knowing the mean volume difference of the potatoes of the two farmers, and having a theoretical model of how potato volume is distributed, one can determine (based on the assumed normal distribution) how likely it is that the difference in potato volume has been observed by chance. (In this case, this would result in an unpaired t-test.) If this is sufficiently unlikely, we reject the hypothesis that the difference has been obtained by chance and argue that we have found evidence in favor of the saying. If the difference in potato size is likely to have been observed by chance, we conclude that we failed to find evidence to support the hypothesis, and that it might have to be abandoned.

In randomization statistics, the first step of the procedure is the same; we establish the test-statistics to compare the potatoes of the two farmers. As above, we can choose to use the difference of mean potato volume, which we will call observed difference. Now the second step of the analysis is different from classical statistics: in order to judge whether the obtained difference in mean potato volume was due to the foolishness of one of the farmers or due to chance, we artificially produce differences in mean potato volume that are due only by chance, and are therefore instances of the null hypothesis. In our example, we take all the potatoes of both farmers, mix them up, redistribute them randomly into their two bags, and re-measure the difference of mean potato volume of the two bags. We will again obtain a difference in mean volume, and we know that this difference is now only due to chance. If the observed effect size (difference of mean potato volume obtained before the randomization) is similar to the effect size we have obtained after mixing, this might suggest that the observed effect size could also have been obtained by chance.

In order to know more precisely how likely it is that the observed effect size is due to chance, a single randomization is not enough, and we have to repeat the randomization and re-measuring procedure many times. This gives us a collection (distribution) of effect sizes obtained under the null hypothesis, i.e. under the assumption that there is no effect of IQ on potato size. Once we have this collection of randomly generated effect sizes, we can estimate the probability that the observed effect size was due to chance. This probability is defined as the number of random effect sizes that are larger than or equal to the observed effect size, divided by the total number of randomizations. In our case, if we had randomly redistributed the potatoes 100 times, and we had obtained random effect sizes larger than or equal to the observed effect size in 43 cases, the probability that the observed effect size is compatible with null hypothesis is 43%, which is large. We would thus typically accept the null hypothesis and conclude that the alternative hypothesis (i.e. the saying) lacks statistical evidence.

The above example illustrates that randomization statistics are conceptually very simple, intuitive, require very little theory, but in exchange a lot of re-measuring. It has been shown that randomization statistics perform in general equally well as (have a similar statistical power to reject the null hypothesis when it is actually false) parametric statistics if the conditions that apply for using parametric statistics are met[16]. They tend to perform better (have higher statistical power) when those conditions are not met[17]. In order to obtain reliable results with randomization, it has been suggested that at least 1000 randomization runs are computed if the critical threshold of the $P$-value is at 5% and 5000 randomizations if the critical $P$-value is at 1%[15]. This computational effort has been a major obstacle for a widespread application of randomization statistics, but is becoming less and less an obstacle with the rapidly increasing computation power of affordable personal computers.

## Applications for scalp field data
### The sample data
The data that we will submit to a series of statistical randomization tests here consist of ERPs of 10 healthy subjects recorded by Stein *et al.*[18]. The subjects were English-speaking exchange students living in Switzerland for one year, and they naturally learned some German during this time. The subjects were recorded twice, once at the beginning of their stay (day 1), when they had a basic German language proficiency, and in the middle of their stay (day 2), when their German language proficiency had improved. The subjects performed a so-called N400 experiment, where German sentences were visually presented word by word. The sentences ended either with a congruent word (The wheel is ROUND), or with an incongruent word (The garden is SHY). It is well known that the violation of the semantic expectancy generated by the first part of the sentence ("The garden is") produces an ERP component in the last word ("shy") called N400 that is proportional to the degree of violation of the semantic expectancy of the subject[19].

The data presented here consist of four ERPs per subject; counting the correct sentence endings at day 1, the false sentence endings at day 1, and the correct and false sentence endings at day 2. The ERPs were recorded from 74 scalp locations with a 250 Hz sampling rate, lasted from stimulus onset to 1000 ms post-stimulus and were low-pass filtered at 8 Hz. The grand mean ERP maps of the four conditions are shown in Figure 8.1. Besides the ERP data, all subjects had performed language tests at day 1 and day 2, and an overall score of language proficiency increase from day 1 to day 2 was available.

### Overview of the analyses
In the following analyses, we will address the following questions with randomization statistics:

- *Definition of the analysis window.* We want to know during which time intervals there is evidence that across subjects at least partially similar generators were active. Since similar generators imply similar topographies, we will test, for each time point of the ERP, whether there is a consistent topography across subjects. The null hypothesis that needs to be tested is thus whether the mean topography across subjects may have been observed by chance.

- *Test for topographic differences between conditions across time.* We would like to know whether parts of the ERPs' differences between conditions are due to the design of the

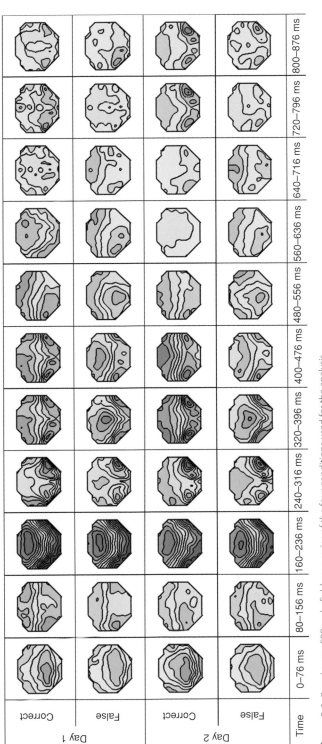

**Figure 8.1** Grand mean ERP scalp field map series of the four conditions used for the analysis.

experiment, i.e. due to the effect of presenting correct or false sentence endings, due to the effect of recording the ERPs at day 1 or day 2, or due to an interaction of both factors. The null hypothesis here is that these differences have been obtained by chance. We will apply this test moment for moment, and address the problem of multiple testing over time in the next step.

- *Test for the frequency and duration of significant effects.* Given that the previous analysis yielded time periods with significant topographic differences between conditions, is the number of significant time points and the duration of these significant periods larger than what we could expect by chance? The null hypothesis is thus that the number and duration of significant effects are compatible with results obtained in randomized data.

- *Partial least squares.* Can we identify factors in the data that are associated with the design of the experiment? How are these factors distributed across time, electrodes and conditions, and how likely is it that we may have observed factors with similar magnitude by chance?

- *Test for correlations with language proficiency increase.* We would like to know whether some of the inter-individual variance in the recorded ERPs can be explained by the variance in language proficiency increase. The null hypothesis is thus that the ERP variance that can be explained by the proficiency increase may have been observed by chance.

- *Test for differences in microstate assignment across conditions.* Given that a microstate analysis of the grand-mean data suggests that there are differences of microstate assignment between conditions, how likely is it that these differences could have occurred by chance?

Since the aim of this chapter is to outline the possible statistical tests that can be used for the analysis of multichannel ERP data and not a complete exploration of a dataset, we will not perform all tests necessary for a full understanding of the data, but merely demonstrate how such tests can be applied and what their results imply.

## Testing the topography consistency across subjects

A test for consistency of topography across subjects can be based upon the following arguments: The GFP of a grand mean ERP across subjects at one moment in time depends on the GFP of the individual ERPs and on the consistency of the topography over subjects in a very simple way: if the GFP of the grand mean across subjects is considerably lower than the mean GFP across subjects, this indicates that there is a relatively high variance of the topography across subjects and that some of the individual signals cancel during the averaging. On the other side, if the GFP of the grand mean is only slightly lower than the average of the individual GFP values, this indicates that there is little cancellation due to variance across subjects, and that the individual topographies are therefore similar. We can thus use the GFP of the grand mean as our measure of effect size.

In order to test whether the observed effect size (the GFP of the grand mean) may also have been observed by chance, we have to destroy the assumed structure of the data, i.e. the spatial configuration of the field that is assumed to be consistent across subjects. This is achieved by shuffling the measured potentials across electrodes in each individual ERP map. This preserves the GFP values of the individual ERPs, but destroys the topographic consistency across subjects. The null hypothesis is thus that the GFP of the grand mean before shuffling is about equally large as after shuffling. We can reject the null hypothesis of no consistent ERP topography across subjects if we can show that the GFP of the grand mean

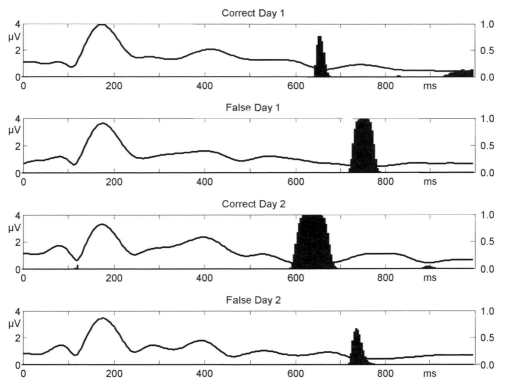

**Figure 8.2** Global field potential of the grand-mean event-related potentials of the four conditions and the result of the test for consistent topography (the height of the black areas indicate the *P*-values, scale to the right, range 0–1).

ERP is consistently larger when the channels are in the correct order opposed to when they are in randomized order. More precisely, the probability of the null hypothesis is defined as the number of randomization runs yielding a GFP larger than or equal to the GFP obtained with the correct channel order.

As an algorithm, the procedure looks as follows.

For a given time point:

(1) Compute the grand mean across subjects.

(2) Compute the GFP of the grand mean.

(3) Separately for each subject, randomly shuffle the measurements across channels.

(4) Compute the grand mean using the randomly shuffled data of the individuals.

(5) Compute the GFP of the randomized grand mean and retain it as one instance of the GFP under the null hypothesis.

(6) Repeat steps 3–5 a sufficient number of times (5000).

(7) Compute the percentage of cases where the GFP obtained after randomization is equal to or larger than the GFP obtained in the observed data. This is the probability of the null hypothesis.

The results of the moment by moment test of map consistency are shown in Figure 8.2. It is apparent that from the beginning of stimulus onset on, there is evidence for activation common across subjects lasting until the end of the analysis period, with interruptions between 600 ms and 800 ms. It is also evident that the significance level of the test is inversely related to the GFP of the ERP. This is to some degree trivial, because the GFP of the grand mean is the measure of effect size that we have been testing against the assumption of randomness. We will use the information obtained here when we apply microstate clustering, excluding time periods from the analysis where we have no evidence for a consistent topography.

## Comparison of map differences between conditions

In order to explain randomization tests for topographical differences, we will first outline the simplest case of just comparing two conditions[13,20]. We will then continue to develop a general scheme that allows testing for effects between several conditions and interactions between several factors. Tests for comparisons of map differences between conditions have previously been called TANOVA (topographic analysis of variance[13,21]).

The procedure to compare two conditions is as follows: first, the scalp field maps are averaged separately for both conditions and the difference map is computed, yielding two condition-wise grand-mean maps. The GFP of this difference map indicates the strength of the difference and will serve as our measure of effect size. Note that if we normalize the two condition-wise grand-mean maps, the GFP of the difference map is the global map dissimilarity described in Chapter 2. Next, samples of the effect size under the null hypothesis are constructed: we shuffle the individual ERPs randomly between the two conditions (either within subject, for paired designs, or across subjects, for unpaired designs). Then we recompute the grand means of the two conditions and compute the GFP of the difference map between the two grand means again. The GFP of the difference maps obtained after randomizing is thus one instance of the GFP compatible with the null hypothesis. In order to estimate how likely it is that the observed GFP of the difference map is compatible with the null hypothesis, the computation of GFP values under the null hypothesis is repeated many times. The probability that the observed GFP difference was obtained by chance is then defined as the percentage of observations where this GFP was smaller than or equal to the GFP of the randomly obtained difference maps[13,20].

Such a test can be applied moment by moment, or on maps averaged across a time period. In the present example, we could employ this test to compare the conditions of interest, e.g. we could ask whether and when there are differences between the processing of the correct sentence endings between day 1 and day 2, or we could ask whether the difference between correct and false sentence endings is different between day 1 and day 2. However, having only paired tests at hand makes it complicated to understand more complex designs, because the number of tests to compute and interpret increases rapidly.

So if the design contains more than two conditions, but we would like to start with a single test across all conditions, we need a test statistic that is more general than the GFP of the difference map. Such a test statistic can be obtained by the variance of the condition-wise grand-mean maps after the grand-mean map across all conditions has been subtracted[21]. We will call maps obtained after subtraction of a mean map residual maps. If all conditions look similar, they also are very similar to the grand mean across all conditions; the residual maps have thus low amplitudes and the variance of the residual maps is small. If the conditions are very different, the grand mean across conditions will only have low amplitudes and the sum of the GFP of the residual maps will be large. We will thus define a general effect size measure for topographic differences as follows:

$$s = \sum_{i=1}^{c} \sqrt{\frac{\sum_{j=1}^{n} (\bar{v}_{ij} - \bar{\bar{v}}_j)^2}{n}} \qquad (1)$$

Where $c$ is the number of conditions, $n$ is the number of electrodes, $\bar{v}_{ij}$ is the grand mean across subjects of the voltage of condition $i$ at electrode $j$, and $\bar{\bar{v}}_j$ is the grand mean across subjects and conditions of the voltage at electrode $j$, and all data are against the average reference. (Note that this general formulation includes the case with only two conditions, where the GFP of the difference map has been used to assess the effect size as a special case.) We will call this measure "generalized dissimilarity." With this general measure of effect size, we can now proceed to test for significance in the same way as we did in the case with two conditions.

As an algorithm, this looks like this:

(1) Compute the grand mean across all conditions.

(2) Subtract this grand mean across all conditions from the ERPs of all subjects and all conditions/groups to obtain the individual residual maps.

(3) For a within-subject factor, compute the grand means of the residual maps for each condition; for a between-group factor, compute the grand means of the residual maps for each group.

(4) Compute the observed effect size as the generalized dissimilarity based on the condition- or group-wise grand means.

(5) For a within-subject factor, randomly shuffle the residual maps across conditions in each subject, for a between-group factor, randomly shuffle the residual maps across the groups.

(6) Recompute the condition- or group-wise grand means of the residual maps after randomization.

(7) Use these grand means to compute and retain an instance of the effect size under the null hypothesis as was done for the observed data in step (4).

(8) Repeat steps (5) to (7) a sufficient number of times (5000).

(9) Compute the percentage of cases where the effect size obtained after randomization is equal to or larger than the effect size obtained in the observed data. This is the probability of the null hypothesis.

In our case, we could use this procedure to test, at a given time instance, whether or not the ERPs of the four conditions are significantly different. A significant result would however be of limited use, because we know that presenting correct and false sentence endings makes consistent ERP differences, so given that the test turns out to be significant, we still would not know whether there is an effect of correctness of sentence endings or of recording day, which is what we are interested in. As in classic ANOVAs, it would be convenient to test the data (a) for an effect of recording day, disregarding whether the sentences were correct or false (main effect of day), (b) for the effect of presenting correct or false sentence endings, independent of the recording day (main effect of correctness), and (c) of the interaction of the two, i.e. effects that depend both on the day of recording and the correctness of the sentence ending and that cannot be explained by the main effects alone (interaction of day and correctness).

In order to address these types of question, we can employ a sequential approach, where we compute the effect size of one factor (e.g. of recording day), remove this effect from the data under test by subtraction, proceed to test the effect of the following factor (e.g. the effect of sentence ending correctness), remove the effect of this factor, and continue this way until we have assessed the effect size of all factors of interest[21]. In order to assess the effect of an interaction of two factors, the effect size is assessed using all possible combinations of the factors as conditions. If the design of the experiment is such that the factors are orthogonal (which is usually the case) this procedure is independent of the sequence of factors to be assessed, as long as the assessments of the main effects precede the assessment of interactions.

The algorithm to perform such an analysis is thus an extension of the algorithm described above:

(1) Compute the grand mean across all conditions.

(2) Subtract this grand mean across all conditions from the ERPs of all subjects and all conditions/groups to obtain the individual residual maps.

(3) For each factor of interest

    a. Compute the grand means of the residual maps for each group or condition.

    b. Compute the observed effect size of the factor.

    c. Remove the grand means of the residual maps obtained in a. from the individual data.

(4) In the data obtained in (2) randomly shuffle the residual maps across conditions within each subject, and across groups if there are any.

(5) Apply the procedure of step (3) to the randomized data, and retain the obtained effect sizes as instances of effect sizes obtained under the null hypothesis.

(6) Repeat step (4) and (5) a sufficient number of times (5000).

(7) Compute the percentage of cases where the effect sizes obtained after randomization were equal to or larger than the effect size obtained in the observed data. These are the probabilities of the null hypotheses of the different factors.

The results of the time-point by time-point analysis of our data with the main, two-level factor day (day 1 vs. day 2), the main, two-level factor correctness (correct vs. false sentence endings), and the four-level interaction (with all four combinations of the two main factors) are shown in Figure 8.3.

## Test for the frequency and duration of effects of the design

The results shown in Figure 8.3 are useful to show at what time periods it is reasonable to continue to compare specific conditions, but there is still a problem of multiple testing, such that there is not yet proper statistical evidence; some of the significant results may simply have occurred because we computed 750 tests. On the other hand, a Bonferroni correction with a factor of 750 is likely to be overly conservative, because many of the tests may have measured the same effect, such that a correction factor of 750 is too large. In order to solve this issue, we can continue to analyze the results of the randomization statistics computed above. For a global statement about the significance of the results shown in Figure 8.3, we can ask how likely it is that we have obtained the number of significant results shown in

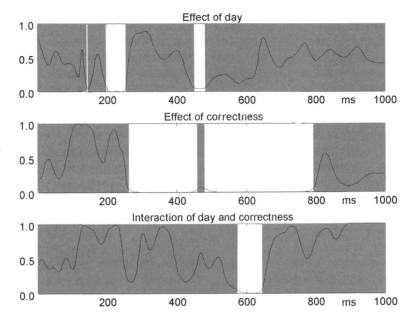

**Figure 8.3**
Significance of the
main effects of day
(upper graph),
correctness (middle
graph) and the
interaction of day
and correctness
(lower graph) as
function of time
(x-axis). White areas
indicate time periods
with $P < 0.05$.

Figure 8.3 by chance, and we can ask how likely it is that we have obtained continuous periods of significance for an equal or longer time than in our observed data by chance.

The information on the count and duration of significant results under the null hypothesis is contained in the collection of observed and randomly obtained effect sizes obtained in the analysis that yielded Figure 8.3. In order to obtain one instance of the count of results significant at a particular $P$-level and under the null hypothesis, we pretend that the first randomization run has actually been our observed data, and compute for each time point a "pseudo-significance" i.e. the percentage of all other effect sizes that were larger than or equal to the effect size of the first randomization run. (We call it pseudo-significance because it is by definition part of the null hypothesis.) We can then count the number of pseudo-significant results at a significance level (e.g. 5%), and we can also record how long each period of pseudo-significance was. By doing this for all randomization runs, we obtain, for a chosen significance level, the distribution of the number of pseudo-significant results under the null hypothesis, and we obtain the distribution of the duration of pseudo-significant results under the null hypothesis. Once we have these distributions, we can ask how often we had observed an equal or larger number of pseudo-significant results compared with the number of significant results in our initial tests. Furthermore, we can ask how often we observed pseudo-significant results that were equally long or longer than the duration of significant effects in our initial tests.

Figure 8.4 shows the histogram of the duration of the count of pseudo-significant results of the two main effects and the interaction. The three graphs look very similar and peak at a value of around 12.5, which is the theoretically expected number because we would expect 5% of all 250 tests in the histogram to be pseudo-significant at a $P$-level of 5%. Now for the effect of day, we have actually observed 35 time points with significant results, which is by far larger than any of the counts obtained by randomization. The probability that we would obtain 35 significant time points by chance is thus, with 5000 randomization runs, smaller than 1/5000,

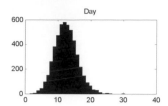
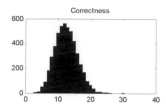
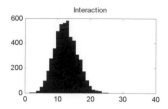

**Figure 8.4** Number of observations (vertical axis) as a function of count of pseudo-significant results (horizontal-axis) for the effect of day (left), correctness (center) and the interaction (right).

or 0.0002. The same holds for the effect of correctness, where we counted significant effects at 160 time points. However, for the interaction, we have counted only 15 time points with significance, and there were 1387 randomization runs that yielded equal or larger counts. Dividing 1387 by 5000 gives 0.277, such that we have to accept the null hypothesis that we have not observed more significant effects than we would have expected by chance in the analysis of the interaction of day and correctness.

Before we stop looking at the interaction, let us have a look at the duration of the effect. In the randomization runs, 99% of all periods of pseudo-significance lasted between 4 and 8 ms (one or two time points). The shortest duration of significance in the observed data was however 24 ms (or 6 time points). From that point of view, we can reject the null hypothesis that significant effects of the observed duration have occurred by chance.

## Post-hoc tests

The randomization tests that we have employed above have used global measures of effect size that subsume effects across an often large amount of data by a single effect-size measure. This has the important advantage that we can reduce the number of tests that we perform and can effectively avoid correcting our statistical results for multiple testing. The disadvantage of global measures is of course that rejecting a null hypothesis based on such an unspecific measure of effect size merely informs us that there is a difference, but is uninformative about the distribution of the difference. Given that we have been able to reject the null hypothesis, the typical procedure is thus to make further post-hoc tests, and use the results of these post-hoc tests as indices of the distribution of signal-to-noise ratios rather than as statistical evidence in the strict sense; this evidence is already given by the global tests and does not need replication. In the current example, we have chosen to compute electrode-by-electrode t-tests of mean maps across particular time intervals, comparing conditions of interest during time periods where the global test was significant.

Because there was a main effect of day in an early time interval we have computed the mean voltages across the time interval of interest and across both conditions and compared these mean maps across subjects with electrode-wise paired t-tests. The result is shown in Figure 8.5.

Furthermore, because there was an interaction of recording day and correctness in a late time period, we have computed t-maps displaying the effects of recording day separately for correct and false sentence endings, the effect of correctness separately for day 1 and day 2, and a t-map comparing the difference of day 2 and day 1 in the correct condition with the difference of day 2 and day 1 in the false condition. The results are shown in Figure 8.6. An inspection of Figure 8.6 suggests that responses to false sentence endings change little from day 1 to day 2, while there is a change for the correct sentence endings. This change

**Figure 8.5** Mean maps of the ERPs at day 2 (left) and day 1 (right) for the early (upper row) and late (lower row) time interval where the global tests indicated significant effects of day. The middle column shows the t-maps comparing day 2 with day 1.

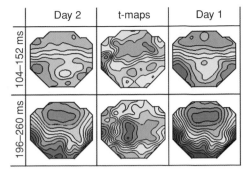

**Figure 8.6** Left and right column, upper and lower row: Mean maps of the four conditions in the time interval from 608 to 628 ms. Middle columns and rows show t-maps comparing the mean maps.

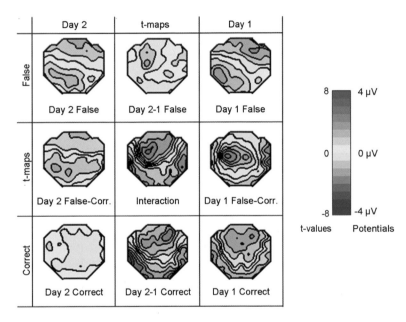

looks very similar to and therefore is also likely to account for the interaction that we have observed.

## Partial least squares

In the above sections, we have begun our analysis with tests that worked across all electrodes at once, but were applied time-instant by time-instant. We then explored the data further by using electrode-by-electrode t-tests. We may also choose to take a step in the other direction, and ask whether we can identify factors in our data that extend across time and electrodes and relate to the design of the experiment. A well-described method to identify such factors is called partial least squares (PLS)[11,22]. Partial least squares is based on a data matrix that typically contains measurements across all subjects, conditions, time points and electrodes, and a design matrix, that contains the design of the experiment. These matrices are matrix-multiplied, such that a single covariance matrix is obtained that contains information on how the entire design is represented in the entire data. This covariance matrix is then decomposed into a set of factors, or so-called latent variables, using a singular-value-decomposition (SVD). (SVD is a frequently used factorization scheme.) Each of these latent variables contains three elements:

- The so-called electrode saliencies, containing information on how the voltage measurements accounted for by the latent variable are distributed across the scalp and across time. Having applied a SVD to extract the latent variables implies that electrode saliencies of the different latent variables are by definition orthogonal (uncorrelated).
- The design saliencies, containing information on how the measurements accounted for by the latent variable are distributed across the different conditions. Having applied a SVD to extract the latent variables implies that the design saliencies of the different latent variables are by definition orthogonal (uncorrelated).
- The singular values, containing information on how much variance is explained by each latent variable.

The test for statistical significance of the resulting latent variable is again based on randomization. As a measure of effect size, singular values are being used, because they directly indicate the amount of variance explained by each latent variable. The aim is thus to obtain samples of singular values under the null hypothesis, which is achieved by random permutations of the design matrix for each subject, and recomputing the PLS. The significance of each latent variable is defined by the number of cases where the singular value of the latent variable obtained after randomization was larger than or equal to the singular value obtained with the correct design. For details on the computation of PLS in ERP data, we refer to Lobaugh et al.[11], where a useful link to a Matlab implementation of PLS is given. For a discussion on orthogonality, we refer to Chapter 5.

In order to demonstrate the method, we have submitted the data already analyzed above to an analysis with PLS. The randomization test indicated that the first two of the obtained latent variables were significant ($P < 0.0002$ for the latent variable 1, and $P < 0.016$ for the latent variable 2, with 5000 randomizations). Further tests estimated the standard error of the electrode saliencies of the latent variables for all channels and electrodes (see Lobaugh et al.[11] for a detailed description) in order to obtain an index of the time intervals at which the electrode saliencies of the latent variables were different from 0. We show the results of our PLS analysis in Figures 8.7 and 8.8.

The results indicate that PLS identified a first latent variable that is clearly associated with the correctness of the sentence endings, because the design saliencies for the false and correct conditions are opposed and differ little between day 1 and day 2. The latency range where there is a good signal-to-noise ratio in the electrode saliencies is in the N400 time range and largely coincident with the time range where we had observed a significant effect of correctness in the TANOVA. The second latent variable reflects differences between day 1 and day 2, mostly in the correct, but to a lesser degree also in the false condition. The time interval where there is a good signal-to-noise ratio in the electrode saliencies covers both an early time window, where we had previously observed a main effect of recording day, and a late effect, where we had observed the interaction. The topographic distribution of the electrode saliencies of the latent variable 2 looks similar to the post-hoc t-maps of the TANOVA main effect of day in the early time interval, and to the post-hoc t-maps of the TANOVA interaction in the late time interval. It therefore appears that the second latent variable is a mixture of the main effect of day and the interaction observed in the TANOVA.

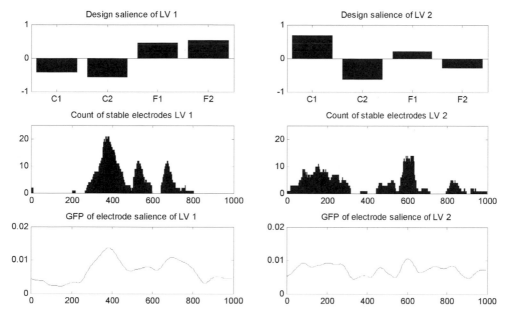

**Figure 8.7** Distribution of the latent variables (left: latent variable 1, right: latent variable 2) obtained by PLS across conditions (upper graph) and across time (middle and lower graph). The middle graph shows the count of significances across electrodes, the lower graph shows the GFP of the latent variables (vertical axes, in μV) as a function of time (horizontal axes, in ms).

## Test for correlations with language proficiency increase

So far, we have treated our data as if all subjects just had learned German. However, when looking at the change of language proficiency from day 1 to day 2, we note that there are considerable differences between subjects. We will now investigate whether the ERPs at day 1 have a predictive value for the increase of language proficiency from day 1 to day 2. For this purpose, we employ a method called TANCOVA[10], that allows us to obtain ERP correlates of an external predictor and test these correlates for significance. The rationale of the TANCOVA is that because ERP fields are additive, the existence of a source that is active proportionally to an external variable results in a single topography that is added to the ERP, proportionally to the external variable. In order to retrieve the topography that is proportional to the external variable, we can compute, across subjects, the covariance of the external variable with the potentials at each electrode. (This is the same idea as using PLS, and it can be shown that the TANCOVA is a special case of PLS.) The obtained covariance map represents the map corresponding to the generators that activate proportionally to the external variable. Similar to the tests performed above, the GFP of this covariance map is a convenient and reference independent measure of effect size. In order to obtain the significance of an observed effect size, we can repeatedly shuffle the individual ERP topographies among subjects, and recompute the GFP of the covariance maps obtained after randomization. The significance of our effect is then again determined by the proportion of randomly obtained effect sizes that are larger than or equal to the effect size observed. Figure 8.9 shows the result of computing moment-by-moment TANCOVAs of the ERPs with the increase of language proficiency. It turns out that the ERP of the correct condition at day 1 is most capable of predicting the students' learning success.

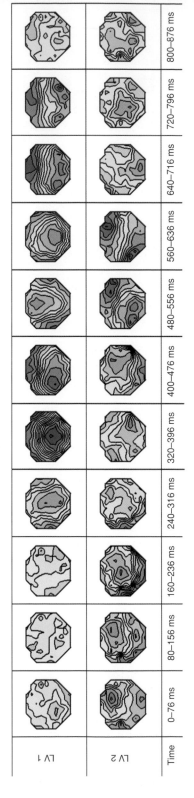

**Figure 8.8** Spatial distribution of the two latent variables across time.

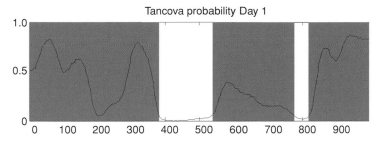
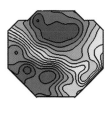

Day 1: 400–500 ms

**Figure 8.9** Significance of the TANCOVA of the ERPs after correct sentence endings at day 1 and language proficiency increase. The vertical axis shows the *P*-value, the horizontal axis indicates time in ms. The map shows the mean covariances in time interval from 400 to 500 ms.

# Randomization tests on microstate assignment

For a further understanding of the data, we have continued to apply a microstate clustering on the grand means of the four conditions. The results, employing 10 clusters and disregarding time periods with inconsistent topography across subjects, are shown in Figure 8.10.

As expected, we observe different microstate classes in our grand-mean ERPs depending on the correctness of the sentence ending and recording day. How can we test whether the microstate assignment is significantly different between two conditions? One possibility is to use the fitting tests described in Chapter 6. Alternatively, one can again use randomization tests[23]. In the following, we will outline how such randomization tests for microstate assignments may be constructed. As above, we will employ a two-step procedure: first, we will apply a single, global test to find out whether there is evidence that somewhere in the data there are differences in microstate assignment between conditions that are unlikely to have occurred by chance. Given that this is the case, we proceed to more specific tests to obtain statistically sound interpretations.

A simple and global measure of effect size for microstate assignment is the count of time points where the microstate assignment was not identical across the grand means of the different conditions. As before, the observed effect size is first computed based on the actual grand-mean ERPs of the different conditions. In order to obtain samples of our measure of effect size under the null hypothesis, we randomly exchange the ERPs of the different conditions within subjects and average each condition across subjects to obtain grand mean ERPs of the different conditions under the null hypothesis[23]. A random sample of our measure of effect size is then obtained by making a microstate assignment to the random-condition grand means and counting the time points where this assignment was not identical across conditions. Note that the same procedure can also be used for group comparisons, but in this case, the randomization has to be a random reassignment of the ERPs to the different groups. The significance of our test is given by the count of randomly obtained effect sizes that are larger than or equal to the observed effect size.

In order to adapt the above procedure to test more specific hypotheses, we can easily modify the measure of effect size to fit our specific needs. We can, for example, define the effect size as the onset-latency difference of a specific microstate class within a specific analysis window (i.e. the time difference between the moments a microstate class is observed for the first time in the analysis window), which yields a test for microstate latency differences. Alternatively, we can count the number of time points a specific microstate class has been observed in a time interval and use the difference of this count between two conditions as a

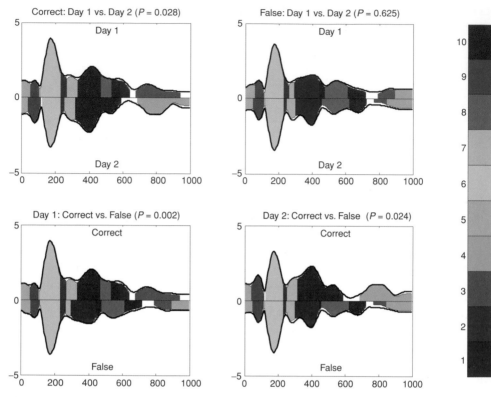

**Figure 8.10** Comparison of the microstate assignment of the four conditions. The vertical axis indicates GFP (in µV), the horizontal axis indicates time (in ms), the colors code the different microstate classes. The P-values indicate the significance of the global test for differences in microstate assignment.

measure of effect size. This allows us to test whether the occurrence of the specific microstate class is associated with a particular condition. Once the measure of effect size has been set, we can apply the same randomization procedure as above.

In our example, we have computed four global tests, comparing the ERPs of day 1 with day 2, separately for the correct and false sentence endings, and comparing correct and false sentence endings separately for days 1 and 2. These global tests were significant ($P < 0.05$) for the comparisons between correct and false sentence endings on both days, and for the comparison of days 1 and 2 using the correct sentence endings, but not the false sentence endings. As one example of a post-hoc test, we have tested, on the ERPs of day 2, the observation that microstate class 1 is apparently associated with the false, but not the correct condition (see Figure 8.10). As a measure of effect size, we therefore compared the number of time points microstate class 1 was observed in the correct and the false condition, in a time window from 256 to 500 ms. The observed effect size was 35 time points (140 ms), and 52 out of 5000 randomization runs yielded random effect sizes that were equal or larger. The probability of the null hypothesis is therefore 1%, and we conclude that there is significant evidence that microstate class 1 is associated with the processing of false sentence endings on day 2. We might continue to test for other discrepancies at other time periods and conditions, but since the aim of this chapter is to outline the possible solutions to EEG-specific statistical questions, we omit an exhaustive analysis of the data here.

# Concluding remarks

All of the above statistics have been based on scalp measurements and not on voxel-based inverse solutions. This does not imply that this is necessarily the best choice. We have chosen to demonstrate statistics at the level of electrodes, because this is described and discussed less extensively than voxel-based statistics, and the problem is smaller in terms of the amount of numbers to include and results to display. The statistics used for voxel-based inverse solution are essentially those that are commonly used in other voxel-based neuroimaging methods such as PET and fMRI, and there is an abundant amount of literature and software for this purpose[24-26].

Electrode- and voxel-based analyses have a conceptual difference that needs to be taken into account when choosing, discussing and comparing statistical results. Electrode-based comparisons emphasize features of the data different from comparisons based on voxel-wise inverse solutions, and make different assumptions: the scalp-potentials differences observed at the level of electrodes reflect both differences of source localization and source orientation, while source orientation is typically not considered in voxel-wise statistics of inverse solutions. Although this is rarely discussed, source orientation seems to be a very robust feature of ERP data: whenever we compute an average evoked potential by averaging scalp potentials, we assume not only that the amplitudes of the sources that make the evoked potential are constant, but their orientations are too. The interpretation of orientation differences remains unclear, however. On one hand, it is not possible for neurons to change orientation. A change of source orientation therefore necessarily implies that different neurons have been active, which is something that we typically want to show. However, unless elaborate individual head models are used, it is often not possible to translate changes of source orientation into chances of source location, such that the interpretation of orientation differences often remains elusive. Furthermore, the scalp field changes induced by a change of orientation are often more drastic than changes of source position, such that our measures of scalp field differences are overemphasizing changes of sources that include changes of source orientation.

On the other hand, statistics based on inverse solutions obviously depend on the correctness of the assumptions of the inverse model, for example that there is a good signal-to-noise ratio, that the real (and unknown) current density distribution is compatible with the distribution assumed by the model, and that the real current density distribution is part of the solution space of the inverse solution. Because we do not know the real current density distribution, it is often difficult to argue whether the data complies with the assumptions.

We thus have the choice of (a) using the scalp data for statistics, which requires very few assumptions, but probably overemphasizes orientation and does not directly localize, or (b) using inverse solution, which typically relies heavily on assumptions, and usually ignores orientation. For an in-depth analysis of a given dataset, it is probably optimal to explore both possibilities before coming to a conclusion.

Another choice that needs to be made when doing statistics is whether or not to use normalization. Normalization at the level of electrodes means that all voltages of a scalp field are divided by the GFP (or some equivalent) before being analyzed further. On the voxel level, normalization means that the voxel-wise current density estimates are divided by the overall current density. Using normalization before doing statistical tests changes the interpretation of the results: if an effect is mainly observed because similar generators have different amplitudes, tests done without normalization will eventually become significant, while a normalization of the data before statistics will eliminate these differences, such that nonsignificant results are obtained. Tests computed without prior normalization will thus test for differences of source orientation, distribution and strength, while normalizing the data before statistics will yield tests that are sensitive only to differences in source orientation and or distribution. Tests done with normalized data are thus typically complemented by tests of global amplitude such as GFP.

The advantage of using normalization is that one obtains a clear separation of effects of source distribution and/or orientation from effects of source amplitude, which may facilitate and sharpen the interpretation of the data. The disadvantage of normalization is that maps with little amplitude and often low signal-to-noise ratios are magnified, which leads to an inflation of noise. As with the issue of whether one should use electrode-based or voxel-based statistics, we think that the choice often depends on the various (and often unknown) features of the data and their interaction with the hypotheses under investigation, such that general recommendations cannot be made.

Statistics on experimental neurophysiological data may be done on the individual level or on a group level (as in the examples given in this chapter). If individual statistical results are available from several subjects, they can be combined to yield second-level group statistics. Such types of analyses are called hierarchical. If randomization tests are being employed in hierarchical analyses, it is important to consider how the data are organized and how the randomization is done, because this affects the generalizability of the results. It is thus important to consider whether the independent variables of the design are equal for all subjects (so-called fixed effects) or have an assumingly continuous distribution in the general population (so-called random effect). For a detailed discussion on this issue, see Friston et al. 2005[27].

# References

1. Gevins A, Le J, Martin NK et al. High resolution EEG: 124-channel recording, spatial deblurring and MRI integration methods. Electroencephalography and Clinical Neurophysiology 1994;**90**:337–358.

2. Michel CM, Thut G, Morand S et al. Electric source imaging of human brain functions. Brain Research. Brain Research Review 2001; **36**:108–118.

3. Tucker DM. Spatial sampling of head electrical fields: the geodesic sensor net. Electroencephalography and Clinical Neurophysiology 1993;**87**:154–163.

4. Duffy FH, Bartels PH, Burchfiel JL. Significance probability mapping: an aid in the topographic analysis of brain electrical activity. Electroencephalography and Clinical Neurophysiology 1981;**51**:455–462.

5. Steger J, Imhof K, Steinhausen H, Brandeis D. Brain mapping of bilateral interactions in attention deficit hyperactivity disorder and control boys. Clinical Neurophysiology 2000;**111**:1141–1156.

6. Vasey MW, Thayer JF. The continuing problem of false positives in repeated measures ANOVA in psychophysiology: a multivariate solution. Psychophysiology 1987;**24**:479–486.

7. Galan L, Biscay R, Rodriguez JL, Perez-Abalo MC, Rodriguez R. Testing topographic differences between event related brain potentials by using non-parametric combinations of permutation tests. Electroencephalography and Clinical Neurophysiology 1997;**102**:240–247.

8. Greenblatt RE, Pflieger ME. Randomization-based hypothesis testing from event-related data. Brain Topography 2004;**16**:225–232.

9. Karniski W, Blair RC, Snider AD. An exact statistical method for comparing

topographic maps, with any number of subjects and electrodes. *Brain Topography* 1994;**6**:203–210.

10. Koenig T, Melie-Garcia L, Stein M, Strik W, Lehmann C. Establishing correlations of scalp field maps with other experimental variables using covariance analysis and resampling methods. *Clinical Neurophysiology* 2008;**119**:1262–1270.

11. Lobaugh NJ, West R, McIntosh AR. Spatiotemporal analysis of experimental differences in event-related potential data with partial least squares. *Psychophysiology* 2001;**38**:517–530.

12. Maris E. Randomization tests for ERP topographies and whole spatiotemporal data matrices. *Psychophysiology* 2004;**41**: 142–151.

13. Strik WK, Fallgatter AJ, Brandeis D, Pascual-Marqui RD. Three-dimensional tomography of event-related potentials during response inhibition: evidence for phasic frontal lobe activation. *Electroencephalography and Clinical Neurophysiology* 1998;**108**:406–413.

14. Edgington ES, Onghena P. *Randomization Tests*. 4th edn. Boca Raton: Chapman & Hall/CRC; 2007.

15. Manly BFJ. *Randomization, Bootstrap, and Monte Carlo Methods in Biology*. 3rd edn. Boca Raton, FL: Chapman & Hall/ CRC; 2007.

16. Hoeffding W. The large sample power of tests based on permutations of observations. *Annals of Mathematical Statistics* 1952;**23**:169–192.

17. Kempthorne O, Doerfler TE. The behaviour of some significance tests under experimental randomization. *Biometrika* 1969;**56**:231–248.

18. Stein M, Dierks T, Brandeis D *et al.* Plasticity in the adult language system: a longitudinal electrophysiological study on second language learning. *Neuroimage* 2006;**33**:774–783.

19. Kutas M, Hillyard SA. Brain potentials during reading reflect word expectancy and semantic association. *Nature* 1984;**307**:161–163.

20. Kondakor I, Pascual-Marqui RD, Michel CM, Lehmann D. Event-related potential map differences depend on the prestimulus microstates. *Journal of Medical Engineering and Technology* 1995;**19**:66–69.

21. Wirth M, Horn H, Koenig T *et al.* The early context effect reflects activity in the temporo-prefrontal semantic system – evidence from electrical neuroimaging of abstract and concrete word reading. *Neuroimage* 2008;**42**:423–436.

22. McIntosh AR, Lobaugh NJ. Partial least squares analysis of neuroimaging data: applications and advances. *Neuroimage* 2004;**23 Suppl 1**:S250–S263.

23. Schumacher R, Wirth M, Perrig W *et al.* ERP correlates of supraordinate category activation. *International Journal of Psychophysiology*, 2009; in press.

24. Friston KJ, Holmes A, Poline JB, Price CJ, Frith CD. Detecting activations in PET and fMRI: levels of inference and power. *Neuroimage* 1996;**4**:223–235.

25. Nichols TE, Holmes AP. Nonparametric permutation tests for functional neuroimaging: a primer with examples. *Human Brain Mapping* 2002;**15**:1–25.

26. Worsley KJ, Taylor JE, Tomaiuolo F, Lerch J. Unified univariate and multivariate random field theory. *Neuroimage* 2004;**23 Suppl 1**:S189–S195.

27. Friston KJ, Stephan KE, Lund TE, Morcom A, Kiebel S. Mixed-effects and fMRI studies. *Neuroimage* 2005;**24**:244–252.

# Chapter 9

# State space representation and global descriptors of brain electrical activity

Jiří Wackermann and Carsten Allefeld

The methods introduced in this chapter aim at a comprehensive assessment of the brain's functional state via a small number of "global" quantitative descriptors. Unlike the approaches presented in the preceding chapters, the objective of the global approach is not a mapping of the brain's functions within the real (physical) three-dimensional space, but rather a mapping of the variety of the brain's functional states into an abstract (mathematical) multidimensional space. Nevertheless, the global methodology shares with the other methods the focus on the spatial configuration of brain electrical fields, is closely related to microstate analysis, and as such belongs in the context of functional brain topography and electrical neuroimaging.

## The state space representation
### The notion of state space

The state, or temporary condition, of a given system is characterized by observations, usually in the form of measurements. For example, the weather situation at a given place and time may be assessed by measuring the temperature $\theta$, the relative humidity $h$ and the air pressure $p$. A convenient representation of the momentary state, which is characterized by three quantities, is a single point within a three-dimensional *state space*, located at coordinates $(\theta, h, p)$. The state space representation is useful in many cases because it gives an overview over all possible states of the system at once. Moreover, the evolution of the state over time appears as a movement within this space, or, disregarding time measure, as a path consisting of successive state points, the *state space trajectory*.

Depending on the kind and number of measured quantities used, the state of the same system may be characterized in a variety of ways, including different degrees of detail. Concerning the relation between two state descriptions, such that states of one description correspond to extended areas within the second state space, one may speak of macro- and microstates, respectively. Note that such a difference in detail generally also leads to different relevant time scales, because less precisely defined states tend to persist over longer periods of time[1]. For example, a fair weather period lasts for days up to weeks, while exact temperature measurements reveal changes on the time scale of minutes.

In the case of a spatially extended system, its state may be assessed using multiple measurements of the same quantity, taken at different places within the system simultaneously;

*Electrical Neuroimaging*, ed. Christoph M. Michel, Thomas Koenig, Daniel Brandeis, Lorena R.R. Gianotti and Jiří Wackermann. Published by Cambridge University Press. © Cambridge University Press 2009.

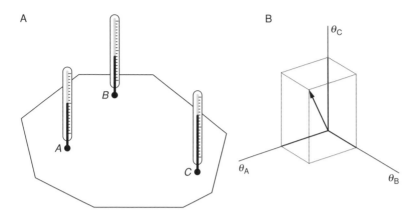

**Figure 9.1**
Simultaneous measurements of the same quantity – for example, temperature – at three locations (A) determine a point in a "thermometric state space" (B).

for example, the air temperature measured in three cities (Figure 9.1A). A triplet of temperatures $(\theta_A, \theta_B, \theta_C)$ gives a snapshot of the weather situation in the region, or, its "momentary thermometric state." These measurements can be seen as separately characterizing the situation at different places, in which case they may be graphically presented on a topographic map of that region. Or the combined measurements $\boldsymbol{\theta} \equiv (\theta_A, \theta_B, \theta_C)$ may be conceived as defining the state of the entire extended system, which again can be represented as a single point within a state space (Figure 9.1B).

Continuously evolving quantities can practically only be measured at a certain number $N$ of time instants $t_n$ (where $n = 0, 1, \ldots, N - 1$), that is, "sampled" in time, thus yielding a "time series," a sequence of measurements of the same quantity. Usually a constant sampling step $\Delta t$ is used, such that $t_n = n \, \Delta t$. In the following we will use the term "trajectory" for the continuous path as well as for the series of samples. Where the temporal order of measurements does not play a role, we simply refer to the set of points in the state space as a "data cloud."

These concepts directly apply to the assessment of brain electrical activity via multi-channel electroencephalography (EEG), which is a time series $\boldsymbol{u}_n \equiv \boldsymbol{u}(t_n)$ of $m$-tuples $\boldsymbol{u} \equiv (u_1, \ldots, u_m)$, consisting of voltages measured at $m$ spatially distributed loci – for example, electrodes displaced on the scalp surface, or elements of an intracranial electrode grid. (In the following $m$ always denotes the number of EEG channels.) Equivalently, we may consider each $m$-tuple as coordinates of a point in an $m$-dimensional space $\mathbb{R}^m$; individual points of this state space indicate instantaneous electrical field distributions, which characterize the momentary brain state. Later we will go on to introduce the lower-dimensional state space of global descriptors $(\Sigma, \Phi, \Omega)$ as a comprehensive characterization of the current brain state; these quantities will be defined based on the properties of short sections of the trajectory in the EEG state space.

It is sometimes said that we "construct" the state space trajectory from EEG data, but this phrase is somewhat misleading. In the present approach, we assume that the state space trajectory is generated by the system under study, i.e. it is *given*; the EEG data result from the observation of the system. The spatial distribution of the measurement loci (EEG electrodes) determines one particular choice of the coordinate system; hence the emphasis on properties of data which are invariant with respect to particular conditions of observation.

# Structure of the EEG state space

## Vector space structure

The elements of a state space defined on the basis of measurements are generally specified by $m$-tuples of real numbers. However, this numeric representation does not necessarily imply that the familiar arithmetic operations are meaningfully defined.

For the EEG state space we may assume the algebraic structure of a linear *vector space*, for the following reasons: EEG measurements are voltages, i.e. differences within the electric potential distribution generated by the brain (see Chapter 1). Voltages generated by the combination of several independent field sources add up, while a differently strong activation of the same field source leads to multiplication of voltages by a common factor. These physical processes are captured by the vector space operations of (element-wise) addition of data vectors and multiplication by a real number.

The elements $u$ of an $m$-dimensional vector space can be represented with respect to a set of linearly independent basis vectors $e_1, e_2, \ldots, e_m$ by $m$-tuples $(u_1, u_2, \ldots, u_m)$ of real numbers such that $u = u_1 e_1 + u_2 e_2 + \cdots + u_m e_m$. For EEG, the original data vectors already have this form, which can be interpreted as their representation in the standard basis $e_1 = (1, 0, \ldots, 0)$, $e_2 = (0, 1, \ldots, 0)$, etc.

## Metric structure

The structure of the EEG state space can be further enriched by introducing a binary operation between vectors, called *inner product*, resulting in a real number; we choose it as the "dot product" of data vectors

$$u \cdot v := \sum_{i=1}^{m} u_i v_i \tag{1}$$

Based on this, a measure of the magnitude of a vector, usually called its *norm*, is defined as

$$\|u\| := \sqrt{u \cdot u} \tag{2}$$

The norm of a difference between two vectors, or equivalently, the distance between state space points, $u$ and $v$, is then

$$\|u - v\| = \sqrt{\sum_{i=1}^{m} (u_i - v_i)^2} \tag{3}$$

The distance in the state space thus naturally provides a single-valued measure of the global difference between momentary electrical brain states represented by data vectors $u, v$.

A given vector $u$ defines a *direction* in the state space; the set of all multiples $au$ (where $a > 0$) constitutes a *ray* in the direction of $u$. Since the magnitude of a vector is irrelevant for the direction, it is meaningful to represent directions by the normalized vector

$$\tilde{u} := \frac{u}{\|u\|}, \quad (\text{for } u \neq 0) \tag{4}$$

whose magnitude is unity. Then, for two non-zero vectors $u, v$, the inner product

$$\tilde{u} \cdot \tilde{v} = \frac{u \cdot v}{\|u\| \, \|v\|} \tag{5}$$

attains a value from $-1$ to $+1$. A number $\phi \in [0, \pi]$ such that $\cos \phi = \tilde{u} \cdot \tilde{v}$ is the *angle* between the vectors $u$ and $v$ (or, generally, between their respective directions). For two vectors pointing into directions perpendicular to each other, the inner product becomes $u \cdot v = 0$; those vectors are called *orthogonal*.

In contrast to the vector space structure of EEG data, which is immediately motivated by the physical properties of EEG measurements, the metric structure introduced via the inner product has to be seen as a heuristic choice which is justified by its utility for the further analysis and characterization of data. In particular, normalization (Eqn 4) allows a separation of the shape and the strength of an electric field distribution, while the definition of angle and distance facilitates a comparison of the shape of different distributions.

An important aspect of this choice is the fact that the definition of norm and angle via the dot product of EEG data vectors implies a dependence on the *reference* underlying the voltage measurements. While it is true that the "landscape" of each single field distribution, as defined in terms of relative differences between measurement loci, is not altered by a change of the reference by an additive term, the geometry of the entire data-set with respect to the inner product *is* changed by the transformation. In the following we assume that the EEG data have been transformed to the average reference (Chapter 2).

## Relation to topographical analysis

There is a one-to-one correspondence between the algebraic–geometrical notions introduced above, and the standard terminology of topographic analysis (see Chapter 2). The "Global field power" (GFP)[2,3] of a field map is proportional to the norm of the data vector

$$\mathrm{gfp}(u) = \frac{1}{\sqrt{m}} \|u\| \tag{6}$$

Data transformation to $\mathrm{gfp}(u) = 1$ is thus equivalent to the normalization to unity, except for a constant multiplicative factor $\sqrt{m}$.

Accordingly, topographies of scalp fields can be identified with directions in the state space, so that topographic global measures are functions of normalized data vectors. Topographic dissimilarity[2,3] between two field maps is defined via the distance

$$\mathrm{diss}(u, v) = \|\tilde{u} - \tilde{v}\| \tag{7}$$

whereas topographic correlation[4] is defined by the inner product of normalized vectors

$$\mathrm{cor}(u, v) = \tilde{u} \cdot \tilde{v} = \frac{u \cdot v}{\|u\| \, \|v\|} \tag{8}$$

An elementary calculation shows that the two measures are related as follows:

$$\tfrac{1}{2} \left( \mathrm{diss}(u, v) \right)^2 = 1 - \mathrm{cor}(u, v) \tag{9}$$

The dissimilarity measure (Eqn 7) has a certain "beauty defect," namely, an asymmetry with respect to the change of the field polarity. Consider two vectors, $u$ and $v$; then $\mathrm{diss}(u, v)$ is in the range from 0 to 2, with the extreme values attained for $v = u$ (identical topography) and $v = -u$ (reversed polarity), respectively. However, if $v$ is orthogonal to $u$, which is arguably a "mid-way case" between the two extremes, then $\mathrm{diss}(u, v) = \sqrt{2}$, and not 1! This inconvenience is avoided by using the similarity measure (Eqn 8), yielding values from the range $-1$ to $+1$, fulfilling the intuitive identity $\mathrm{cor}(u, -v) = -\mathrm{cor}(u, v)$ and yielding $\mathrm{cor}(u, v) = 0$ for orthogonal vectors.

**Figure 9.2** A. Parallel projection of points $K, L, M \in \mathbb{R}^2$ in the direction of line $p$ onto line $l$. B. Central projection of points $P, Q, R \in \mathbb{R}^2$ onto a unit circle $k$.

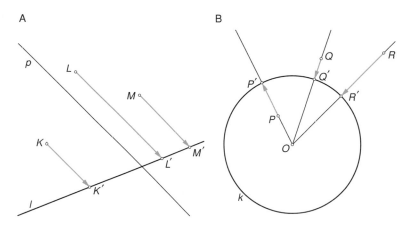

**Figure 9.2** A. Parallel projection of points $K, L, M \in \mathbb{R}^2$ in the direction of line $p$ onto line $l$. B. Central projection of points $P, Q, R \in \mathbb{R}^2$ onto a unit circle $k$.

## Linear transformations

A function $A$ which maps each element of a vector space, $x \in \mathbb{R}^m$, onto another element $y \in \mathbb{R}^m$, $y = A(x)$, and which fulfills the conditions

$$A(u + v) = A(u) + A(v) \tag{10}$$

$$A(cu) = c\,A(u) \quad (c \in \mathbb{R}) \tag{11}$$

is called a linear transform. In terms of the vector components, the transform attains the form of a linear combination

$$y_i = \sum_{j=1}^{m} a_{ij} x_j \tag{12}$$

which can be written in shorter form using matrix notation as $y = \mathbf{A}x$, where $\mathbf{A} \equiv [a_{ij}]_{i,\,j=1,\ldots,m}$. If the columns of $\mathbf{A}$ are normalized and mutually orthogonal vectors, the same holds for the columns of the transposed matrix $\mathbf{A}^{\mathrm{T}} \equiv [a_{ji}]$, and the transform is called orthogonal. Such a transformation corresponds to a rigid rotation; i.e. lengths and angles are preserved. In the language of EEG measurements, a linear transform recombines the originally measured data channels into a new set of artificially defined measurements, or "virtual electrodes."

## Projections

In the following sections we often speak about "projections" of data clouds or trajectories. Usually we refer to linear projections from $\mathbb{R}^m$ into $\mathbb{R}^k$, where $k < m$; this can be intuitively understood as a parallel projection of an $m$-dimensional object to its $k$-dimensional "shadow" (Figure 9.2A). A trivial example of a linear projection is a choice of the $i$th channel from EEG data, i.e. a reduction of the original $m$-dimensional data to a one-dimensional time series (single-channel EEG). Another instance of linear projection is transformation of EEG data to the average reference, by which the EEG data cloud is projected onto an $(m-1)$-dimensional subspace defined by the condition $\sum_{i=1}^{m} u_i = 0$; one dimension is thus lost. Algebraically, a linear projection $\mathbb{R}^m \rightarrow \mathbb{R}^k$ can be expressed as multiplication by a $k \times m$ matrix.

As a broader notion, any transformation $P$ which is "idempotent," i.e. $P(P(x)) = P(x)$ for any $x$, is called projection. Such transforms may be generally nonlinear; an example of a nonlinear projection is the normalization to unity, given by Eqn 4. Geometrically, this corresponds to the projection of data onto the surface of a unit sphere (Figure 9.2B).

The aim of the preceding paragraphs was to introduce the main algebraic concepts as far as they are necessary to specify the structure of the EEG state space. For further details, refer to any standard textbook on linear algebra.

# Principal component analysis
## Principal components

Consider a collection of $N$ EEG data points $\boldsymbol{u}_0, \boldsymbol{u}_1, \ldots, \boldsymbol{u}_{N-1} \in \mathbb{R}^m$. Let $u_{i,n}$ denote the $i$th component of vector $\boldsymbol{u}_n$, so that $u_i \equiv (u_{i,0}, u_{i,1}, \ldots, u_{i,N-1})$ is the time series recorded in the $i$th channel. In the following, we assume that the data has been centered over time, i.e. $\langle u_i \rangle = 0$ for all $i$, where $\langle \cdot \rangle$ denotes the arithmetic mean over the observation epoch $n = 0, \ldots, N - 1$.

Strictly speaking, the subtraction of the time average leads to a shift in the EEG state space, slightly altering norms of data vectors and angles between them. However, since EEG data are oscillatory in nature and usually already "DC-corrected" during recording, the change induced by this is practically negligible.

The power (variance) of the signal $u_i$ – geometrically, the dispersion of the data cloud in the direction of the $i$th axis – is then

$$V_i = \operatorname{var} u_i := \langle u_{i,n}^2 \rangle \tag{13}$$

and

$$W = \sum_{i=1}^{m} V_i \tag{14}$$

is the total variance summed across all channels. Substituting Eqn 13 in Eqn 14 and swapping the order of summation gives

$$W = \langle \|\boldsymbol{u}_n\|^2 \rangle \tag{15}$$

Put in words, the total variance of a data-set is proportional to the integral of the global field power over the measurement epoch.

A linear transformation of EEG channels into new data channels, $x_n = \mathbf{F} \boldsymbol{u}_n$, generally leads to new channel variances $\operatorname{var} x_i$. However, if $\mathbf{F}$ is an orthogonal transform, the sum $\sum_{i=1}^m \operatorname{var} x_i = W$ is preserved. In other words, such a transform induces just a *redistribution* of data variance among the channels, while the total power remains invariant.

Using the column vectors of the transposed transformation matrix, $\mathbf{F}^{\mathrm{T}} = (\boldsymbol{f}_1, \boldsymbol{f}_2, \ldots, \boldsymbol{f}_m)$, the new channels resulting from an orthogonal transform can be written as $x_i = \boldsymbol{f}_i \cdot \boldsymbol{u}$. It can be shown that for a given data-set at least one – and, in most cases, exactly one – transform has the following extremal property: $\operatorname{var} x_1$, where $x_1 = \boldsymbol{f}_1 \cdot \boldsymbol{u}$, attains the maximum value among all possible choices of $\boldsymbol{f}_1$; $\operatorname{var} x_2$, where $x_2 = \boldsymbol{f}_2 \cdot \boldsymbol{u}$, attains the maximum value among all possible choices of $\boldsymbol{f}_2$ which are orthogonal to $\boldsymbol{f}_1$; etc. The directions of the vectors $\boldsymbol{f}_i$ are then so-called "principal axes" of the data cloud in the state space, and the new data channels $x_i$ are referred to as "principal components." Practically, the *principal component analysis* (PCA)[5] is performed by the so-called eigenvalue decomposition[6] of the covariance matrix $\mathbf{C} \equiv [C_{ij}]$,

$$C_{ij} = \text{cov}(u_i, u_j) := \langle u_{i,n} u_{j,n} \rangle \tag{16}$$

into the eigenvectors $\boldsymbol{f}_i$ and associated eigenvalues $\lambda_i$, which specify the variance accounted for by the $i$th principal component. From the preservation of the total variance and Eqn 14 it follows that

$$\sum_{i=1}^{m} \lambda_i = \sum_{i=1}^{m} V_i . \tag{17}$$

A direction in the state space corresponds to a definite "field map," i.e. a topographic distribution of the brain's electrical field over the observed scalp region. Therefore, PCA performed on EEG data is sometimes referred to as "spatial PCA," and the field topographies corresponding to the eigenvectors as "spatial modes." Sorting the eigenvalues in descending order, $\lambda_1 \geq \lambda_2 \geq \cdots \geq \lambda_m$, and numbering the eigenvectors accordingly, we obtain a transformed data-set such that, for any $l < m$, the projection of the data cloud into a subspace spanned by $\boldsymbol{f}_1, \ldots, \boldsymbol{f}_l$, i.e. the collection of principal components $x_1, \ldots, x_l$, provides the best possible representation of the given data-set within an $l$-dimensional space.

## Phenomenology of EEG trajectories

The results of this section are illustrated (Figure 9.3) using a 21-channel EEG data-set (2 seconds) comprising $N = 256$ scalp field samples. In Figure 9.3B, C, the global field power and the signals assigned to the three major principal components (i.e. accounting for the highest portion of the total variance) are plotted.

For the same EEG data, a reconstruction of the trajectory in a subspace spanned by the three principal axes is shown in Figure 9.4, together with the respective spatial modes. The state space trajectory consists of almost closed orbits of a roughly elliptic shape. This structure reflects the repetition of momentary field topographies, occurring at the dominant frequency of the brain electrical activity[7] – here alpha activity of ~11 Hz, characteristic for the "idling" brain state. Figure 9.5 shows a "view from inside" the EEG trajectory, which is projected onto the surface of the unit sphere. Displayed is the sequence of the momentary states along the projected trajectory; the background shading encodes the probability density of occurrence of a field topography in a given direction.

## Source model and spatial modes

Generally, we can assume a linear model of EEG in the form

$$\boldsymbol{u}(t) = \sum_{i=1}^{s} y_i(t) \boldsymbol{g}_i \tag{18}$$

where $\boldsymbol{g}_1, \ldots, \boldsymbol{g}_s$ are field distributions generated by the sources, and $y_i$ is the time-varying strength or, in other words, the signal driving the $i$th source. (For the sake of unique representation, we always assume that the field vectors are normalized to unity.)

Principal component analysis results in a decomposition of the EEG data in the form

$$\boldsymbol{u}(t) = \sum_{i=1}^{m} x_i(t) \boldsymbol{f}_i \tag{19}$$

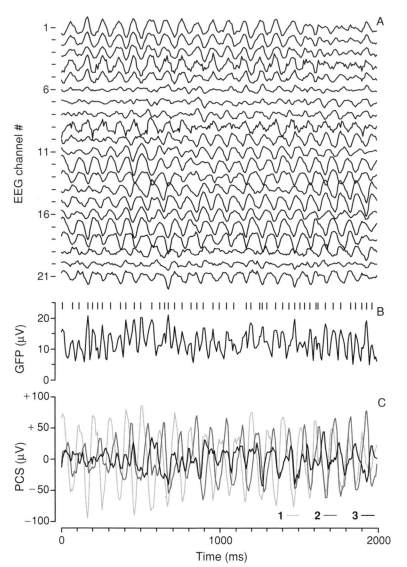

**Figure 9.3** A. Two seconds of 21-channel EEG data (10/20-system), sampled at 128 data vectors/second ($N = 256$). Displayed data are transformed to the average reference and zero mean over time. B. Global field power (GFP) as a function of time; the vertical ticks indicate local maxima of the GFP curve. C. The three major principal components as a function of time, i.e. the "signals" driving the source topographies displayed in Figure 9.4C.

where $f_1, \ldots, f_m$ are the spatial modes, and $x_i$ is, formally, the "signal" driving the $i$th mode. These topographies and signals must not be interpreted in terms of brain physiology[8]; they are just results of a mathematically convenient data representation. Principal component analysis identifies a subspace, usually of a relatively low dimension, to which a major portion of the total variance is confined.

Computation of the eigenvalues and eigenvectors of the covariance matrix $\mathbf{C}$ leads to a diagonalization procedure,

$$\mathbf{FCF}^{\mathrm{T}} = \mathbf{\Lambda} = \mathrm{diag}(\lambda_1, \ldots, \lambda_m) \tag{20}$$

Principal component analysis thus leads not only to a redistribution of the total power in the sense of the above-stated extremal property, but also to a de-correlation of signals assigned

A

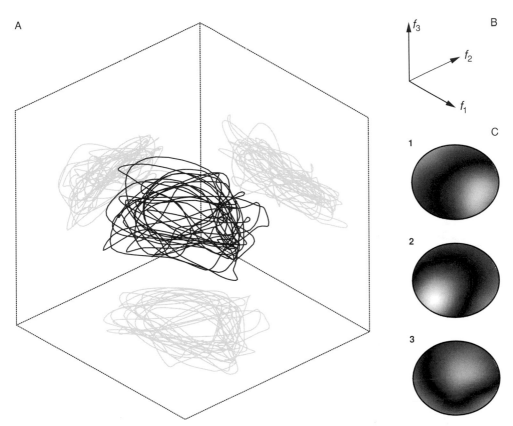

B

C

**Figure 9.4** A. Three-dimensional reconstruction of the EEG state space trajectory for the data shown in Figure 9.3, upsampled by a factor 4 to obtain a smoother picture. Two-dimensional projections of the trajectory onto the lateral planes (gray "shadows") added for easier visual inspection of the trajectory. B. Directions of eigenvectors $f_1, f_2, f_3$, i.e. principal axes in A. C. Field topographies corresponding to the eigenvectors $f_1, f_2, f_3$ (red: positive, blue: negative polarity).

to the spatial modes. The PCA solution can thus be seen as decomposition into "linearly independent components," while in the independent component analysis (ICA) the independence is defined in terms of higher-order moments (see Chapter 5).

The identification of the representational subspace is not sufficient for an unambiguous identification of sources. This is easily seen in the case of a two-source, single-frequency model

$$\boldsymbol{u}(t) = y_1(t)\boldsymbol{g}_1 + y_2(t)\boldsymbol{g}_2 \qquad (21)$$

where $\boldsymbol{g}_1, \boldsymbol{g}_2$ are non-colinear – but not necessarily orthogonal – normalized topographies of two sources, which are driven by harmonic signals at a single frequency $\omega$

$$y_i(t) = a_i \sin(\omega t + \phi_i) \qquad (i = 1, 2) \qquad (22)$$

This model generates an elliptic trajectory in the state space, similar to the orbits seen in the example given above of EEG data. The shape and orientation of the orbits are determined by the amplitude ratio $a_2/a_1$, the (relative) signal phase $\phi_2 - \phi_1$ and the angle $\gamma$ between the topography vectors, such that $\cos \gamma = \boldsymbol{g}_1 \cdot \boldsymbol{g}_2$; the latter may be called a "topographic phase."

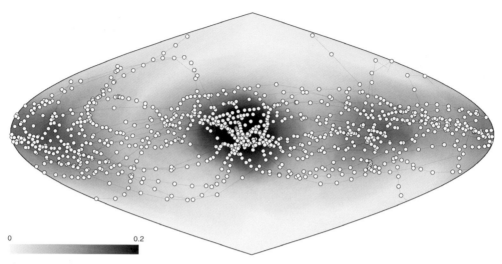

0                              0.2

**Figure 9.5** "Sky-map plot" of the same EEG trajectory as in Figure 9.4, upsampled by a factor 4 and projected onto the unit sphere. The equator is the intersection of the plane ($f_1$, $f_2$) with the sphere, while the poles correspond to points $\pm f_3$. Projections of individual samples (effective frequency = 512/s) marked by small open circles. Background shading indicates the density of the data distribution in different topographic directions; see the gray-scale at the left bottom.

As illustrated in Figure 9.6, different combinations of these three parameters produce orbits of exactly the same shape and orientation.

So, neither the source topographies nor the driving activities are uniquely determined by the observed data – a consequence of the topography–signal phase indeterminacy[9]. For a uniquely determined solution, additional constraints regarding properties of the source topographies and/or the driving activities are necessary (see Chapter 3). However, the approach presented in the following section is different: our objective is a quantitative characterization of geometric properties of the EEG trajectory, which are unequivocally determined by the data.

## Global descriptors
## Principle of dimensional simplicity

Meaningful descriptions of reality always imply a reduction of primary (observed) data, and a separation of qualities into different descriptive dimensions. For example, a book may for many practical purposes be described just in terms of size and weight; that is, the description consists of four numbers, three for the dimensions (e.g. in centimetres) plus one for the weight (e.g. in grams). Statistical dependencies between those qualities with respect to some "typical ensembles" of such objects do not play any role in the description; spatial extensions are separated from the body's mass, in spite of the fact that larger books are usually also heavier, etc. We call this a principle of dimensional simplicity.

## Integral field strength ($\Sigma$) and generalized frequency ($\Phi$)

A single-channel EEG record can be seen (a) as a continuous curve in the plane; or, if digitized, (b) as a series of values $u_n$ assigned to time instants $t_n$; or (c) as an object which is

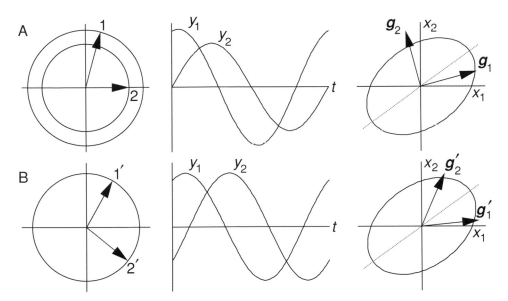

**Figure 9.6** Topography–signal phase indeterminacy. Two pairs of oscillators operating at the same circular frequency (left), generating sine-wave signals with different signal phase differences and different amplitude ratios, and driving sources of different topographies (right). Source configurations A and B generate in the state space an elliptic orbit of exactly the same shape and orientation, and are thus observationally not distinguishable. Note that the major principal axis (dotted line) of the orbit is not identical to any of the real sources.

globally (even if roughly) described by only two values, assessing its typical amplitude and frequency.

Similarly, a dimensionally simple description of a trajectory in the $m$-dimensional EEG state space is provided by two descriptors[10], assessing the average extent of the data cloud, and the average speed of change between two successive states. For this purpose, we define

$$M_0 := \langle \| \boldsymbol{u}_n \|^2 \rangle, \qquad M_1 := \langle \| \dot{\boldsymbol{u}}_n \|^2 \rangle \qquad (23)$$

where

$$\dot{\boldsymbol{u}} := \frac{\boldsymbol{u}_n - \boldsymbol{u}_{n-1}}{\Delta t} \qquad (24)$$

is the vector of change of the field in the $n$th sampling step. Further, we define the *integral field strength*

$$\Sigma := \sqrt{\frac{M_0}{m}} \qquad (25)$$

and the *generalized frequency*

$$\Phi := \frac{1}{2\pi} \sqrt{\frac{M_1}{M_0}} \qquad (26)$$

Since the physical units of the quantities $M_0$ and $M_1$ are, $\mu V^2$ and $\mu V^2 \cdot s^{-2}$, respectively, the units for the two descriptors are $[\Sigma] = \mu V$ and $[\Phi] = s^{-1}$, as expected. In fact, these descriptors are multidimensional analogs of Hjorth's[11,12] descriptors of "activity" and "mobility." It is easy to see that $\Sigma^2$ is the mean squared global field power – compare Eqns 23 and 25.

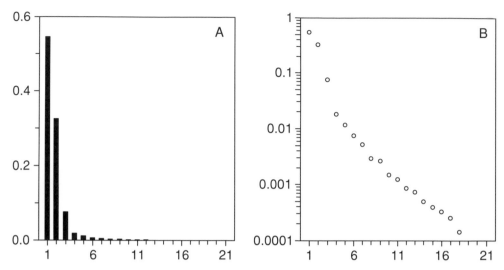

**Figure 9.7** Spectrum of eigenvalues of the covariance matrix for the data shown in Figure 9.3, on a linear scale (A) and a logarithmic scale (B). The three largest eigenvalues account for ~89% of the total power. The logarithmic plot provides a better overview of the distribution of eigenvalues. The three smallest eigenvalues $\lambda_{19,20,21} = 0$ are not shown in the pictures; this partial degeneracy of the spectrum is due to two of 21 channels being linearly interpolated, and the data being transformed to the average reference.

## Measure of spatial complexity ($\Omega$)

In the preceding section we have seen that PCA yields an *optimal* representation of a given data-set within a space of lower dimension. The relative portion of the total variance represented by the $i$th spatial mode is

$$\lambda'_i \equiv \lambda_i / W, \quad \text{where } W = \sum_{i=1}^{m} \lambda_i \qquad (27)$$

The set $\{\lambda'_1, \ldots, \lambda'_m\}$ is called a (normalized) $\lambda$-spectrum of the covariance matrix **C**. As seen from Eqn 27, all possible forms of $\lambda$-spectra are bound by the condition $\sum_i \lambda'_i = 1$ (partition of unity). A graphic representation of the $\lambda$-spectrum, sorted in descending order, provides a comprehensive picture of the efficiency of PCA for a given data-set. Since the $\lambda'_i$-values may vary over several orders of magnitude, it is convenient to plot $\log \lambda'_i$ vs. $i$ (see Figure 9.7).

For a numerical characterization of the dimensional reducibility of EEG data we need a function, assigning to a partition of unity a real number. Especially, we require that the function

- is symmetrical, i.e. invariant under re-ordering of its arguments;
- attains a minimum value in the case $\lambda'_k = 1$ for some $k$ (and thus $\lambda'_i = 0$ for $i \neq k$); and
- attains a maximum value for $\lambda'_1 = \lambda'_2 = \cdots = \lambda'_m = 1/m$.

The standard choice is the Shannon entropy $H$, leading to a definition

$$\log \Omega := H(\lambda'_1, \ldots, \lambda'_m) = -\sum_{i=1}^{m} \lambda'_i \log \lambda'_i \qquad (28)$$

$\Omega$ is taken as a measure of spatial complexity of a given EEG set[10]. It attains values from the interval 1 to $m$, with $\Omega = 1$ if the data consists of exactly one spatial mode, and $\Omega = m$ for data with the total variance uniformly distributed across all $m$ modes. $\Omega$ is, of course, a dimensionless quantity.

A measure similar to $\Omega$, "linear complexity," was defined via eigenvalues of the correlation matrix of EEG data by Paluš *et al.*[13]; a measure identical to $\Omega$ except for a different scaling was independently published by Pézard *et al.*[14], and later "reinvented" again[15,16]. A common precursor of these parallel approaches seems to be Morgera's work on "covariance complexity"[17]. There is an analogous situation with respect to the frequency domain, where conceptually similar measures were proposed – for example "spectral entropy"[18], "wavelet entropy"[19] – with a common predecessor dating some decades ago[20]. Obviously, all cited measures have been based on the same general principle, that is, the decomposition of total data variance with respect to an orthonormal basis over the domain of interest (space, time, frequency), and the single-valued characterization of the variance distribution by a suitable "entropic" function[9].

## Three-dimensional representation of global functional states

The three quantities defined by Eqns 25–28, integral field strength $\Sigma$, generalized frequency $\Phi$, and spatial complexity $\Omega$, constitute a three-dimensional system of global descriptors of the brain's electrical activity. Since EEG sensitively reflects the global functional state of the brain, the global descriptors can be used, jointly or individually, to characterize brain functional states[10,21].

The descriptors $\Sigma$, $\Phi$ and $\Omega$ are evaluated for data segments of a constant duration (typically 1–4 seconds), obtained either in a regular sequence or as a sliding window from the original EEG record. This leads to a considerable data reduction: $N \times m$ simultaneous measurements are transformed into just three numbers. Therefore, the method is of particular interest in studies of relatively slowly changing brain functional states as a function of time, assessed by long-term continuous EEG recordings[21,22].

A triplet ($\Sigma$, $\Phi$, $\Omega$), obtained from a given EEG segment, can be represented as a point in a three-dimensional *macrostate space*. This technique can be used in different experimental designs and for various purposes. The following example illustrates the concept of the macrostate space of the global descriptors, using a continuous whole-night EEG recording from a single sleeping subject. Each point in Figure 9.8 corresponds to a segment of 60 s of EEG. The data cloud is confined to a relatively thin manifold of a hyperboloid shape, also known as "sleep shell"[10]. The trajectory traverses this hyperboloid structure several times during the night, in a roughly periodic course, as seen from Figure 9.9 where the three global descriptors are plotted as a function of time starting from the beginning of the EEG recording (light off). The periodic pattern corresponds to repeated sleep cycles, otherwise known from classic "hypnograms"; indeed, a discrimination function constructed upon the three global descriptors distinguishes well between sleep stages[23].

## Transformations in the $\Sigma$-$\Phi$-$\Omega$ space

The restriction of the sleeping brain's macrostates to a two-dimensional manifold is mainly due to an inverse relation between descriptors $\Sigma$ and $\Phi$, which can be expressed as

$$\Sigma \Phi \approx k \qquad (29)$$

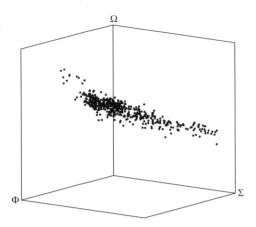

**Figure 9.8** Three-dimensional view of ($\Sigma$, $\Phi$, $\Omega$) data obtained from an individual whole-night sleep EEG recording. Global descriptors were calculated from 2-second epochs; each point represents median values for a block of 30 consecutive epochs = 60 s. Scales: $\Sigma$ from 0–22.5 $\mu$V; $\Phi$ from 0–15 Hz; $\Omega$ from 0–7.5. The variety of sleep EEG macrostates is confined to a hyperboloid "sleep shell."

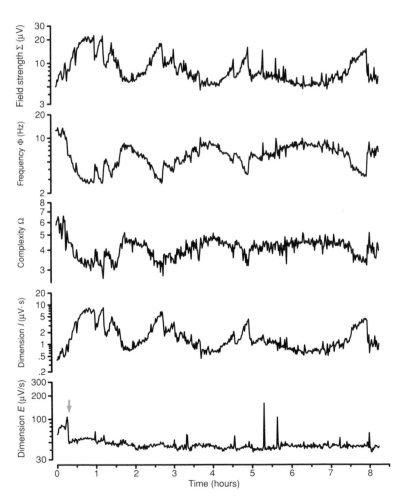

**Figure 9.9** The same data as in Figure 9.8, plotted as a function of time from the beginning of the EEG recording ($t = 0$). The top three curves show time series of the three global descriptors, $\Sigma$, $\Phi$, $\Omega$, on logarithmic scales. Below, time series of the two derived macrostate variables $I$ and $E$ (logarithmic scale) are shown. The course of $I$ reflects repeated passages through the sleep stages, and is inversely correlated with $\Omega$. Note the abrupt drop of the $E$-curve at sleep onset (gray arrow), and the sharp peaks at $t > 5$ h indicating the subject's spontaneous awakenings.

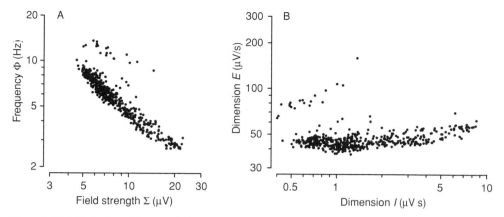

**Figure 9.10** A. Projection of the sleep EEG macrostates onto the (log $\Sigma$, log $\Phi$)-plane. Time resolution as in Figure 9.8, i.e. each point corresponds to a 60 s epoch. B. The same data in the rotated coordinates (log $I$, log $E$).

where $k$ is a constant. Taking logarithms of both sides of Eqn 29 gives

$$\log \Sigma + \log \Phi \approx \log k \qquad (30)$$

which suggests the following transformation:

$$\log I = \log \Sigma - \log \Phi \qquad (31)$$
$$\log E = \log \Sigma + \log \Phi \qquad (32)$$

Geometrically this corresponds to a rotation in the (log $\Sigma$, log $\Phi$)-plane (Figure 9.10). In this way, the common factor underlying the correlation of the descriptors $\Sigma$ and $\Phi$ is separated in the new macrostate variable $I$. The macrostate variable $E$ varies minimally during sleep, but it sensitively reflects the transition between the waking state and sleep (Figure 9.9). In other words, log $I$ reflects the course of the sleep cycle, and is related to sleep stages, while log $E$ − log $k$ may serve as an individual measure of vigilance.

Individual $\Sigma$-$\Phi$-$\Omega$ portraits of sleep EEG from different subjects show generally the same form, expressed by Eqn 29, but with individual constants $k$, and with individual peculiarities concerning the distribution of sleep stages within the sleep shell. These varieties of higher-order macrostates provide good examples of "idioversal laws"[24], regulating the functioning of an individual neural system. Further re-parameterizations or transformations of the idioversal laws may be required to obtain the form of a truly universal law; merely averaging the individual data does not serve this purpose.

## Extensions and modifications

Since its introduction in the 1990s, the $\Sigma$-$\Phi$-$\Omega$ system has been subject to various modifications, mostly concerning the measure of spatial complexity.

### Regional measures

The attribute "global" implies that the three descriptors are evaluated for brain electrical data recorded from a full-scalp electrode array. However, the same descriptors can also be calculated for EEG recorded from circumscribed scalp regions – e.g. above the left and right cerebral hemispheres – provided that the electrode array is dense enough. This modification was mostly utilized in neuropsychiatric and neuropharmacological studies[25–28].

A
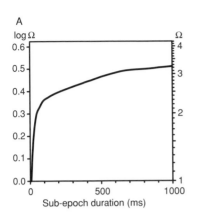

B
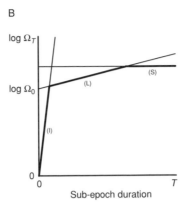

**Figure 9.11**
Determination of the
"complexity production
rate". A. Plot of $\log \Omega_T$
vs. $T$ for the data shown
in Figure 9.3, with
sub-epoch duration $T$
varied from 1/64 to 1 s.
B. Schematic
approximation of the
initial (I), linear scaling (L)
and saturation (S) region
in the plot of $\log \Omega_T$ vs.
$T$. The L-region is fitted
by Eqn (33) with $\Omega_0 =$
2.25 and $\beta = 0.52$ s$^{-1}$.

## Local complexity differentials

This method[29] consists in calculation of $\Omega$ complexity for the full-scalp coverage ($m$ electrodes) and for all $m$ possible subsets of $m-1$ electrodes, with the $i$th channel ($i = 1, \ldots, m$) left out. The differences between the partial-array and full-array complexity measures assess contributions of locally measured activities to global spatial complexity. These differences can be positive ("moderating" activities) or negative ("dominating" activities).

## $\Omega$ complexity as a function of frequency

In some applications, evaluation of spatial complexity within selected frequency bands may be of interest and clinical relevance[30]. Alternatively, $\Omega$ can be calculated from $\lambda$-spectra of cross-spectral matrices, obtained separately for each frequency point via Fourier transform[31].

## $\Omega$ complexity production rate

The global descriptors are usually evaluated for EEG epochs of a few seconds duration. With too short data epochs ($T < 1$ s), $\Omega$ is underestimated as there are not enough data points to provide a representative portrait of the EEG trajectory. Using too long data epochs ($T > 10$ s) is not recommended, either: different source configurations may be mixed up within a single data epoch, which leads to overestimation of spatial complexity.

In systematic studies of $\Omega$ as a function of the epoch duration $T$, we usually distinguish three regions in $\log \Omega_T$-vs.-$\log T$ plots (Figure 9.11): an initial steep increase (I), a linear-scaling region (L), and a saturation plateau (S). The L-region can be approximated by the regression equation

$$\log \Omega_T = \log \Omega_0 + \beta T \tag{33}$$

where $\Omega_0$ is the spatial complexity extrapolated to zero epoch duration, and the coefficient $\beta$ is the "complexity production rate" (CPR)[32], measured in s$^{-1}$. $\Omega_0$ can be used to disambiguate findings on spatial complexity obtained in studies with different epoch durations. The CPR may serve as an additional global descriptor, differentiating between states which are undistinguishable solely by means of $\Omega$.

## $\Omega$ complexity from correlation matrices

Pei et al.[33] used $\Omega$ as a measure of synchronization between two locally measured signals and suggested a normalization of input signals to unit variance, to avoid an alleged dependence of $\Omega$ on the signal power. But it is easily shown[9] that epoch-wise normalization of EEG data

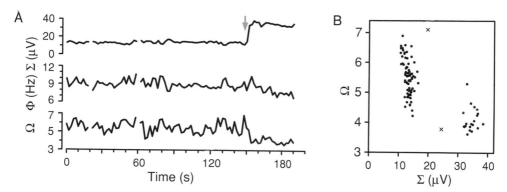

**Figure 9.12** Global description of an about 3 minutes long, 19-channel EEG record, with a transition to a regular 3 s$^{-1}$ spike–wave activity (*petit mal* seizure). A. Time series of descriptors, $\Sigma$, $\Phi$, $\Omega$, calculated for consecutive 2-s epochs. The onset of paroxysmal activity marked by a gray arrow. B. Projection of the macrostate space onto the ($\Sigma$, $\Omega$)-plane, where the two functional states (non-paroxysmal, paroxysmal) are neatly separated. Artifact-contaminated EEG epochs are omitted from A and marked by × in B.

implies a re-scaling of the original axes of the state space by different factors, thus modifying the geometry of the data cloud, and is therefore alien to the original idea of $\Omega$ complexity.

### Record-wise variance normalization

Examination of Pei *et al.*'s criticism elicited further studies to investigate effects of data inhomogeneities (superimposed artifacts) on estimates of spatial complexity. A compromise strategy has been proposed, consisting of equalization of variance across the entire ensemble of EEG epochs, that is, record-wise. This modification still allows comparisons in terms of $\Omega$ between epochs, but makes the analysis more robust against artifacts[9,34].

## Selected applications
## Sleep stages and vigilance variations

Szelenberger *et al.*[23] studied co-variations of the global descriptors with sleep stages. Portraits of single subject's whole-night sleep EEG data in the $\Sigma$-$\Phi$-$\Omega$ space usually reveal a typical "sleep shell" structure of a roughly hyperboloid-cylindric shape (see Figure 9.8). Logarithmic transformation (see Eqns 31, 32) of the global descriptors maps this structure to a more or less planar data cloud, allowing a clean discrimination of sleep stages. Data from individual multiple sleep latency tests[35] projected into the $\Sigma$-$\Phi$-$\Omega$ space show transitions from the waking state to the sleep plane[21].

## Epilepsy and paroxysmal brain activity

Episodes of paroxysmal electrical activity, which are easily recognized visually in EEG records, also show characteristic state shifts in the $\Sigma$-$\Phi$-$\Omega$ space: increased $\Sigma$, decreased $\Phi$ and decreased $\Omega$ due to preponderance of one spatial mode (Figure 9.12).

For diagnostic purposes, however, subtle changes of inter-ictal EEG and their characterization by means of the global descriptors are of more interest. Kondákor *et al.*[28] found reduced $\Omega$ complexity (global as well as regional) in patients with idiopathic generalized epilepsy (IGE) vs. healthy controls. Furthermore, they described a shift of the inter-regional $\Omega$ gradient in IGE patients toward normal values as an effect of chronic anticonvulsive therapy with valproate.

## Neuropathology, neuropsychiatry

Szelenberger et al.[25] described deviations of interhemispheric $\Omega$ complexity gradients in depressed patients vs. normal controls. Saito et al.[26] found increased regional $\Omega$ complexity in frontal areas in schizophrenic patients vs. normal controls. Tóth et al.[36] reported interhemispheric $\Omega$ asymmetry in reaction to gustatory stimuli in anorectic patients. Yoshimura et al.[37] found increased global $\Omega$ complexity in patients with a mild form of Alzheimer's disease; the same effect has been reported by Czigler et al.[38]. Irisawa et al.[39] reported increased $\Omega$ complexity along with decreased microstate duration in nonmedicated schizophrenic patients. Molnár et al.[30] studied differences of $\Omega$ complexity between eyes-open and eyes-closed conditions, and reported reduced reactivity of $\Omega$ to eyes opening in a patient with a sub-cortical ischemic stroke.

## Effects of neuroactive substances

Yagyu et al.[40] reported effects of the active substance of green tea, theanine, on global $\Omega$ complexity. Kondákor et al.[41] reported a reduction of $\Omega$ complexity after a single-dose application of piracetam. Kondákor et al.[28] also described effects of valproate on the inter-regional gradient of $\Omega$ complexity (see above, under *Epilepsy*). Neuroleptic medication has reportedly no effect on $\Omega$, while other measures of dimensional complexity are affected[42].

## Developmental changes of EEG

Wackermann[43] studied the three global descriptors as a function of chronological age in a small sample ($N = 40$) ranging from 0.6 to ~80 years. $\Sigma$ decreased and $\Phi$ increased monotonically with age, both descriptors reaching a plateau in the early adulthood. $\Omega$ showed a steep increase during the early childhood, reaching a peak at about 5–6 years, and a slower decrease afterwards. Using a larger sample ($N \approx 500$, age range 5–80 years), Koenig and Wackermann (unpublished) obtained parametric developmental equations for the three global descriptors in the form $a + b\,e^{-c\,t}$, where $t$ is chronological age and $a$, $b$, $c$ are adjustable parameters (Figure 9.13). Stam et al.[44] studied $\Omega$ complexity in a sample with age range 0.25–16 years, and suggested that $\Omega$ "might prove to be clinically useful as an objective, quantitative measure of brain maturation." Kim et al.[45] reported a rapid increase of $\Omega$ complexity in newborns within the first 48 hours after birth, and significant differences between different modes of delivery.

## Sensory and motor processes

Kondákor et al.[46] reported increased global $\Omega$ complexity as a response to enabled vs. disabled visual input (eyes-open vs. eyes-closed conditions) and related them to spatial redistribution of intracerebral activation, supported by source localization methods. Stančák and Wackermann[47] described changes of regional $\Omega$ complexity (sensorimotor areas) during preparation and execution of voluntary finger movements. Moreover, Stančák et al.[48] found correlations between limb movement-related changes of $\Omega$ and the trans-sectional area of corpus callosum, suggesting a direct link between spatial complexity and neural connectivity. Müller et al.[49] studied the time course of global $\Omega$ complexity during perception of a bistable visual dynamic stimulus; they found short periods of decreased complexity, preceding the perceptual 'switch' by ~750 ms to 300 ms.

**Figure 9.13**
Developmental curves of global descriptors $\Sigma$, $\Phi$, $\Omega$, obtained from a normative population of $N = 478$ EEG data-sets, recorded in a resting state. The individual values are shown as gray points, to which exponential curves have been fitted. Asymptotes of the developmental curves are marked by dashed horizontal lines. Time constants $c^{-1}$ of the three exponential functions are all in the range 8–10 years.

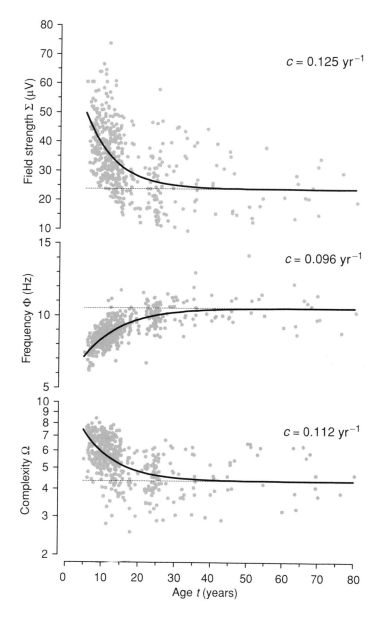

$c = 0.125 \text{ yr}^{-1}$

$c = 0.096 \text{ yr}^{-1}$

$c = 0.112 \text{ yr}^{-1}$

# Miscellaneous topics

Bhattacharya *et al.*[50,51] used $\Omega$ complexity as a measure of long-range synchronization in the gamma frequency band induced by listening to music; they found higher synchronization in musicians than in nonmusician controls. Pizzagalli *et al.*[27] reported reduced interhemispheric $\Omega$ asymmetry in subjects with deviant cognitive processing, manifested by a "strong belief in paranormal phenomena." Isotani *et al.*[52] reported a decrease of $\Omega$ complexity under hypnotically induced relaxation.

A

B

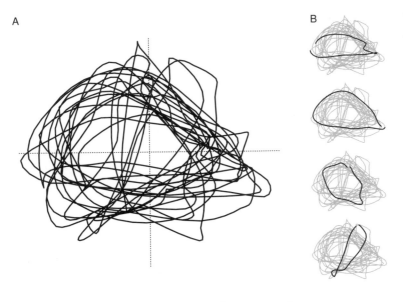

**Figure 9.14** A. Projection of the EEG trajectory shown in Figure 9.4A into the plane spanned by the two major principal axes, showing an approximately periodic structure. B. Four example orbits (black) determined by local GFP maxima, occurring over different time periods within the entire 2-s recording epoch (gray background). This picture shows the "precession" of the main axis of the orbits over time.

## Relations to other analytical approaches
### Microstate models

As seen in the preceding sections, there is a direct correspondence between the geometry of the state space and the spatial analysis of EEG. In fact, many of the notions of topographic analysis are empirically motivated re-inventions of elementary concepts of vector algebra.

One of the key notions of spatial analysis is that of the electrical *microstate*, which was defined as a period of relatively stationary scalp field topography[53] (see Chapter 6). The aim of microstate analysis is the identification of these stable topographies, a decomposition of the stream of EEG data into a sequence of microstates ("segmentation"), and a statistical characterization of the distribution of microstate dwell-times and other parameters. (In this section, we are dealing exclusively with microstate analysis of on-going EEG activity, not with transient responses to a stimulus or a cognitive event.) Field topographies correspond to directions in state space; therefore, a microstate would correspond to a period of time for which the EEG trajectory is confined to a relatively narrow bi-cone in the state space; or, equivalently, to a circumscribed region on the unit sphere surface (Figure 9.5). The transitions between microstates would then reflect sudden changes in the central direction of the bi-cone.

A visual inspection of EEG state space projections reveals that real EEG trajectories consist of ellipsoidal orbits, repeatedly entering topographies but never oscillating along exactly the same line. The main axis of the orbits changes its orientation over time, in a kind of "precession motion" (Figure 9.14). This typical feature of EEG trajectories was utilized by early strategies of microstate analysis, focusing on field topographies at times of local GFP maxima. As local maxima are quite vulnerable to noise and other perturbations of the data, the main axis of the elliptic orbits – determined, for example, by PCA over one orbital period – may provide a more robust topographic description.

In either case, this strategy implies a preliminary reduction of the EEG data to selected field maps. This step could be called "tokenization" of the EEG data stream, since the intention of microstate analysis has been described as a "parsing" of EEG data. The discontinuous structure of brain electrical activity, as revealed by the segmentation procedures, is thus conditioned by the data preprocessing strategy, which is based on the microstate model. Although it may be tempting to interpret the momentarily dominant topographies in realistic terms, as signatures of momentarily active sources, we must remember the fact of topography–signal phase indeterminacy. The same orbit, and thus the same direction of the main axis, may be generated by an infinite variety of different activation patterns – a strong argument for not taking the "source realism" too far and for staying with the global, phenomenological description of EEG data.

On a larger time scale, the diversity of dominant topographies occurring in the stream of EEG data is revealed by the increase of $\Omega$ complexity with increasing duration of the observation epoch. Therefore, the CPR analysis may provide an alternative way to assess essentially the same features of brain electrical activity as those aimed at by the traditional microstate analysis, without postulating a strictly discrete microstate structure and/or abrupt transitions between the microstates[54].

## Synchronization measures

The measure of $\Omega$ complexity has occasionally been interpreted as a measure of synchronization of the EEG[33,50,51], just as other measures quantifying linear signal interdependence like the correlation coefficient, coherence, and measures derived thereof. While the interpretation of a decreased value of $\Omega$ as indicating an increased level of global synchronization may be justified in certain contexts, it has to be noted that this quantity has neither been designed as a synchronization measure, nor is it particularly well suited for this purpose.

Synchronization is defined generally as the adjustment of the rhythms of two or more self-sustained oscillators due to coupling[55]. It has therefore to be distinguished, firstly, from signal similarity that arises where observable signals are varying mixtures of source signals, as is presumably the case with EEG. Secondly, synchronization is to be distinguished from covariation in terms of signal amplitudes, as opposed to their phase component that corresponds to the rhythmic (oscillatory) character of the process.

## Summary

The global approach sketched in this chapter presents a "third way" in addition to topographic analysis of brain electrical fields in the two-dimensional scalp space (traditionally known as "brain mapping") and to identification of sources in the three-dimensional intracranial space (modern "electrical neuroimaging"). The global approach circumvents the problem of identification of the "real" sources; its specific objective is to aggregate information on the brain functional state in a few numerical descriptors, that is, macroscopic state variables of well-defined physical meaning. For this reason the global approach has been described as "phenomenological neurophysics"[9]. The identification of functional macrostates of the brain achieved via the global descriptors may provide a context for interpretation of findings obtained on more detailed scales, that is, with a higher spatial and/or temporal resolution.

This approach is particularly useful in studies that focus on trait differences or slow state-shifts, as for example neurophysiological correlates of states of consciousness (vigilance, sleep, hypnosis), neuro- and psycho-pharmacological studies, or developmental/degenerative changes. A particularly promising area of research is the study of global properties of the brain's electrical activity in relation to structural conditions of its functioning, e.g. intracortical connectivity or other macroscopic properties of the neural substrate.

## Acknowledgements

The authors wish to thank the following persons for EEG data which were used as illustrative examples in this chapter: Dietrich Lehmann, Zurich (Figures 9.3–5, 9.7, 9.11, 9.14), Peter Achermann, Zurich (Figures 9.8, 9.9), Vladimír Krajča and S. Ebu Petránek, Prague (Figure 9.12) and Thomas Koenig, Berne (Figure 9.13).

## List of symbols

| | |
|---|---|
| $:=$ | defines |
| $\equiv$ | denotes |
| $\in$ | element of |
| $\mathbb{R}$ | real numbers |
| $\mathbb{R}^m$ | $m$-dimensional real vectors |
| $a, b, \ldots, z$ | scalar values |
| $\boldsymbol{a}, \boldsymbol{b}, \ldots, \boldsymbol{z}$ | vectors |
| $\boldsymbol{u} \cdot \boldsymbol{v}$ | inner product of vectors $\boldsymbol{u}, \boldsymbol{v}$ |
| $\|\boldsymbol{u}\|$ | norm of vector $\boldsymbol{u}$ |
| $\tilde{\boldsymbol{u}}$ | unit vector in the direction of $\boldsymbol{u}$ |
| $\langle x \rangle$ | mean value of $x$ |
| $\mathrm{gfp}(\boldsymbol{u})$ | global field power |
| $\mathrm{diss}(\boldsymbol{u}, \boldsymbol{v})$ | topographic dissimilarity |
| $\mathrm{cor}(\boldsymbol{u}, \boldsymbol{v})$ | topographic correlation |

## References

1. Allefeld C, Atmanspacher H, Wackermann J. Mental states as macrostates emerging from EEG dynamics. *Chaos* 2009;**19** in press.

2. Lehmann D, Skrandies W. Reference-free identification of components of checkerboard-evoked multichannel potential fields. *Electroencephalography and Clinical Neurophysiology* 1980;**48**:609–621.

3. Lehmann D. Principles of spatial analysis. In Gevins AS, Rémond A, eds. *Methods of Analysis of Brain Electrical and Magnetic Signals*. Amsterdam: Elsevier; 1987, pp. 309–354.

4. Brandeis D, Naylor H, Halliday R, Callaway E, Yano L. Scopolamine effects on visual information processing, attention and event-related potential map latencies. *Psychophysiology* 1992;**29**:315–336.

5. Jolliffe, IT. *Principal Component Analysis*. 2nd edn. New York: Springer; 2002.

6. Golub GH, Van Loan CF. *Matrix Computations*. Baltimore: John Hopkins University Press; 1983.

7. Lehmann D. Multichannel topography of human alpha EEG fields. *Electroencephalography and Clinical Neurophysiology* 1971;**31**:439–449.

8. Silberstein R, Cadusch PJ, Schier MA. Volume conduction effects on spatial principal components analysis of scalp recorded brain electrical activity. *Brain Topography* 1990;**3**:273–274.

9. Wackermann J, Allefeld C. On the meaning and interpretation of global descriptors of brain electrical activity. Including a reply to X. Pei *et al. International Journal of Psychophysiology* 2007;**64**:199–210.

10. Wackermann J. Beyond mapping: estimating complexity of multichannel EEG recordings. *Acta Neurobiologiae Experimentalis* 1996;**56**:197–208.

11. Hjorth B. EEG analysis based on time domain properties. *Electroencephalography and Clinical Neurophysiology* 1970;**29**: 306–310.

12. Hjorth B. The physical significance of the time domain descriptors in EEG analysis. *Electroencephalography and Clinical Neurophysiology* 1973;**34**:321–325.

13. Paluš M, Dvořák I, David I. Remarks on spatial and temporal dynamics of EEG. In

Dvořák I, Holden AV, eds. *Mathematical Approaches to Brain Functioning Diagnostics.* Manchester: Manchester University Press; 1991, pp. 369–385.

14. Pézard L, Nandrino JL, Renault B *et al.* Depression as a dynamical disease. *Biological Psychiatry* 1996;**39**:991–999.

15. James CJ, Lowe D. Extracting multisource brain activity from a single electromagnetic channel. *Artificial Intelligence in Medicine* 2003;**28**:89–104.

16. Carmeli C, Knyazeva MG, Innocenti GM, De Feo O. Assessment of EEG synchronization based on state-space analysis. *Neuroimage* 2005;**25**:339–354.

17. Morgera SS. Information theoretic complexity and its relation to pattern recognition. *IEEE Transactions on Systems, Man, and Cybernetics* 1985;**15**:608–619.

18. Inouye T, Shinosaki K, Sakamoto H *et al.* Quantification of EEG irregularity by use of the entropy of the power spectrum. *Electroencephalography and Clinical Neurophysiology* 1991;**79**:204–210.

19. Rosso OA, Blanco S, Yordanova J *et al.* Wavelet entropy: a new tool for analysis of short duration brain electrical signals. *Journal of Neuroscience Methods* 2001;**105**:65–75.

20. Powell, CE, Percival IC. A spectral entropy method for distinguishing regular and irregular motion of Hamiltonian systems. *Journal of Physics A* 1979;**12**:2053–2071.

21. Wackermann J. Towards a quantitative characterisation of functional states of the brain: from the non-linear methodology to the global linear description. *International Journal of Psychophysiology* 1999;**34**: 65–80.

22. Wackermann J. State space representation and global descriptors of the brain's electrical activity. In *Training Course Textbook.* Awaji Island: International Pharmaco-EEG Society; 2006, pp. 39–48.

23. Szelenberger W, Wackermann J, Skalski M, Niemcewicz S, Drojewski J. Analysis of complexity of EEG during sleep. *Acta Neurobiologiae Experimentalis* 1996;**56**:165–169.

24. Wackermann J. Rationality, universality, and individuality in a functional conception of theory. *International Journal of Psychophysiology* 2006;**62**:411–426.

25. Szelenberger W, Wackermann J, Skalski M, Drojewski J, Niemcewicz S. Interhemispheric differences of sleep EEG complexity. *Acta Neurobiologiae Experimentalis* 1996;**56**:955–959.

26. Saito N, Kuginuki T, Yagyu T *et al.* Global, regional and local measures of complexity of multichannel EEG in acute, neuroleptic-naive, first-break schizophrenics. *Biological Psychiatry* 1998;**43**:794–802.

27. Pizzagalli D, Lehmann D, Gianotti L *et al.* Brain electric correlates of strong belief in paranormal phenomena: intracerebral EEG source and regional Omega complexity analyses. *Psychiatric Research and Neuroimaging* 2000;**100**:139–154.

28. Kondákor I, Tóth M, Wackermann J *et al.* Distribution of spatial complexity of EEG changed in idiopathic generalised epilepsy and restored by chronic valproate therapy. *Brain Topography* 2005;**18**:115–123.

29. Wackermann, J. Unfolding the global complexity: topographies of complexity differentials of multi-channel EEG. In *NOLTA2002, Symposium on Non-Linear Theory and Its Applications.* Xi'an; October 2002, pp. 319–322.

30. Molnár M, Csuhaj R, Horváth S *et al.* Spectral and complexity features of the EEG changed by visual input in a case of subcortical stroke compared to healthy controls. *Clinical Neurophysiology* 2006;**117**: 771–780.

31. Wackermann J, Pütz P, Gäßler M. Unfolding EEG spatial complexity as a function of frequency. *Brain Topography* 2003;**16**:124.

32. Wackermann J. Global characterisation of brain electrical activity by means of the $\Omega$ complexity production rate. *Brain Topography* 2005;**18**:135.

33. Pei X, Zheng C, Zhang A, Duan F, Bin G. Discussion on "Towards a quantitative characterisation of functional states of the brain: from the non-linear methodology to the global linear description" by J. Wackermann. *International Journal of Psychophysiology* 2005;**56**:201–207.

34. Allefeld C, Wackermann J. Omega complexity: effects of different normalization strategies. *Brain Topography* 2007;**20**:51–52.

35. Carskadon MA, Dement WC. Effects of total sleep loss on sleep tendency. *Perception and Motor Skills* 1979;**48**:495–506.

36. Tóth E, Kondákor I, Túry F *et al*. Nonlinear and linear EEG complexity changes caused by gustatory stimuli in anorexia nervosa. *International Journal of Psychophysiology* 2004;**51**:253–260.

37. Yoshimura M, Isotani T, Yagyu T *et al*. Global approach to multi-channel EEG analysis for diagnosis and clinical evaluation in mild Alzheimer's disease. *Neuropsychobiology* 2004;**49**:163–166.

38. Czigler B, Csikós D, Hidasi Z *et al*. Quantitative EEG in early Alzheimer's disease patients – power spectrum and complexity features. *International Journal of Psychophysiology* 2008;**68**:75–80.

39. Irisawa S, Isotani T, Yagyu T *et al*. Increased Omega complexity and decreased microstate duration in nonmedicated schizophrenic patients. *Neuropsychobiology* 2006;**54**:134–139.

40. Yagyu T, Wackermann J, Kinoshita T *et al*. Effects of chewing gum flavor onto global complexity of EEG activity. *Neuropsychobiology* 1997;**35**:46–50.

41. Kondákor I, Michel CM, Wackermann J *et al*. Single-dose piracetam effects on global complexity measures of human spontaneous multichannel EEG. *International Journal of Psychophysiology* 1999;**34**:81–87.

42. Waltinger T, Lehmann D, Faber PL *et al*. Global dimensionality of multichannel EEG in schizophrenic patients is reduced by neuroleptic medication. *Neuropsychobiology* 2007;**55**:62.

43. Wackermann J. From microstates to macrostates: assessment of electrical dynamics of the brain by global descriptors. In *8th World Congress of ISBET*. Zurich; March 1997, p. 5.

44. Stam CJ, Hessels-van der Leij EM, Meulstee J, Vliegen JH. Changes in functional coupling between neural networks in the brain during maturation revealed by omega complexity. *Clinical Electroencephalography* 2000;**31**:104–108.

45. Kim HR, Jung KY, Kim SY *et al*. Delivery modes and neonatal EEG: spatial pattern analysis. *Early Human Development* 2003;**75**:35–53.

46. Kondákor I, Brandeis D, Wackermann J *et al*. Multichannel EEG fields during and without visual input: Frequency domain model source locations and dimensional complexities. *Neuroscience Letters* 1997;**226**: 49–52.

47. Stančák A, Wackermann J. Spatial EEG synchronisation over sensorimotor areas in brisk and slow self-paced index finger movements. *Brain Topography* 1998;**11**:23–33.

48. Stančák A, Lücking CH, Kristeva-Feige R. The size of corpus callosum and functional connectivities of cortical regions in finger and shoulder movements. *Cognitive Brain Research* 2002;**13**:61–74.

49. Müller TJ, Koenig T, Wackermann J *et al*. Subsecond changes of global brain state in illusory multistable motion perception. *Journal of Neural Transmission* 2005;**112**: 565–576.

50. Bhattacharya J. Complexity analysis of spontaneous EEG. *Acta Neurobiologiae Experimentalis* 2000;**60**:495–501.

51. Bhattacharya J, Petsche H, Pereda E. Long-range synchrony in the $\gamma$ band: role in music perception. *Journal of Neuroscience* 2001;**21**:6329–6337.

52. Isotani T, Kinoshita T, Lehmann D, Pascual-Marqui RD, Wackermann J. Spatial configuration of brain electrical activity during positive, neutral and negative emotions. *Methods and Findings in Experimental and Clinical Pharmacology* 2002;**24D**:109–110.

53. Lehmann D, Ozaki H, Pal I. EEG alpha map series: brain micro-states by space-oriented adaptive segmentation. *Electroencephalography and Clinical Neurophysiology* 1987;**67**:271–288.

54. Wackermann J. Continuity and discontinuity in models of brain electrical dynamics. *Brain Topography* 2006;**18**: 223.

55. Pikovsky A, Rosenblum M, Kurths J. *Synchronization: A Universal Concept in Nonlinear Sciences*. Cambridge: Cambridge University Press; 2001.

# Chapter 10

# Integration of electrical neuroimaging with other functional imaging methods

Daniel Brandeis, Christoph M. Michel, Thomas Koenig and Lorena R.R. Gianotti

## Introduction

Integrating evidence from different imaging modalities is important to overcome specific limitations of any given imaging method, such as insensitivity of the EEG to unsynchronized neural events, or the lack of fMRI sensitivity to events of low metabolic demand. Processes that are visible in one modality may be related in a nontrivial way to other processes visible in another modality and insight may only be obtained by integrating both methods through a common analysis. For example, brain activity at rest seems to be at least partly determined by an interaction of cortical rhythms (visible to EEG but not to fMRI) with sub-cortical activity (visible to fMRI, but usually not to EEG without averaging). A combination of EEG and fMRI data during rest may thus be more informative than the sum of two separate analyses in both modalities.

Integration is also an important source of converging evidence about specific aspects and general principles of neural functions and their dysfunctions in certain pathologies. This is because not only electrical, but also energetic, biochemical, hemodynamic and metabolic processes characterize neural states and functions, and because brain structure provides crucial constraints upon neural functions. Focusing on multimodal integration of functional data should not distract from the privileged status of the electric field as the primary direct, noninvasive real-time measure of neural transmission.

The preceding chapters illustrate how electrical neuroimaging has turned scalp EEG into an imaging modality which directly captures the full temporal dynamics of neural activity in the brain. However, despite major advances regarding distributed source solutions and realistic head models (Chapter 3), the methods still depend on assumptions and constraints for adequate neuroanatomical resolution. Here we build on these results to cover the advantages and limitations of integrating electrical neuroimaging and other forms of neuroimaging to multimodal imaging. To this end, we discuss the often implicit concepts of integration, the limited sensitivity of the EEG to detect or distinguish some specific aspects of neural activity, and then turn to the strength and weakness of each specific method's combinations.

Integration may take different forms. It can range from direct integration or fusion over indirect integration through modeling and through probabilistic Bayesian approaches to discussions of converging evidence, depending on the degree of overlap of sensitivity to the same aspects of activation in the same neural networks[1,2]. Combinations such as EEG and MEG reflect measures that are closely coupled through basic physics. They are sensitive to the same

*Electrical Neuroimaging*, ed. Christoph M. Michel, Thomas Koenig, Daniel Brandeis, Lorena R.R. Gianotti and Jiří Wackermann. Published by Cambridge University Press. © Cambridge University Press 2009.

**Table 10.1** The sensitivity profiles of different imaging methods

|       | Depth | Shape | 3D-Direction | Timing |
|-------|-------|-------|--------------|--------|
| EEG   | XX    | X     | XXX          | XXX    |
| MEG   | X     | X     | XX           | XXX    |
| PET   | XXX   | XX    |              | X      |
| fMRI  | XXX   | XXX   |              | XX     |
| NIRS  | X     | X     |              | XX     |

neurophysiological processes and similar networks, exhibit overlapping temporal and spatial resolution, and are thus particularly suitable for direct integration[1]. This may not always be possible for other measures such as EEG and fMRI, which are related by more complex physiological cascades rather than simple physical principles. Combinations are typically considered useful if they complement each other in terms of temporal and spatial resolution, and more generally in terms of sensitivity profiles (Table 10.1). The current treatment also emphasizes the importance of overlap in this resolution and sensitivity space and with regard to the neural processes being measured[3].

Combinations can be based on sequential or simultaneous recordings. Sequential studies are typically done using counterbalanced cross-over designs with the same subjects to control order effects and avoid interindividual variability. There are no constraints upon the equipment and no compromises regarding data quality in each imaging modality, but keeping conditions and subject states constant over different sessions and settings is a major difficulty. Most importantly, a number of phenomena like variability due to fluctuating states or processes, rapid learning or repetition effects, and particularly unpredictable EEG-defined events such as epileptic activity cannot be studied properly through sequential recordings. Such variable, unpredictable EEG-defined events are the domain of simultaneous recordings.

Combinations of imaging modalities are usually challenging in terms of data-size. In unimodal neuroimaging studies, the large data stream coming from the physiological measurements is confronted with a stream of information coming from the experimental design. Good experiments often keep the stream of design information as small as possible to maintain the complexity of the results at a comprehensible level and to preserve statistical power. On the other hand, one generally tries to increase the stream of physiological data to obtain results with a good resolution. If both modalities measure signals that are tightly connected by physical or physiological mechanisms, one can accommodate both data streams in a common, a-priori defined model through direct integration[1]. The main benefit of such common models is usually a better resolution of the results in time and/or space[4-6].

However, in many cases, the relation among the signals from the different measurement modalities is not known a priori. In these cases, we are faced with two large, physiological data streams that may interact in various and nontrivial ways, such that the complexity of the results increases exponentially if no countermeasures are taken. For the understanding of such data, it is thus often vital to do a feature extraction on the data before combined statistics are computed. The lack of an a-priori model that accommodates both modalities is thus compensated by an a-priori choice of features to extract. It is thus obvious that the relevance of the obtained results is limited by the relevance and interpretability of the features that were extracted. The proper extraction of features is thus critical, but we hope that for the part of EEG feature extraction, this book has made a useful contribution. In the existing literature, there are two kinds of features that are extracted. One possibility is to focus on features that have previously proven to be of interest, such as representations of ERP components with fixed topography in the continuous EEG[7,8], or EEG montages that are known to be sensitive to specific processes[9]. Other studies have used factorizations of time- or frequency-domain EEG data as primary feature extraction[10,11].

## Combining EEG and MEG

Neural currents in the brain give rise to closely coupled electrical and magnetic fields, rotated to each other by 90 degrees (see Chapter 1). When measured at a distance across the skull at the scalp as in EEG, or about 4 cm above the scalp as in MEG, the close coupling remains dominant, but important differences in terms of sensitivity emerge. In brief, the MEG provides a more limited and selective view than the EEG upon activity in the same networks: the MEG is insensitive ("blind") to fields generated by radial currents or dipoles (as illustrated in Chapter 1), less sensitive to deep sources, and not attenuated by the skull due to its insensitivity to conductivity.

Historically, MEG studies of brain function[12-14] started over 40 years after the EEG studies[15] and after introducing dipole modeling to EEG[16]. However, since then MEG work has consistently used spatial information through source localization, partly aided by the greater simplicity of MEG source localization which can neglect radial sources and conductivities. Theoretical models have shown that independent of the number of electrodes, some sources are visible in EEG but not in MEG, as illustrated in Chapter 1, i.e. that the modalities have partially orthogonal null-spaces. Sensors in one modality may thus not simply replace sensors in another modality[17]. Also, in practice it has become clear that there are useful differences between EEG and MEG[18], but no general localization advantages for either method given proper spatial sampling and accurate head and source modeling, except in the case of radial and very deep sources where the insensitivity of the MEG is undisputed. Recent evidence that the attenuation due to the lower conductivity of the skull has been overestimated – particularly for children – suggests that the resolution of the EEG has been underestimated[19] (for a detailed discussion see Chapter 4). Both measures share the genuine millisecond time resolution, but also the limitation that they contain no genuine three-dimensional location information regarding their sources and rely on constraints and inverse solution for localization. However, when combined, their differences in sensitivity to source depth and orientation, and different noise properties[20,21] can be invaluable to disambiguate inverse solutions. Intuitively, one may consider the ambiguity which could arise from the superficial similarity between EEG maps due to one tangential source or two opposing radial sources: the insensitivity of the MEG to the latter case would quickly resolve this ambiguity.

In practice, the combination of EEG and MEG is particularly well suited for direct integration due to their physical coupling. Simultaneous recording is also technically unproblematic except that active electrodes which reduce time for skin preparation interfere with MEG recording. In fact, most MEG equipment includes integrated EEG channels. The need to hold the head still inside the large Dewar which encloses the superconducting MEG sensors to cool them, and the sensitivity to magnetic interference, still limits MEG recording flexibility and duration during combined recordings, however. The near instantaneous no-contact recording from several hundred MEG sensors is an advantage if combined with conventional high-density EEG recordings which require considerable time for skin preparation, but the combination with modern high-density EEG systems which allow fast high-impedance recordings with minimal skin preparation no longer makes time a significant factor.

Theoretical and experimental studies show that combining EEG with MEG in a common source and conductor model improves source localization over what is possible with either modality alone, and that the advantage is genuine and independent of the total number of sensors[22,23]. Combined EEG and MEG measurements of known "calibration" sources also allow estimation of conductivities of brain and skull, which critically affect the EEG but not the MEG[22,24]. In cognitive neuroscience, combined EEG and MEG measurements and analyses have helped to disentangle distinct dynamics of attentional modulation in nearby visual cortex sources[25] and have proven important to better detect patterns of epileptic activity[20,26]. In sum, theoretical and experimental work consistently suggests that combining EEG with MEG is particularly suitable for direct comparison, mutual disambiguation and direct fusion, and is highly informative for clinical and cognitive application.

# Combining EEG with fMRI

Combining fast measures of synchronized, directional electrical mass activation with the slower nondirectional hemodynamic data (Chapter 1) is less straightforward than the combination with MEG, because the measurements reflect different aspects of neural function and are represented on primarily incompatible time scales: the typical frequency of EEG is way above the frequencies of the hemodynamic response (HRF) function of the fMRI (that is, the intrinsic temporal low-pass filter of fMRI recordings). On the other hand, oscillating EEG signals would obviously suffer from a massive cancellation of signals if they were just averaged across time or directly convolved with the HRF of the fMRI. Therefore, the polarity of the EEG signals is typically discarded by computing measures of power or strength before the convolution.

## Combining EEG with fMRI using sequential recordings

Correspondence between EEG and hemodynamic data has been established in several ways. For one, a highly correlated response to the intensity of sensory stimulation has been demonstrated in animal studies using invasive intracranial EEG, and local fMRI-based activity measures[27,28]. These results reveal close coupling between local electrophysiological and hemodynamic responses under a wide range of conditions. Importantly, this correlation is strongest for structures and processes involved in EEG generation, such as for local field potentials reflecting synaptic input mainly into cortical layers IV, rather than for spiking multi-unit activity reflecting mainly cortical output. On the other hand, this coupling can also be disrupted, for example through pharmacological manipulation by nitrous oxygen blockers which leave evoked potential unaffected for several minutes after eliminating the BOLD response[27,29].

Correspondence between EEG and fMRI has also been demonstrated noninvasively by comparing visual evoked potential amplitudes and fMRI[30-32] from visual regions, suggesting that these measures are mediated by a similar, nonlinear neural response to the rate or the intensity of stimulation. This close coupling is not limited to the visual modality, since linear relations between sensory evoked potential and fMRI signals are also observed when varying the intensity of auditory[33] or somatosensory stimulation[34]; in some instances electrical source strength may be better related to the extent rather than to the strength of the fMRI activation[33]. Most of these studies have relied on conventional evoked potential measures in separate recording sessions and thus leave open the spatial and temporal specificity of such coupling. However, source localization also demonstrates strong local correlations during simultaneous measurements, at least for visual rate and contrast[32] and for auditory intensity[33]. The logic to demonstrate regional coupling through parametric manipulation has been successfully extended to cognitive stimulus dimensions such as quality of face perception in noise relating the N170 amplitude to fusiform face responses[35] or working memory load relating frontal midline theta to a fronto-parietal network[36].

Combined, sequential EEG–fMRI has revealed detailed and systematic spatial correspondence between fMRI and temporally integrated EEG sources. Some visual studies illustrate particularly well how the temporal sequence of evoked potential sources matches the hierarchy of fMRI-derived retinotopic cortical regions. They also demonstrated that these regions are activated within less than 200 ms[37–39], and how attention may inhibit processing in a retinotopic fashion[40] and modulate re-entrant, later activity in so-called "early" visual areas[41]. This work also confirms that relatively early sensory microstates or components such as the visual P100 already reflect synchronized, extended networks with multiple sources, in line with unimodal electric neuroimaging studies and the microstate concept[42,43]. Combined studies also illustrate that while constraining source analyses can be essential to resolve the temporally overlapping sequence of activations in nearby regions, limiting EEG solutions to regions of fMRI activations is not warranted.

Correspondence is not only found for focal sensory activations but also in unconstrained cases and for distributed cognitive activation patterns. To evaluate such concordance or discordance, distributed source solutions and a probabilistic framework are crucial. For reading related activity, statistical correspondence was significant between distributed ERP source solutions integrated over time and fMRI at an average distance of less than 15–18 mm between corresponding clusters, although correspondence was not significant in every single subject[3], and comparable results are found for auditory cognitive paradigms[44]. The findings also suggest that distributed source solutions imposing strong, global smoothness assumptions on the electrical sources (like LORETA and its variants or relatives; Chapter 3) might not be an optimal match for fMRI activation characterized by multiple distinct but nearby foci.

## Combining EEG with fMRI in developmental populations

There are also important domains and measures where no obvious correspondence can be expected, such as ERP latency measures which directly reflect the hierarchy of processing steps and processing speed in electrical neuroimaging. Such latency changes are particularly prominent in developmental studies, where shorter latencies are interpreted in terms of accelerated processing due to maturation involving regionally specific myelinization trajectories and increased efficiency of connections in gray matter due to use and pruning. These latency decreases continue during adolescence, without corresponding changes in the distribution of the *activation*, i.e. of the task-related ERP source distribution and the fMRI activation pattern, as clarified by recent developmental EEG–fMRI work[45–47]. Instead, late development changed a *deactivation* network in both EEG and fMRI from the same subjects; this network corresponds to the so-called default network[47]. These combined developmental studies led to a model of late "temporal tuning" within the established "spatial boundaries" of specific neural networks, and illustrate how divergence due to different sensitivities of the methods may be particularly useful for theoretical advances. At the same time, these EEG–fMRI studies demonstrate that the convergence between fMRI activation (rather than deactivation)

Semantic incongruency effect

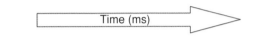

Figure 10.1 Convergence of semantic incongruity effects during sentence reading in children's ERP (Top LAURA, bottom LORETA tomography) and fMRI (center inset). The incongruence effects are computed by contrasting activity for incongruent vs. congruent sentence endings.[48] $N = 52$ children for ERP analyses, mean age 11.5 years, $*: P < 0.05$, $+: P < 0.01$, LORETA and LAURA using the same standard adult head model (see Chapter 4). Subgroup of $N = 37$ children for fMRI analyses, $P < 0.001$ uncorrected, red for positive, blue for negative BOLD effect. Modified from Schulz et al.[48]

patterns and the temporally integrated EEG source solutions also holds for 11-year-old children, even when using standard hemodynamic functions for the event-related fMRI, and standard "adult" head models and conductivities for the EEG sources[48]. This is illustrated in Figure 10.1, where the dynamic source sequence of semantic incongruence effects in the EEG covers two microstates in about 500 ms, closely matching the regions of increased activation in the corresponding fMRI.

While the shape of the hemodynamic response function has been reported to undergo only minor changes with development in primary sensory regions in event-related fMRI studies[49,50], recent event-related fMRI work[50] indicates that in a language task, significant delays of more than 1 s may characterize 6-year-old children's frontal language regions when compared with adults. This suggests that latency estimates should not only be obtained for EEG-based neuronal activity (as is common), but also for fMRI-based hemodynamic imaging in order to characterize the full extent of correspondence.

These considerations apply to developmental as well as to clinical and basic research. In fact, estimating rather than assuming the shape of the hemodynamic response functions has already proven to be crucial for understanding correspondence of simultaneous EEG–fMRI in understanding brain function in epilepsy and during rest, as discussed below.

## Combining EEG with fMRI in simultaneous recordings

To safely record the EEG during scanning, special nonmagnetic EEG hardware and additional precautions are needed. False usage of EEG inside an MRI scanner may lead to serious burn injuries of the subject[51]. Safety requires a current-limiting setup[52], and careful selection of scanning sequences with low specific absorption rates (SAR) and a low potential for radio-frequency interactions. The gradient-echo echo planar imaging (EPI) sequences typically used for fMRI usually meet these requirements[53.] Provided that all these technical precautions are taken, safe recordings without a risk of dangerous heating of electrodes has been demonstrated by expert groups using custom-made or commercial MR-approved equipment during fMRI scanning, even at the very high magnetic field strength of 7T[54,55].

During fMRI scanning, two major artifacts exceed the EEG by orders of magnitude and thus obliterate it before post-processing. First, scanning-related voltages are induced by magnetic gradient switching. These range up to 15 mV but are highly replicable and largely independent of the scanner's B0 field strength. They require fast (ideally 5 kHz) sampling and a large input range (around 20 mV) to avoid aliasing and clipping of the signals. Ideally, the sampling clocks of the EEG and fMRI equipment are synchronized to facilitate the subsequent artifact removal[56]. Second, electrocardiogram (ECG) related voltages are due to motion or flow from the ballistocardiogram which is more variable and reaches 150–700 μV at 1.5–7T, proportional to the field strength[57]. Reducing them requires stabilization to minimize movement, and ECG channels for precise triggering. Once these conditions are met, post-processing based on subtraction of scan- and ECG-triggered averages[58,59] routinely yields EEG and ERPs of good quality from up to 64 channels and up to 3T, as documented in recent reviews of clinical[60,61] and cognitive[2] applications. Besides methods that subtract some average artifact, PCA- or ICA-based approaches have also proven to be efficient to isolate and eliminate the ballistocardiogram artifact. To improve the separation of EEG data from the artifacts, it has proven to be useful to include "learning" EEG data in the data that have been recorded under comparable conditions, but outside the scanner[10]. Particularly at high field strength, the signal-to-noise ratio (SNR) still remains lower than for separate sessions. This holds despite considerable further improvements such as hardware synchronization[56,62], and the full use of topographic information through EEG-source-based filtering[63].

## Simultaneous EEG–fMRI in epilepsy

Simultaneous EEG–fMRI combination has become of particular interest for the localization of epileptogenic foci, a clinical application which has in fact driven the technical developments which made simultaneous recordings possible. It has been demonstrated repeatedly that the correlation of the BOLD response with the epileptic discharges detected in the simultaneous EEG allows identification of the epileptogenic focus. Thus EEG–fMRI represents a promising localizing tool with high spatial resolution, in particular in chronic focal epilepsy[64–68]. Recent studies have also demonstrated interesting results in patients with idiopathic generalized epilepsy[69–71], consistently showing patterns of thalamic activations and frontal and parietal lobe deactivations. Variable timing of the hemodynamic response has been reported in several studies, with some results suggesting that hemodynamic changes in the thalamus regions may even preceed the corresponding EEG events[72,73]. The reasons for a negative BOLD response related to epileptic activity are not yet clear. Possible reasons are a steal phenomenon secondary to the increased blood flow, abnormal coupling between blood flow and neuronal activity in the pathological area, or inhibited synaptic activity (for a discussion see Gotman[74]).

Despite some promising results in selected cases, the overall clinical yield of the EEG–fMRI combination in epilepsy is relatively low. The largest prospective study on focal epilepsy with 63 consecutively recruited patients revealed significant BOLD changes that were concordant with electro-clinical results in only 17 patients (27%)[75], corresponding to other reports with lower numbers of patients[76]. A large part of the negative result was due to the impossibility of detecting interictal epileptic discharges (IED) in the scanner. In the study of Salek-Haddadi and colleagues[75], this was the case in 40% of the patients. Whether this is due to distorted EEG despite effective artifact corrections or due to other electromagnetic or physiological factors (e.g. patient is awake and tense, which may reduce epileptic discharges) is unclear. Movement artifacts are another important problem, particularly in small children and retarded subjects. This was the case in four patients in the study of Salek-Haddadi and collaborators[75]. From the remaining 34 patients with spikes in the scanner and without movement artifacts, 11 patients (32%) showed no BOLD changes that significantly correlated with the spike activity, and another six patients showed BOLD changes that were not concordant with the clinical data. Finally, from the 17 cases (27%) with concordant responses, only seven patients showed unambiguous fMRI signals. The remaining ten patients showed activations related to the "real" focus but also additional noncorresponding areas, providing ambiguous results as to which BOLD response is truly significant with respect to primary focus localization.

The reason for multiple areas of spike-correlated BOLD response is the low temporal resolution of the fMRI. Interictal epileptic discharges propagate within a few milliseconds to remote brain areas[77,78]. The temporal blurring of the BOLD response over seconds makes it virtually impossible to separate discharges from the primary focus and those from propagated areas. It is therefore the rule rather than the exception to find multiple areas of BOLD changes, and additional tools are needed to determine their functional–anatomical relationship.

Since this temporal resolution is exactly the strength of the EEG, the most rational approach is to combine EEG–fMRI with EEG source imaging (ESI), as already demonstrated in a case report in 1998[64]: ESI analysis at different time points during the spike-wave complex identified the generators of epileptogenic discharges (left lateral frontal) and differentiated it from areas activated by propagation (mesial frontal bilaterally and right frontal). Surgical resection of the initial left frontal area with subsequent seizure freedom confirmed the correctness of this localization. A more recent study of Boor and colleagues[79] compared multiple dipole analysis (MDA) obtained by 23-channel EEG with EEG–fMRI in 11 patients with benign childhood epilepsy with centrotemporal (rolandic) spikes. In all patients, MDA correctly located the spike sources in the rolandic face or hand region. In 10 of the 11 patients, a second (or even a third) dipole was found in remote areas with delays of about 20 ms, most likely representing propagation. Again, only in 4 of the 11 patients (36%) did the fMRI provide useful results. In these four patients the expected rolandic areas showed increased BOLD response, but also additional areas in the central cortex, the sylvian fissure and the insula. Most of these areas (but not all) corresponded to the propagated dipoles as identified by the ESI. These examples underline the importance of combining different imaging modalities with different spatial and temporal properties in the evaluation of epileptic patients. Figure 10.2. illustrates such a combination in a case of a presurgical epilepsy evaluation.

However, the studies[64,79] discussed above, and similar other studies[52,80,81] used the EEG recorded outside the scanner to compare with the BOLD response, assuming that the spatiotemporal behavior of the spikes are the same inside and outside the magnet. It is well known in clinical practice that the propagation behavior of single spikes is quite variable, even in patients known for stable unifocal epilepsy. Since very powerful correction algorithms are currently available, so that artifact-reduced high density EEG (more than 64 channels) can be retrieved inside the magnet[82], ESI analysis can now be performed on the same spikes that are associated with the BOLD response[83,84]. This will allow more direct combination of the two techniques in the future. Most interesting in this respect will be studies on epileptic networks that include both sub-cortical and cortical structures[74].

Advanced use of the simultaneously recorded EEG has been demonstrated[10]. The study used an ICA to decompose the EEG data and could identify factors that displayed the typical temporal dynamics and spatial distributions of interictal activity. The time course of such factors was then used as a continuous predictor for the fMRI signal. This technique improves the sensitivity of the method and extends its application to cases where there are indices of

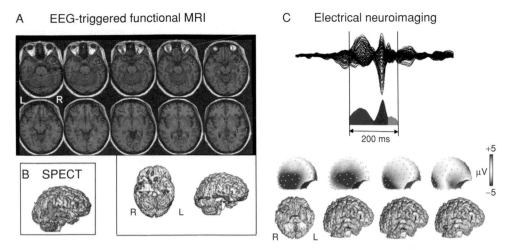

A    EEG-triggered functional MRI

C    Electrical neuroimaging

B   SPECT

**Figure 10.2** Multimodal imaging in presurgical epilepsy evaluation: data from a 43-year-old woman suffering from pharmaco-resistant epilepsy for 12 years. Structural MRI as well as hippocampal volumetry were normal. Video-EEG suggested a right mid- to posterior temporal focus; PET revealed right anterior temporal hypometabolism while ictal SPECT indicated right posterior lateral temporal blood flow increase (B). The EEG-triggered functional MRI showed several areas of spike-correlated BOLD responses (A) in the right temporal lobe, including the anterior pole as well as mid- and posterior areas. The electric neuroimaging based on 128-channel recordings of interictal spikes revealed a fast propagation of the activity from the anterior temporal pole to middle and posterior temporal areas (C). The figure shows the LAURA inverse solution for the four maps that were identified by a functional microstate analysis (see Chapter 6). The subsequent intracranial recordings confirmed the initiation of the seizures in the anterior of the right temporal pole with fast propagation to posterior parts of the temporal lobe. Surgical resection of the anterior temporal lobe led to seizure freedom.

interictal epileptiform EEG activity in the absence of spikes. An example of results obtained with this method is given in Figure 10.3.

## Simultaneous EEG-fMRI in resting state recordings

Electroencephalography and fMRI have also been used to investigate the resting state activity of the brain and its fluctuations. The initial investigations of resting states focused on combinations of EEG with other imaging methods allowing for absolute measurements of activation such as positron emission tomography (PET). Occipital alpha band power with eyes open was correlated positively with thalamic activity, and negatively with occipital activity across subjects in PET studies[85,86]. On the other hand, changes of cortical source distribution of the alpha band at rest were found to be closely related to changes in the corresponding PET activation pattern, with the more anterior alpha sources and PET distribution in patients with Alzheimer's disease illustrating the clinical significance[87].

Subsequently, the focus has shifted towards correlating fluctuations of EEG spectral amplitudes during resting state recordings with corresponding fluctuation of the fMRI signal in the same subject and session. Such combined resting EEG–fMRI has become an essential source of information about the neural networks correlated with specific frequency bands. Alpha-band power has been shown to be positively correlated to fMRI–BOLD signals from the insula and from sub-cortical, namely thalamic regions[9,88,89]. These regions had previously been hypothesized to be the pace-makers of the alpha rhythm. The positive correlation of intra-individual occipital alpha power fluctuations with thalamic activity hold for different resting states[9,88–91]. They thus confirm and extend previous findings despite some

A

B

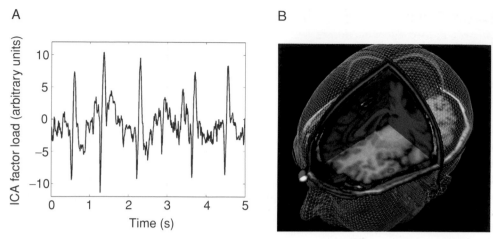

**Figure 10.3** Combining EEG and fMRI for the localization of interictal epileptiform activity. A. A time segment showing the typical dynamics of factor load of an ICA factor that isolated the epileptiform EEG activity. The absolute value of this factor load was convolved with a hemodynamic response function and correlated with the simultaneously measured fMRI–BOLD signals. The location of significant correlation between the epileptiform EEG activity and the BOLD signal is shown in B. The location of the correlation matched well with the clinical symptoms that were characterized by transient motor aphasia during the interictal spikes.

exceptions[92,93]. On the other hand, alpha-band power often showed negative BOLD correlations in posterior cortical regions, where the EEG generators of the alpha rhythm are predominantly located. There is thus a nontrivial relation between oscillating EEG sources and neural oxygen consumption. It suggests (in agreement with the large knowledge base on resting EEG alone) that EEG oscillations may indicate idling of specific neural networks, and that activation of these networks may induce more desynchronized patterns of neural firing, resulting in increased oxygen consumption, but reduced EEG scalp signals. Interestingly, different temporal lags were found for the correlation between alpha power and thalamic versus occipital fMRI activity, suggesting that hemodynamic changes in the thalamus may even precede the increases in oscillatory alpha activity[88].

Since then, fMRI studies have also discovered that fluctuations during rest consistently identify the so-called "default networks," i.e. that fluctuations spontaneously form consistently correlated (or anticorrelated) clusters of brain regions that are co-active during rest, and that these default networks are also more active during rest than in active tasks. Findings from EEG–fMRI studies regarding the relation between EEG frequency modulations and these default networks have been less consistent, with different studies relating default networks to beta activity[94], frontal theta activity[95], or to thalamo-cortical networks involving multiple frequencies clustered by statistical means[91].

Since most of these studies are based on EEG analyses of only a few selected scalp channels despite multichannel recordings, the added regional specificity through source localizing or topographic clustering remains open. Grouping subjects according to their alpha EEG power map topographies has shown that these topographic differences also correspond to differently distributed hemodynamic response patterns[92], but systematic investigations utilizing variations of microstate structure along with distributed source imaging in the same subjects promise a much more detailed and better-interpretable picture of the dynamic patterns correspondence.

# Further simultaneous EEG–fMRI applications

A particularly challenging domain for simultaneous EEG–fMRI studies are single trial analyses which capture the variability of task-related brain functions over time. Topographic decomposition (ICA) and source imaging have successfully demonstrated that not only the mean response but its trial-by-trial variability co-localizes to the fMRI localizations for error- and target-related activity[7,8,96].

Finally, the combination of simultaneous EEG and fMRI has also proven essential in recent attempts at direct MR-based neural current imaging. Unlike conventional BOLD fMRI, these approaches are based on the presumed sensitivity of the fMRI to subtle magnetic field distortions due to the magnetic field generated by the neural currents, using fast current-sensitive MR sequences sampling at $> 20\,Hz$[62,97]. Most results have so far been mainly negative for the relatively small sensory-evoked activity, and for the large-amplitude alpha activity[62], even though the equivalent current dipoles in the latter case clearly exceed the 10 nA detectability limit. An important conclusion from these findings is that the single dipole approximation of EEG sources may not be appropriate at the local "voxel" level[97–99].

# The EEG and transcranial magnetic stimulation

Transcranial magnetic stimulation (TMS) uses an electromagnetic coil which is placed against the subject's head to induce an electric field in the underlying nervous tissue. This stimulation of the cortical neurons usually leads to a disruption of the normal pattern of neuronal activity. Transcranial magnetic stimulation is an important tool in neuroscience because it can demonstrate causality. In fact, applying TMS to a specific cortical region and studying its consequences on task performances enables researchers to deduce about the importance of the disrupted cortical region on a specific behavior.

The instantaneous neuronal TMS-evoked effects are strongest underneath the coil, but TMS also has effects on remote regions that are interconnected with the stimulated area. The concurrent EEG recording enables the temporal and spatial tracing of the spreading of the TMS-evoked neuronal activity, thus mapping corticocortical effective connectivity. Importantly, the combination of the two methods dissociates effective connectivity (or causal interactions), defined as "the influence that one neural system exerts over another either directly or indirectly" from functional connectivity, defined as "temporal correlations between spatially remote neurophysiological events"[100]. Compared with the experimental manipulation of neuronal activity in the form of sensory stimulation, the perturbation of the normal pattern of neuronal activity with TMS has some advantages. First, the stimulation is under explicit experimental control and can therefore be located precisely in time and space. Second, since direct cortical stimulation does not activate the formatio reticularis, its effects are unconfounded by peripheral effects. Finally, observed changes in the neuronal activity are not confounded by the subject's ability to perform a task or by the strategy used. Using this approach, Massimini et al.[101] mapped the TMS-evoked activity in the premotor area during quiet wakefulness and during NREM sleep in healthy subjects and found a lack of propagation beyond the stimulation site during sleep, providing evidence for a breakdown in corticocortical effective connectivity during sleep. Based on similar reports, Komssi and Kähkönen[102] suggested that the online combination of EEG and TMS "may provide a window to plastic changes in cortical connectivity, e.g. after brain injuries, and could be used for diagnostic as well as for prognostic purposes" (p. 187), due to the relatively repeatable and spatially specific connectivity patterns in healthy subjects.

Another important domain of application of the online combination of EEG and TMS is the investigation of cortical reactivity, usually based on the amplitudes of event-related potentials, in relation to a certain disease or to medication. In a series of studies, Kähkönen and coauthors illustrated, for instance, the effects of alcohol on TMS-evoked potentials at frontal areas[103,104].

The combination of the two methods also opens a new avenue of research into the functional significance of the spontaneous fluctuations in different frequency bands. This has, for example, been crucial to establish a close link between the level of posterior alpha-band activity and the excitability of the visual cortex, predicting stimulus perception[105].

## Other combinations and conclusions

A number of other combinations will be touched upon only briefly. The combination of structural imaging such as MRI or diffusion tensor imaging (DTI) is partly addressed in the chapter on source localization. Structural MRI data are now routinely used for source imaging by constraining the solution space to a realistic boundary element model of gray matter in the brain. The results of theoretical and experimental studies suggest a considerable advantage of realistic or anatomically constrained models over spherical models, but the advantage for using individual rather than averaged realistic brain models is less well documented[106-108]. Structural, MRI-based measures of brain structure and connectivity are also starting to augment electrical neuroimaging beyond simply serving to constrain the EEG source space. An intriguing example is the recent finding that regional white matter measures correlate with ERP latencies. Faster latencies of the cognitive P3b ERP component were found to be moderately correlated with larger thalamic, callosal and precentral white matter volumes[109], and faster latency of a saccade-related visual MEG response was strongly correlated with white matter anisotropy of parietal and frontal regions modulating visual activity[110]. There is clearly an increasing need for research and modeling which include latency and frequency-specific connectivity (coherence), where such combinations of measures are likely to be highly predictive.

In conclusion, the increasingly accepted status of electrical field recordings as a genuine neuroimaging method also offers ample opportunities for combinations to validate results and clarify their functional significance. Combinations are often based on at least partial convergence or overlap. These can only be determined if the limited localizing power of electrical neuroimaging and the limited time resolution of metabolic methods are optimally used. As a consequence, the use of innovative spatio-temporal methods and integration frameworks is mandatory. Also a critical, explicit approach to the assumptions and weaknesses inherent in each individual approach, such as constant maximal spatial smoothness or constant hemodynamic responses, is essential for further progress.

## References

1. Horwitz B, Poeppel D. How can EEG/MEG and fMRI/PET data be combined? *Human Brain Mapping* 2002;**17**:1–3.

2. Laufs H, Daunizeau J, Carmichael DW, Kleinschmidt A. Recent advances in recording electrophysiological data simultaneously with magnetic resonance imaging. *Neuroimage* 2008;**40**:515–528.

3. Vitacco D, Brandeis D, Pascual-Marqui RD, Martin E. Correspondence of event-related potential tomography and functional magnetic resonance imaging during language processing. *Human Brain Mapping* 2002;**17**:4–12.

4. Babiloni F, Carducci F, Cincotti F et al. Linear inverse source estimate of combined EEG and MEG data related to voluntary movements. *Human Brain Mapping* 2001;**14**:197–209.

5. Trujillo-Barreto NJ, Martínez-Montes E, Melie-García L, Valdés-Sosa PA. A symmetrical Bayesian model for fMRI and EEG/MEG neuroimage fusion. *International Journal of Bioelectromagnetism (online journal).* 2001;**3**.

6. Wagner M, Fuchs M. Integration of functional MRI, structural MRI, EEG, and MEG. *International Journal of Bioelectromagnetism (online journal).* 2001;**3**.

7. Debener S, Ullsperger M, Siegel M, Engel AK. Single-trial EEG-fMRI reveals the dynamics of cognitive function. *Trends in Cognitive Sciences* 2006;**10**:558–563.

8. Debener S, Ullsperger M, Siegel M et al. Trial-by-trial coupling of concurrent electroencephalogram and functional magnetic resonance imaging identifies the dynamics of performance monitoring. *Journal of Neuroscience* 2005;**25**:11730–11737.

9. Goldman RI, Stern JM, Engel J, Jr., Cohen MS. Simultaneous EEG and fMRI of the alpha rhythm. *Neuroreport* 2002;**13**:2487–2492.

10. Jann K, Wiest R, Hauf M et al. BOLD correlates of continuously fluctuating epileptic activity isolated by independent component analysis. *Neuroimage* 2008;**42**:635–648.

11. Martinez-Montes E, Valdes-Sosa PA, Miwakeichi F, Goldman RI, Cohen MS. Concurrent EEG/fMRI analysis by multiway Partial Least Squares. *Neuroimage* 2004;**22**:1023–1034.

12. Cohen D. Magnetoencephalography: detection of the brain's electrical activity with a superconducting magnetometer. *Science* 1972;**175**:664–666.

13. Hamalainen MS, Hari R, Ilmoniemi RJ, Knuutila JE, Lounasmaa OV. Magnetoencephalography-theory, instrumentation, and applications to noninvasive studies of the working human brain. *Review of Modern Physics* 1993;**65**:413–497.

14. Hari R, Levanen S, Raij T. Timing of human cortical functions during cognition: role of MEG. *Trends in Cognitive Sciences* 2000;**4**:455–462.

15. Berger H. Über das Elektroenkephalogramm des Menschen. *Archiv für Psychiatrie und Nervenkrankheiten* 1929;**87**:527–570.

16. Lehmann D, Kavanagh RH, Fender DH. Field studies of averaged visually evoked EEG potentials in a patient with a split chiasm. *Electroencephalography and Clinical Neurophysiology* 1969;**26**:193–199.

17. Riera JJ, Valdes PA, Tanabe K, Kawashima R. A theoretical formulation of the electrophysiological inverse problem on the sphere. *Physics in Medicine and Biology* 2006;**51**:1737–1758.

18. Cohen D, Cuffin BN. Demonstration of useful differences between magnetoencephalogram and electroencephalogram. *Electroencephalography and Clinical Neurophysiology* 1983;**56**:38–51.

19. Malmivuo JA, Suihko VE. Effect of skull resistivity on the spatial resolutions of EEG and MEG. *IEEE Transactions on Biomedical Engineering* 2004;**51**:1276–1280.

20. Ramantani G, Boor R, Paetau R et al. MEG versus EEG: influence of background activity on interictal spike detection. *Journal of Clinical Neurophysiology* 2006;**23**:498–508.

21. de Jongh A, de Munck JC, Goncalves SI, Ossenblok P. Differences in MEG/EEG epileptic spike yields explained by regional differences in signal-to-noise ratios. *Journal of Clinical Neurophysiology* 2005;**22**:153–158.

22. Fuchs M, Wagner M, Wischmann HA et al. Improving source reconstructions by combining bioelectric and biomagnetic data. *Electroencephalography and Clinical Neurophysiology* 1998;**107**:93–111.

23. Sharon D, Hamalainen MS, Tootell RBH, Halgren E, Belliveau JW. The advantage of combining MEG and EEG: comparison to fMRI in focally stimulated visual cortex. *Neuroimage* 2007;**36**:1225–1235.

24. Goncalves S, de Munck JC, Verbunt JP, Heethaar RM, da Silva FH. In vivo measurement of the brain and skull resistivities using an EIT-based method and the combined analysis of SEF/SEP data. *IEEE Transactions on Biomedical Engineering* 2003;**50**:1124–1128.

25. Hopf JM, Luck SJ, Boelmans K *et al.* The neural site of attention matches the spatial scale of perception. *Journal of Neuroscience* 2006;**26**:3532–3540.

26. Bast T, Ramantani G, Boppel T *et al.* Source analysis of interictal spikes in polymicrogyria: loss of relevant cortical fissures requires simultaneous EEG to avoid MEG misinterpretation. *Neuroimage* 2005;**25**:1232–1241.

27. Lauritzen M. Relationship of spikes, synaptic activity, and local changes of cerebral blood flow. *Journal of Cerebral Blood Flow & Metabolism* 2001;**21**:1367–1383.

28. Logothetis NK, Pauls J, Augath M, Trinath T, Oeltermann A. Neurophysiological investigation of the basis of the fMRI signal. *Nature* 2001;**412**:150–157.

29. Burke M, Buhrle C. BOLD response during uncoupling of neuronal activity and CBF. *Neuroimage* 2006;**32**:1–8.

30. Singh M, Kim S, Kim TS. Correlation between BOLD-fMRI and EEG signal changes in response to visual stimulus frequency in humans. *Magnetic Resonance in Medicine* 2003;**49**:108–114.

31. Janz C, Heinrich SP, Kornmayer J, Bach M, Hennig J. Coupling of neural activity and BOLD fMRI response: new insights by combination of fMRI and VEP experiments in transition from single events to continuous stimulation. *Magnetic Resonance in Medicine* 2001;**46**:482–486.

32. Wan X, Riera J, Iwata K, Takahashi M, Wakabayashi T, Kawashima R. The neural basis of the hemodynamic response nonlinearity in human primary visual cortex: implications for neurovascular coupling mechanism. *Neuroimage* 2006;**32**:616–625.

33. Mulert C, Jager L, Propp S *et al.* Sound level dependence of the primary auditory cortex: simultaneous measurement with 61-channel EEG and fMRI. *Neuroimage* 2005;**28**:49–58.

34. Arthurs OJ, Williams EJ, Carpenter TA, Pickard JD, Boniface SJ. Linear coupling between functional magnetic resonance imaging and evoked potential amplitude in human somatosensory cortex. *Neuroscience* 2000;**101**:803–806.

35. Horovitz SG, Rossion B, Skudlarski P, Gore JC. Parametric design and correlational analyses help integrating fMRI and electrophysiological data during face processing. *Neuroimage* 2004;**22**:1587–1595.

36. Meltzer JA, Negishi M, Mayes LC, Constable RT. Individual differences in EEG theta and alpha dynamics during working memory correlate with fMRI responses across subjects. *Clinical Neurophysiology* 2007;**118**:2419–2436.

37. Vanni S, Warnking J, Dojat M *et al.* Sequence of pattern onset responses in the human visual areas: an fMRI constrained VEP source analysis. *Neuroimage* 2004;**21**:801–817.

38. Di Russo F, Martinez A, Sereno MI, Pitzalis S, Hillyard SA. Cortical sources of the early components of the visual evoked potential. *Human Brain Mapping* 2002;**15**:95–111.

39. Liu Z, He B. FMRI-EEG integrated cortical source imaging by use of time-variant spatial constraints. *Neuroimage* 2008;**39**:1198–1214.

40. Hopf J-M, Boehler CN, Luck SJ *et al.* Direct neurophysiological evidence for spatial suppression surrounding the focus of attention in vision. *Proceedings of the National Academy of Sciences, USA* 2006;**103**:1053–1058.

41. Martinez A, Anllo-Vento L, Sereno MI *et al.* Involvement of striate and extrastriate visual cortical areas in spatial attention. *Nature Neuroscience* 1999;**2**:364–369.

42. Morand S, Thut G, de Peralta RG *et al.* Electrophysiological evidence for fast visual processing through the human koniocellular pathway when stimuli move. *Cerebral Cortex* 2000;**10**:817–825.

43. Steger J, Imhof K, Denoth J *et al.* Brain mapping of bilateral visual interactions in

children. *Psychophysiology* 2001;**38**:243–253.

44. Mulert C, Jager L, Schmitt R *et al.* Integration of fMRI and simultaneous EEG: towards a comprehensive understanding of localization and time-course of brain activity in target detection. *Neuroimage* 2004;**22**:83–94.

45. Brem S, Bucher K, Halder P *et al.* Evidence for developmental changes in the visual word processing network beyond adolescence. *Neuroimage* 2006;**29**:822–837.

46. Bucher K, Dietrich T, Marcar VL *et al.* Maturation of luminance- and motion-defined form perception beyond adolescence: a combined ERP and fMRI study. *Neuroimage* 2006;**31**:1625–1636.

47. Halder P, Brem S, Bucher K *et al.* Electrophysiological and hemodynamic evidence for late maturation of hand force control under visual feedback. *Human Brain Mapping* 2007;**28**:69–84.

48. Schulz E, Maurer U, Van Der Mark S *et al.* Impaired semantic processing during sentence reading in children with dyslexia: combined fMRI and ERP evidence. *Neuroimage* 2008;**41**:153–168.

49. Richter W, Richter M. The shape of the fMRI BOLD response in children and adults changes systematically with age. *Neuroimage* 2003;**20**:1122–1131.

50. Brauer J, Neumann J, Friederici AD. Temporal dynamics of perisylvian activation during language processing in children and adults. *Neuroimage* 2008;**41**:1484–1492.

51. Lemieux L, Allen PJ, Franconi F, Symms MR, Fish DR. Recording of EEG during fMRI experiments: patient safety. *Magnetic Resonance in Medicine* 1997;**38**:943–952.

52. Lemieux L, Krakow K, Fish DR. Comparison of spike-triggered functional MRI BOLD activation and EEG dipole model localization. *Neuroimage* 2001;**14**:1097–1104.

53. Lazeyras F, Zimine I, Blanke O, Perrig SH, Seeck M. Functional MRI with simultaneous EEG recording: feasibility and application to motor and visual activation. *Journal of Magnetic Resonance Imaging* 2001;**13**:943–948.

54. Vasios CE, Angelone LM, Purdon PL *et al.* EEG/(f)MRI measurements at 7 Tesla using a new EEG cap ("InkCap"). *Neuroimage* 2006;**33**:1082–1092.

55. Mullinger K, Brookes M, Stevenson C, Morgan P, Bowtell R. Exploring the feasibility of simultaneous electroencephalography/functional magnetic resonance imaging at 7 T. *Magnetic Resonance Imaging* 2008; **26**:968–977.

56. Mandelkow H, Halder P, Boesiger P, Brandeis D. Synchronization facilitates removal of MRI artefacts from concurrent EEG recordings and increases usable bandwidth. *Neuroimage* 2006;**32**:1120–1126.

57. Debener S, Mullinger KJ, Niazy RK, Bowtell RW. Properties of the ballistocardiogram artefact as revealed by EEG recordings at 1. 5, 3 and 7 T static magnetic field strength. *International Journal of Psychophysiology* 2008;**67**:189–199.

58. Allen PJ, Josephs O, Turner R. A method for removing imaging artifact from continuous EEG recorded during functional MRI. *Neuroimage* 2000;**12**:230–239.

59. Allen PJ, Polizzi G, Krakow K, Fish DR, Lemieux L. Identification of EEG events in the MR scanner: the problem of pulse artifact and a method for its subtraction. *Neuroimage* 1998;**8**:229–239.

60. Gotman J, Benar C-G, Dubeau F. Combining EEG and fMRI in epilepsy: a multimodal tool for epilepsy research. *Journal of Magnetic Resonance Imaging* 2006;**23**:906–920.

61. Laufs H, Duncan JS. Electroencephalography/functional MRI in human epilepsy: what it currently can and cannot do. *Current Opinion in Neurology* 2007;**20**:417–423.

62. Mandelkow H, Halder P, Brandeis D *et al.* Heart beats Brain: The problem of detecting alpha waves by neuronal current imaging in joint EEG-MRI experiments. *Neuroimage* 2007;**37**:149–163.

63. Brookes MJ, Mullinger KJ, Stevenson CM, Morris PG, Bowtell R. Simultaneous EEG source localisation and artifact rejection

during concurrent fMRI by means of spatial filtering. *Neuroimage* 2008;**40**:1090–1104.

64. Seeck M, Lazeyras F, Michel CM *et al.* Non invasive epileptic focus localization using EEG-triggered functional MRI and electromagnetic tomography. *Electroencephalography and Clinical Neurophysiology* 1998;**106**:508–512.

65. Krakow K, Woermann FG, Symms MR *et al.* EEG-triggered functional MRI of interictal epileptiform activity in patients with partial seizures. *Brain* 1999;**122**:1679–1688.

66. Lazeyras F, Blanke O, Perrig S *et al.* EEG-triggered functional MRI in patients with pharmacoresistant epilepsy. *Journal of Magnetic Resonance Imaging* 2000;**12**:177–185.

67. Lemieux L. Electroencephalography-correlated functional MR imaging studies of epileptic activity. *Neuroimaging Clinics of North America* 2004;**14**:487–506.

68. Al-Asmi A, Benar CG, Gross DW *et al.* fMRI activation in continuous and spike-triggered EEG-fMRI studies of epileptic spikes. *Epilepsia* 2003;**44**:1328–1339.

69. Gotman J, Grova C, Bagshaw A *et al.* Generalized epileptic discharges show thalamocortical activation and suspension of the default state of the brain. *Proceedings of the National Academy of Sciences USA* 2005;**102**:15236–15240.

70. Aghakhani Y, Bagshaw AP, Benar CG *et al.* fMRI activation during spike and wave discharges in idiopathic generalized epilepsy. *Brain* 2004;**127**:1127–1144.

71. Laufs H, Lengler U, Hamandi K, Kleinschmidt A, Krakow K. Linking generalized spike-and-wave discharges and resting state brain activity by using EEG/fMRI in a patient with absence seizures. *Epilepsia* 2006;**47**:444–448.

72. Hawco CS, Bagshaw AP, Lu Y, Dubeau F, Gotman J. BOLD changes occur prior to epileptic spikes seen on scalp EEG. *Neuroimage* 2007;**35**:1450–1458.

73. Moeller F, Siebner HR, Wolff S *et al.* Changes in activity of striato-thalamo-cortical network precede generalized spike wave discharges. *Neuroimage* 2008;**9**:1839–1849.

74. Gotman J. Epileptic networks studied with EEG-fMRI. *Epilepsia* 2008;**49**:42–51.

75. Salek-Haddadi A, Diehl B, Hamandi K *et al.* Hemodynamic correlates of epileptiform discharges: an EEG-fMRI study of 63 patients with focal epilepsy *Brain Res* 2006;**1088**:148–166.

76. Lantz G, Spinelli L, Menendez RG, Seeck M, Michel CM. Localization of distributed sources and comparison with functional MRI. *Epileptic Disorders* 2001;**Special Issue**:45–58.

77. Alarcon G, Guy CN, Binnie CD *et al.* Intracerebral propagation of interictal activity in partial epilepsy: implications for source localisation. *Journal of Neurology, Neurosurgery and Psychiatry* 1994;**57**:435–449.

78. Lantz G, Spinelli L, Seeck M *et al.* Propagation of interictal epileptiform activity can lead to erroneous source localizations: A 128 channel EEG mapping study. *Journal of Clinical Neurophysiology* 2003;**20**:311–319.

79. Boor R, Jacobs J, Hinzmann A *et al.* Combined spike-related functional MRI and multiple source analysis in the non-invasive spike localization of benign rolandic epilepsy. *Clinical Neurophysiology* 2007;**118**:901–909.

80. Bagshaw AP, Kobayashi E, Dubeau F, Pike GB, Gotman J. Correspondence between EEG-fMRI and EEG dipole localisation of interictal discharges in focal epilepsy. *Neuroimage* 2006;**30**:417–425.

81. Grova C, Daunizeau J, Kobayashi E *et al.* Concordance between distributed EEG source localization and simultaneous EEG-fMRI studies of epileptic spikes. *Neuroimage* 2008;**39**:755–774.

82. Grouiller F, Vercueil L, Krainik A *et al.* A comparative study of different artefact removal algorithms for EEG signals acquired during functional MRI. *Neuroimage* 2007;**38**:124–137.

83. Vulliemoz S, Thornton R, Rodionov R *et al.* The spatio-temporal mapping of epileptic networks: combination of EEG-fMRI and EEG source imaging. *Neuroimage* 2009; in press.

84. Groening K, Brodbeck V, Moeller F *et al.* Combination of EEG-fMRI and EEG source analysis improves interpretation of spike-associated activation networks in paediatric pharmacoresistant focal epilepsies. *Neuroimage* 2009; in press.

85. Sadato N, Nakamura S, Oohashi T *et al.* Neural networks for generation and suppression of alpha rhythm: a PET study. *Neuroreport* 1998;9:893–897.

86. Buchsbaum MS, Kessler R, King A, Johnson J, Cappelletti J. Simultaneous cerebral glucography with positron emission tomography and topographic electroencephalography. *Progress in Brain Research* 1984;62:263–269.

87. Dierks T, Jelic V, Pascual-Marqui RD *et al.* Spatial pattern of cerebral glucose metabolism (PET) correlates with localization of intracerebral EEG-generators in Alzheimer's disease. *Clinical Neurophysiology* 2000;111:1817–1824.

88. Feige B, Scheffler K, Esposito F *et al.* Cortical and subcortical correlates of electroencephalographic alpha rhythm modulation. *Journal of Neurophysiology* 2005;93:2864–2872.

89. Moosmann M, Ritter P, Krastel I *et al.* Correlates of alpha rhythm in functional magnetic resonance imaging and near infrared spectroscopy. *Neuroimage* 2003; 20:145–158.

90. De Jong R, Coles MGH, Logan GD, Gratton G. In search of the point of no return: the control of response processes. *Journal of Experimental Psychology: Human Perception and Performance* 1990; 16:164–182.

91. Mantini D, Perrucci MG, Del Gratta C, Romani GL, Corbetta M. Electrophysiological signatures of resting state networks in the human brain. *Proceedings of the National Academy of Sciences, USA* 2007;104:13170–13175.

92. Laufs H, Holt JL, Elfont R *et al.* Where the BOLD signal goes when alpha EEG leaves. *Neuroimage* 2006;31:1408–1418.

93. Laufs H, Kleinschmidt A, Beyerle A *et al.* EEG-correlated fMRI of human alpha activity. *Neuroimage* 2003;19:1463–1467.

94. Laufs H, Krakow K, Sterzer P *et al.* Electroencephalographic signatures of attentional and cognitive default modes in spontaneous brain activity fluctuations at rest. *Proceedings of the National Academy of Sciences, USA* 2003;100:11053–11058.

95. Scheeringa R, Bastiaansen MCM, Petersson KM *et al.* Frontal theta EEG activity correlates negatively with the default mode network in resting state. *International Journal of Psychophysiology* 2008;67:242–251.

96. Bénar C-G, Schön D, Grimault S *et al.* Single-trial analysis of oddball event-related potentials in simultaneous EEG-fMRI. *Human Brain Mapping* 2007; 28:602–613.

97. Konn D, Gowland P, Bowtell R. MRI detection of weak magnetic fields due to an extended current dipole in a conducting sphere: a model for direct detection of neuronal currents in the brain. *Magnetic Resonance in Medicine* 2003;50:40–49.

98. Blagoev KB, Mihaila B, Travis BJ *et al.* Modelling the magnetic signature of neuronal tissue. *Neuroimage* 2007;37:137–148.

99. Murakami S, Okada Y. Contributions of principal neocortical neurons to magnetoencephalography and electroencephalography signals. *Journal of Physiology* 2006;575:925–936.

100. Lee L, Harrison LM, Mechelli A. A report of the functional connectivity workshop, Dusseldorf 2002. *Neuroimage* 2003;19: 457–465.

101. Massimini M, Ferrarelli F, Huber R *et al.* Breakdown of cortical effective connectivity during sleep. *Science* 2005; 309:2228–2232.

102. Komssi S, Kähkönen S. The novelty value of the combined use of electroencephalography and transcranial magnetic stimulation for neuroscience research. *Brain Research Reviews* 2006; 52:183–192.

103. Kähkönen S, Wilenius J. Effects of alcohol on TMS-evoked N100 responses. *Journal of Neuroscience Methods* 2007;166: 104–108.

104. Kähkönen S, Wilenius J, Nikulin VV, Ollikainen M, Ilmoniemi RJ. Alcohol

reduces prefrontal cortical excitability in humans: a combined TMS and EEG study. *Neuropsychopharmacology* 2003;**28**:747–754.

105. Romei V, Brodbeck V, Michel C *et al*. Spontaneous fluctuations in posterior {alpha}-band EEG activity reflect variability in excitability of human visual areas. *Cerebral Cortex* 2007;**18**:2010–2018.

106. Fuchs M, Kastner J, Wagner M, Hawes S, Ebersole JS. A standardized boundary element method volume conductor model. *Clinical Neurophysiology* 2002;**113**:702–712.

107. Park HJ, Kwon JS, Youn T *et al*. Statistical parametric mapping of LORETA using high density EEG and individual MRI: application to mismatch negativities in schizophrenia. *Human Brain Mapping* 2002;**17**:168–178.

108. Spinelli L, Andino SG, Lantz G, Seeck M, Michel CM. Electromagnetic inverse solutions in anatomically constrained spherical head models. *Brain Topography* 2000;**13**:115–125.

109. Cardenas VA, Chao LL, Blumenfeld R *et al*. Using automated morphometry to detect associations between ERP latency and structural brain MRI in normal adults. *Human Brain Mapping* 2005; **25**:317–327.

110. Stufflebeam SM, Witzel T, Mikulski S *et al*. A non-invasive method to relate the timing of neural activity to white matter microstructural integrity. *Neuroimage* 2008;**42**:710–716.

# Index

acetylcholine 14, 15
adaptive spatial filter
    techniques 64–71
age
  alpha-band synchrony
    153
  combined EEG–fMRI
    developmental studies
    219–220
  functional microstates 114
  global descriptors 208
aliasing 80
$\alpha$ (regularization parameter)
    56, 63–64
alpha rhythms 12–13, 49, 153,
    223–224
Alzheimer's disease 114, 150,
    153, 208
amplitude
  detection limit 6
  multichannel waveform
    analysis 120–121
  spectral amplitude (power)
    maps 105, 107,
    149–150
  see also frequency analysis
anesthesia 7–10
anorexia 208
antipsychotic drugs 114, 208
artifacts, detection and
    correction of 30–32,
    87–89, 129, 220–221
attenuation of signals 5–6

bad data 30–32, 87–89, 129,
    220–221
beamformers (adaptive spatial
    filters) 64–71
Berger, Hans 49
beta-gamma rhythms 14–15
blurring of images
  deblurring methods 36
  effect of regularization
    parameter value 63
  tissue conductivity
    differences 5–6, 82–84
brain, tissue conductivity 5, 71

cardiac artifacts 89, 221
CAT (computerized axial
    tomography) scans 55
centroids of scalp field map
    potential areas 40
cerebellum 5
children
  alpha-band synchronicity
    153
  combined EEG–fMRI
    developmental studies
    219–220
  skull conductivity 6, 82
cluster analysis 102, 106–107
  in frequency analysis 162
  in localization of
    epileptogenic foci 132
  microstate analysis 107,
    115–117, 124–125,
    130
cognitive functions
  neuronal networks 112
  spatial ERP analysis
    126–127
  see also dementia
coherence 105, 155
combinations of different
    imaging methods
    215–217
  EEG and fMRI 111, 218
    developmental studies
    219–220
    identification of
    epileptogenic foci 60,
    131, 221–223
    sequential recordings
    218–219
    simultaneous recording
    220–225
  EEG and MEG 217–218
  EEG and structural MR 226
  EEG and TMS 225–226
computerized axial
    tomography (CAT)
    scans 55
conductivity of tissue types 52,
    71, 218

blurring caused by
    differences in 5–6,
    82–84
consciousness 111–117,
    124
  see also resting (wakeful)
    state
cortical connectivity 225
cortical reactivity 226
cortical sinks and sources of
    EEG activity 2–3
  alpha rhythms 12
  delta rhythms 8–10
  fast (beta-gamma) rhythms
    14–15
cross-spectral matrices
    154–156
cross-validation tests 32, 64
current dipoles 3–6, 51–54,
    72
current source density (spatial
    derivative) 36, 37

deblurring (spatial derivative)
    36
delta dictionary 96–97
  combined with spatial
    elements 104, 106–107
delta rhythms 7–11
dementia 114, 150, 153, 208
depression 114, 208
depth localization errors 57
deviant cognition 209
diazepam 114
dictionaries (time functions)
    95–100
  combined with topographies
    104–107
dictionary learning algorithms
    162
difference maps 42–45, 127,
    169, 176
digitization methods for
    defining electrode
    positions 85
dimensional simplicity 200
dipoles see current dipoles

discrete, 3D distributed, linear tomographies *see* distributed source models

distributed source models 54–61, 102, 219
  dynamic statistical parametric maps 61
  head models and 72
  LAURA 58–61
  LORETA 57–61
  minimum norm solution 57, 59
  regularization parameter ($\alpha$) 56, 63–64
  sLORETA 61–64

driving, in time-frequency analysis 161

dynamic statistical parametric maps (dSPM) 61

effect size 170–171

electric gravity center of scalp field maps 40

electrodes
  faulty 30, 87–89
  number of 79–82, 89, 169
    skull conductivity and 82–84
  position of 30, 84–87

entorhinal complex 12

epilepsy
  EEG frequencies 2
  global descriptors 207
  intracranial recordings 6, 59, 131
  localization of the primary focus 59–60, 130–133, 221–223

event-related potentials (ERP) 118
  example data from healthy subjects 25
  N400 102, 120, 126, 172
  randomization statistics 172–187
  spatial analysis 118–120, 126–127
    field strength/topography 121–123
    microstates 123–125, 134
    single trial analysis 129–130

source 125–126
  waveform 120–121
  time-frequency analysis 159–160

event-related synchronization/desynchronization (ERS/ERD) 160–161

evoked potentials (EP) *see* event-related potentials (ERP)

extrapolation of data 32

extreme potential values 38, 41

eye movement artifacts 88–89

FFT (fast Fourier transformation) *see* Fourier analysis

field strength analysis *see* global field power

finite element model (FEM) 72

fMRI (functional magnetic resonance imaging), combined with EEG 111, 215, 218
  developmental studies 219–220
  in localization of epileptogenic foci 60, 131, 221–223
  sequential recordings 218–219
  simultaneous recording 220–225

forward problem/solution 5, 93, 100
  *see also* lead field

Fourier analysis (FFT) 95, 97–99, 146, 156–157
  combined with spatial elements 105

frequency analysis 145–146, 163–165
  combined EEG–fMRI in the resting state 223–224
  combined EEG–TMS 226
  Fourier analysis 95, 97–99, 146, 156–157
  frequency domain analysis (FFT-based) 146, 156–157
    cross-spectral matrices 154–156
    inverse solutions 156

phase synchrony 150–154
  power maps 105, 107, 149–150
  references and 146–148, 150, 154
  several sources 148
  single source 148
  $\Omega$ complexity and 206

wavelets (time-frequency analysis) 99, 145, 156–163
  combined with spatial elements 105–107
  *see also* rhythms

functional magnetic resonance imaging *see* fMRI

functional microstates 106–107, 133–134
  ERP analysis 123–125, 134
  randomization statistics 174, 185–187
  single-trial 130
  spontaneous EEG analysis 112–117, 134
  state-dependent information processing 127–129
  state space representation and 210–211

Gabor functions 99, 106, 145, 158

gamma rhythms 14–15

generalized dissimilarity 177

generalized frequency ($\Phi$) 201, 203–205, 208

generators of EEG activity 1–6, 50–51
  spatial extent 6–7
  waveforms 7–15

GEV (global explained variance) 115

GFP *see* global field power

GFS (global field synchronization) 106, 153–154

glial cells 10, 15

global descriptors ($\Sigma$, $\Phi$, $\Omega$) 200–207, 211
  in specific conditions 207–209
  synchronization and 106, 211

*see also* state space
representation
global explained variance
(GEV) 115
global field power (GFP)
41–42, 45
ERP field strength/
topography differences
123–124, 174–176
spontaneous EEG 117
state space representation
and 194, 197
global field synchronization
(GFS) 106, 153–154
global map dissimilarity
(GMD) 45, 176
ERP topography differences
123
functional microstates
115–117
global spectral amplitude
153
GMD *see* global map
dissimilarity
gradient (spatial derivative) 35,
37
gravity center of scalp field
maps 40

harmonic motion *see* Fourier
analysis
head volume conductor models
53, 71–72
hippocampus 5, 12
hypnosis 114, 209

independent component
analysis (ICA) 89, 101,
129–130
infants, skull conductivity 6,
82
inner product of vectors 67,
193
integral field strength ($\Sigma$) 153,
201, 203–205, 208
integration of different imaging
methods 215–217
EEG and fMRI 111, 218
developmental studies
219–220
identification of
epileptogenic foci 60,
131, 221–223

sequential recordings
218–219
simultaneous recording
220–225
EEG and MEG 217–218
EEG and structural MR
226
EEG and TMS 225–226
interpolation of data 30–32, 87
intracellular recordings 1–2, 7,
10, 12
intracranial recordings 2–3, 5
in epilepsy 6, 59, 131
inverse problem/solution
CAT scans 55
constraints 49–51, 72
cross-spectral matrices
155
difference maps and 43
dipole models 52–54
distributed source models
electrode-based statistical
analysis compared with
187
frequency analysis 155–156
head volume models 71–72
spatial filters 64–71
isopotential lines in scalp field
maps 27–30, 32

K-means cluster analysis *see*
cluster analysis

latent variables in
randomization statistics
181–182
LAURA (local autoregressive
average) 58–61, 132
lead field 53, 55, 71, 93,
148
in MEG 65
lexical decision tasks,
pre-stimulus microstate
and 127–128
"linear complexity" 203
linear projections (in state
space) 195
linear transformations (in state
space) 195–196
localization of sources
EEG and fMRI 60, 131,
221–223
EEG and MEG 217–218

EEG and structural MR 226
electrode position and
85–87
of epileptogenic foci 59–60,
130–133, 221–223
errors
depth of source 57
insufficient spatial
sampling 80–82
spatial ERP analysis
125–126
validation of inverse
solutions 59–61
LORETA (low resolution
electromagnetic
tomography) 57–61,
132
*see also* sLORETA

macrostate space 203–205
magnetic resonance imaging
(MRI) 86, 226
*see also* fMRI (functional
magnetic resonance
imaging)
magnetoencephalograms
(MEG)
adaptive spatial filter
techniques 64–71
combined/compared with
EEG 3, 5, 217–218
distributed source models
56
MANOVA (multivariate
analysis of variance)
170
map descriptors of scalp field
maps 38
GFP *see* global field power
GMD 45, 115–117, 123, 176
spatial descriptors 38–41
MEG *see* magnetoencephalograms
metric structure (in state
space) 193–194
microstates *see* functional
microstates
minimum norm solution 57,
59
as non-adaptive spatial filter
66
minimum-variance spatial
filter 67–71

models for analysis of EEG
data 93–96
combined methods 104–107
representation bases
103–104
spatial elements 95,
100–103
temporal elements 95–100
motor processes 14, 208
MRI (magnetic resonance
imaging) 86, 226
*see also* fMRI (functional
magnetic resonance
imaging)
multimodal imaging *see*
integration of different
imaging methods
multiple testing corrections
121, 123
multivariate statistical analysis
MANOVA 170
randomization statistics
170–172
music 209

N400 ERP 102, 120,
126
worked example using
randomization statistics
172–187
neural activity index 68
neuroactive substances, effects
of 114, 208, 226
neuronal workspace hypothesis
111–112
*see also* functional
microstates
neurotransmitters 14, 15
noise *see* signal-to-noise ratio
noise-normalized current
density method
(dynamic statistical
parametric maps) 61
non-adaptive spatial filters
66–67
normalization 44–45, 87,
187–188
null hypothesis 170
Nyquist rate 80

Ω (omega) *see* spatial
complexity
orthogonality

representation bases
103–104
vectors 194–196

partial least squares (PLS)
analysis 101, 174,
181–182
perceptual ambiguity tests,
pre-stimulus microstate
and 128
PET (positron emission
tomography) 59, 223
phase resetting 130, 160
$\Phi$ (phi) (generalized
frequency) 201,
203–205, 208
photogrammetry for
measurement of
electrode position 86
piracetam 208
PLS (partial least squares)
analysis 101, 174,
181–182
polarity, mapping 105,
117
polarization/depolarization of
neurons 4–6, 10
positron emission tomography
(PET) 59, 223
power maps (spectral
amplitude maps) 105,
107, 149–150
pre-stimulus baseline 127–129
corrections 43, 127
principal component analysis
(PCA) 101, 196–200,
202
projections (in state space) 195
PROMS weighting method 57
pseudo-significance in
randomization statistics
179–180

randomization statistics
electrode- vs voxel-based
statistics 187
general theory 170–172
hierarchical analysis and
188
scalp field data (N400 test
worked example)
data set and hypotheses
tested 172–174

effect of experimental
design 174, 181–182
effect of increase in
language proficiency
174, 183
electrode-by-electrode
t-tests 180–181
frequency and duration of
significant effects 174,
178–180
microstate differences
174, 185–187
topographic consistency
174–176
topographic differences
172, 176–178
redundancy of data 161,
169
reference electrodes
amplitude and phase
analysis 146–148, 150,
154
average reference 35,
148
spatial analysis 25, 32–35,
56, 79, 100
regularization parameter ($\alpha$)
56, 63–64
representation bases 103–104
residual maps 176
resistivity of tissue types *see*
conductivity of tissue
types
resting (wakeful) state 111–112
combined EEG–fMRI 215,
223–224
functional microstates in
spontaneous EEGs
112–117, 134
power maps 149–150
rhythms 12, 14, 49
state-dependent effects on
post-stimulus activity
127–129
time-frequency analysis
161–163
rhythms 7
alpha 12–13, 49, 153,
223–224
beta-gamma (fast) 14–15
delta (slow) 7–11
sigma (spindle) 10, 13
theta 11–12

scalar spatial filter 66
scalp field maps
    basic construction 25–30
    difference maps 42–45, 127, 169, 176
    interpolation of scalp potentials 30–32
    map descriptors 38–41
    GFP see global field power
    GMD 45, 115–117, 123, 176
    reference electrodes 25, 32–35
    spatial derivatives 35–37
    summation of sources 3, 93, 148
    see also randomization statistics
schizophrenia 114, 208
semantic tests
    in children using EEG–fMRI 220
    N400 ERP 102, 120, 126, 172
    pre-stimulus microstate and 127–128
sensory stimuli
    using combined EEG–fMRI 218–219
    see also visual stimuli
(Σ) (sigma) (integral field strength) 153, 201, 203–205, 208
sigma (spindle) rhythms 10, 13
signal-to-noise ratio
    in the analysis of phase 152, 160
    interpolation of data and 30
    regularization parameter value and 64
sinewave (sinusoidal) dictionary 97–99
    combined with spatial elements 105–107
single channel analysis 100
    combined with temporal elements 104–105
single photon emission computed tomography (SPECT) 59
sinks of electrical activity 2–3, 51

skull conductivity 5–6, 71, 82–84
sleep
    corticocortical connectivity 225
    delta rhythms 8–10
    global descriptors 203–205, 207
    spindle rhythms 13
sLORETA (standardized low resolution electromagnetic tomography) 61–64
    as nonadaptive spatial filter 67
SMAC (spherical head model with anatomical constraints) 72
somatosensory evoked potentials (SSEP) 70–71, 80
sources 2–3, 6, 50–51
    localization see localization of sources
spatial analysis
    evoked potentials/ERPs 118–127
    interictal activity 130–133
    single-trial data 129–130
    spontaneous EEG 111–117
spatial buffering 10
spatial cluster analysis see cluster analysis
spatial complexity (Ω) 153, 202–207, 211
    age and 208
    in epilepsy 207
    neuroactive drugs and 208
    psychiatric disorders 208
    sensory/motor processes 208
    synchronization and 106, 211
spatial derivatives 35–37
spatial distributions (topographies) 95–96, 100–103
    combined with temporal elements 104–107
spatial factor analysis 100–101
    combined with temporal elements 106
spatial filters 64–71, 102

spatial map descriptors 38–41
spatial outliers, detection of 88
spatial sampling
    electrode numbers 79–82, 89
    skull conductivity and 82–84
    electrode position 84–85
    measurement of 85–87
    normalization 87
spatio-temporal dipole model 54
SPECT (single photon emission computed tomography) 59
spectral amplitude (power) maps 105, 107, 149–150
spherical head models 71–72
spindle (sigma) rhythms 10, 13
spline interpolations 30–32
spontaneous EEG see resting (wakeful) state
state space representation 191–192
    as applied to EEG 41, 44, 192, 211
    microstates and 210–211
    PCA 196–200, 202
    structure of the state space 193–196
    synchronization and 211
    see also global descriptors
sulpiride 114
synchronization 150–154
    coherence 105
    ERS/ERD 160–161
    GFS 106, 153–154
    spatial complexity (Ω) 211
    spatial extent of 2, 3, 6, 51

TANCOVA (topographic analysis of covariance) 183
TANOVA (topographic analysis of variance) 176–178
TCR (topographic component recognition) 102, 125
    combined with temporal elements 107

temporal dynamics 93–94
  dictionaries 95–100
    combined with
      topographies 104–107
  functional microstates
    112–117,
    123–125
  *see also* time-frequency
    analysis
thalamus 7, 221
  alpha rhythms 223,
    224
  beta-gamma rhythms
    14, 15
  delta rhythms 8
  spindle rhythms 13
theanine 208
theta rhythms 11–12
Tikhonov regularization
  parameter 56, 63–64
time-frequency analysis
  (wavelets) 99, 145,
    156–163

combined with spatial
  elements 105–107
  *see also* temporal dynamics
TMS (transcranial magnetic
  stimulation)
    225–226
topographic analysis 121–123,
  126
  randomization statistics
    172–174
  TANCOVA 183
  TANOVA 176–178
  test for topographic
    consistency
    174–176
  state space 194
  *see also* scalp field maps
topographic component
  recognition (TCR) 102,
    125
  combined with
    temporal elements
    107

topographies (spatial
  distributions) 95–96,
    100–103
  combined with temporal
    elements 104–107
transcranial magnetic
  stimulation (TMS)
    225–226

valproate 208
vectors in state space
  representation 193–194
visual cortex 12
visual stimuli 14, 126, 208, 218,
  219

waveform analysis 120–121
wavelet analysis 99, 145,
  156–163
  combined with spatial
    elements 105–107
  *see also* temporal dynamics
white matter 2, 226